Shell-Shock and Medical Culture in First World War Britain

Shell-Shock and Medical Culture in First World War Britain is a thought-provoking reassessment of medical responses to war-related psychological breakdown in the early twentieth century. Dr Loughran places "shell-shock" within the historical context of British psychological medicine to examine the intellectual resources doctors drew on as they struggled to make sense of nervous collapse. She reveals how medical approaches to "shell-shock" were formulated within an evolutionary framework which viewed mental breakdown as regression to a level characteristic of earlier stages of individual or racial development, but also ultimately resulted in greater understanding and acceptance of psychoanalytic approaches to human mind and behaviour. Through its demonstration of the crucial importance of concepts of mind–body relations, gender, will-power, and instinct to the diagnosis of "shell-shock", this book locates the disorder within a series of debates on human identity dating back to the Darwinian revolution and extending far beyond the medical sphere.

TRACEY LOUGHRAN is a Senior Lecturer in the Department of History at Cardiff University.

Studies in the Social and Cultural History of Modern Warfare

General Editor

Jay Winter, *Yale University*

Advisory Editors

David Blight, *Yale University*

Richard Bosworth, *University of Western Australia*

Peter Fritzsche, *University of Illinois, Urbana-Champaign*

Carol Gluck, *Columbia University*

Benedict Kiernan, *Yale University*

Antoine Prost, *Université de Paris-Sorbonne*

Robert Wohl, *University of California, Los Angeles*

In recent years, the field of modern history has been enriched by the exploration of two parallel histories. These are the social and cultural history of armed conflict, and the impact of military events on social and cultural history.

Studies in the Social and Cultural History of Modern Warfare presents the fruits of this growing area of research, reflecting both the colonization of military history by cultural historians and the reciprocal interest of military historians in social and cultural history, to the benefit of both. The series offers the latest scholarship in European and non-European events from the 1850s to the present day.

This is book 48 in the series, and a full list of titles in the series can be found at: www.cambridge.org/modernwarfare

Shell-Shock and Medical Culture in First World War Britain

Tracey Loughran
Cardiff University

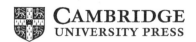

CAMBRIDGE
UNIVERSITY PRESS

University Printing House, Cambridge CB2 8BS, United Kingdom

Cambridge University Press is part of the University of Cambridge.

It furthers the University's mission by disseminating knowledge in the pursuit of education, learning and research at the highest international levels of excellence.

www.cambridge.org
Information on this title: www.cambridge.org/9781107128903

© Tracey Loughran 2017

First published 2017

Printed in the United States of America by Sheridan Books, Inc.

A catalogue record for this publication is available from the British Library

Library of Congress Cataloging-in-Publication Data
Names: Loughran, Tracey.
Title: Shell-shock and medical culture in First World War Britain / Tracey Loughran (Cardiff University).
Description: Cambridge, United Kingdom ; New York, New York : Cambridge University Press, 2016. | Series: Studies in the social and cultural history of modern warfare; 48 | Includes bibliographical references and index.
Identifiers: LCCN 2016011209 | ISBN 9781107128903 (Hardback)
Subjects: LCSH: War neuroses–Great Britain–History–20th century. | Soldiers–Mental health–Great Britain–History–20th century. | Veterans–Mental health–Great Britain–History–20th century. | War neuroses–Treatment–Great Britain–History–20th century. | Military psychiatry–Great Britain–History–20th century. | Social medicine–Great Britain–History–20th century. | World War, 1914-1918–Veterans–Great Britain. | World War, 1914-1918–Medical care–Great Britain. | World War, 1914-1918–Health aspects–Great Britain.
Classification: LCC RC550 .L68 2016 | DDC 616.85/212–dc23 LC record available at http://lccn.loc.gov/2016011209

ISBN 978-1-107-12890-3 Hardback

For Matthew, always

Contents

Acknowledgements

People often talk about the 'lone scholar' model in the humanities. As I consider all the people who have helped with this project, this seems not only mistaken but also a ludicrous way to think about History. I owe much, not least my ability to make a living in the discipline I love, to so many people.

This book originated as a PhD thesis. I was extremely fortunate in having two supervisors who supported and encouraged me, and made me have faith in my own abilities. I remain grateful to Michèle Barrett for all her help and support in those intellectually and financially precarious years. I first met Daniel Pick in 2000 when I was a second-year undergraduate. Since then, he has remained a constant source of guidance and inspiration. Sally Alexander and John Forrester were excellent external examiners, and John Forrester's kindness and willingness to provide references at short notice meant that I called upon his generosity far more often than was right.

In my immediate postdoctoral period, I spent two years at the University of Manchester. I was fortunate enough to meet many supportive colleagues there. Max Jones was extremely helpful to someone settling down in a strange department. Hannah Barker was a marvellous mentor and gave me the best single piece of advice about academic writing I am ever likely to receive. Peter Gatrell was more generous with his time than I had any right to expect, and he remains my model of what an academic should be like.

It took me a long time to stop missing London after I left in 2006. It is testament to the many strengths of my colleagues in the History Department at Cardiff University that when I moved away from the city in 2013, I felt even more heartbroken than when I departed my first hometown. Bill Jones and Val Davidge deserve special thanks for making a strange city feel like home. Stephanie Ward's wit, warmth, and wisdom make her an excellent colleague and an even better friend. Lloyd Bowen is a constant source of support in matters large and small and probably has no idea just how much I have relied on him since I joined the

Department. Federica Ferlanti's kindness, patience, and generosity make it easier to get through long days. Lisa Watkins' sterling administrative support has also made my working life easier in so many ways.

Many people offered their time and expertise as I completed the book. Alice Tomic's communications about her grandfather Millais Culpin were extremely helpful and made me think about the doctors I had studied for many years in a new way. Keir Waddington read earlier drafts of some chapters. His knowledge of the history of medicine and psychiatry in the late nineteenth and early twentieth centuries, especially medical education, has greatly improved the earlier parts of the book. Kevin Passmore went above and beyond the call of duty in reading the entire manuscript. It is much better for his thoughtful observations. Mike Roper also read a full draft of the book. His perceptive and supportive comments gave me much food for thought and helped to clarify some knotty problems with which I had long struggled.

My parents spent a lifetime working and struggling to ensure that their children had opportunities which were not open to them; I have a life that makes me happy now because they sacrificed much, and because they encouraged me along unfamiliar paths. This is my greatest debt. My sister Jennie Morgan has been a rock over the past decade. When I felt lost and lonely after I moved out of London, she never failed to phone, put a card in the post, and to provide a warm welcome when we visited. I don't know what I would have done without her. Many thanks are also due to my brother-in-law Lee Morgan and to my two funny, clever, and beautiful nieces Chloe Morgan and Emily Morgan. They always cheer me up and make me laugh. My older brother Simon Loughran has always protected and looked out for me; I know now, as I've known since I was born, that I can always rely on him. And, too late, I wish I could have done more for my younger brother Gary, who died, far too young, while this book was in press. I hope he knew how much I loved him. I will always miss him.

Eileen and Joe Grant have made me feel one of the family and have helped us out in ways small and large over the years. Many thanks too to Marney Loughran, June and David Thurkle, and Jim Johnson for too many things to list. My nan Georgina Johnson always has tea and Tunnocks on hand. Her house still feels like home, even without my much-missed granddad Joe Johnson. To my friends Katy Bell, Helen Birtwistle, Anna Cureton, Kate Hart and Kristina Heiduk-Spix: thank you. Matthew Eggerton deserves special mention for putting up with me as a houseguest, numerous brilliant impressions, and always knowing when to open a bottle of red wine. Finally, my deep gratitude to J.D.B., S.M., N.W., and R.E. as they continue to shock, awe, and inspire me.

I have also been fortunate enough to receive financial support from many organizations over the years, without which this book would not have been written. The Arts and Humanities Research Council funded my studies at Master's and PhD levels; the Scouloudi Foundation provided a six-month grant to help me complete my thesis; and I benefitted from an Economic and Social Research Council Postdoctoral Fellowship, a scheme now sadly defunct, which almost certainly kept me in academia. I also owe thanks to many librarians and archivists, but especially those at the British Library and the King's College London Archives.

Finally, to Matthew Grant: ever since I walked into that building in the Mile End Road in November 2003 and bumped into you, I haven't been able to believe my luck. Since then we've pulled out of too many towns to count, with the window down and the wind blowing back our hair. Tramps like us are born to run. This book is for you, with all my love.

Abbreviations

ANP	*Archives of Neurology and Psychiatry*
BEF	British Expeditionary Force
BMJ	*British Medical Journal*
BPS	British Psychological Society
EMJ	*Edinburgh Medical Journal*
GHMSA	Guy's Hospital Medical School Archive
JMS	*Journal of Mental Science*
KCHMSA	King's College Hospital and Medical School Archive
KCHR	*King's College Hospital Reports*
M-PA	Medico-Psychological Association
NYDN	Not Yet Diagnosed Nervous
PRSM	*Proceedings of the Royal Society of Medicine*
PTSD	Post-Traumatic Stress Disorder
RAFMS	Royal Air Force Medical Services
RAMC	Royal Army Medical Corps
RMO	Regimental Medical Officer
RSM	Royal Society of Medicine
RWOCESS	*Report of the War Office Committee of Enquiry into "Shell-Shock"*
SBHA	St Bartholomew's Hospital Archives
SBHR	*St Bartholomew's Hospital Reports*
TMW	*The Medical World*

Introduction
"Shell-Shock" and Medical Culture in First World War Britain

Even now, the First World War resists easy comprehension. No less than the generations to follow, those who lived through this colossal disaster struggled to make sense of it. War in the heart of Europe undermined cherished myths of western intellectual and moral superiority and spurred urgent reassessments of the status of "civilization" long after the ink had dried on the Treaty of Versailles.[1] In late 1915, when Sir William Osler (1849–1919), Regius Professor of Medicine at Oxford University, addressed a new intake of medical students on the relation of science and war, he captured the prevalent mood of doubt about what "progress" now meant. Osler set out to determine whether science was a force for good or evil in the contemporary world. On the one hand, science had enabled men to wage a war of unprecedented scale and destruction; on the other, modern medicine had managed to stem the resultant flow of suffering and death to an extent unimaginable only fifty years previously. On balance, Osler decided, 'the wounded soldier would throw his sword into the scale for science and he is right'.[2] He spoke to an audience shocked to its core by successive revelations of German 'savagery' in warfare: the 'barbarism' of chlorine gas, the murder of civilians by U-boats, the atrocities in Belgium, and the spectacle of Zeppelins above British towns. Osler's lecture responded to widespread fears that the demonic mix of bestial nature, wicked imagination, and technological achievement now revealed to lurk behind the façade of *Kultur* might destroy "civilization". Little

---

[1] A. Gregory, *The Last Great War: British Society and the First World War* (Cambridge and New York: Cambridge University Press, 2008), pp. 40–69; R. Overy, *The Morbid Age: Britain and the Crisis of Civilization, 1919–1939* (London: Penguin, 2010), especially pp. 9–49.

[2] W. Osler, 'An Address on Science and War', *Lancet*, 9 October 1915, 801. The death of Osler's son at Passchendaele severely challenged this commitment to medical benevolence and, he confessed, rage 'changed me into an ordinary barbarian': A. Carden-Coyne, *Reconstructing the Body: Classicism, Modernism, and the First World War* (Oxford: Oxford University Press, 2009), p. 42.

wonder, then, if his final endorsement of the benevolent power of science rang hollow even in Osler's own ears.

Osler did not flinch from brutal truths: he detailed the horrors of submarine warfare, aerial bombardment, and high-explosive munitions. Yet in the standard manner of eminent physicians addressing their apprentices, the manifest content of his lecture also reaffirmed the noble values and achievements of the medical profession. In only one place did Osler's profound anxieties about the future surface with full force:

I had a dream not long since that explorers in Central Africa had accidentally opened a vein of deadly radium which flowed slowly but imperceptibly like an unseen lava over the surface of the earth, killing by the exhalation of an irrespirable gas. It had crossed beneath the Mediterranean, swept through Europe, and had reached England. Convocation had been summoned by the Chancellor and the members of the University in full academics awaited the end of all things. On came the irresistible and deadly vapour, swept down the ranks, reached me, and I awoke – gasping for breath.[3]

Osler made little of this dream, only using it to dramatically introduce his discussion of Germany's 'diabolical' use of chemical warfare. At the distance of a century, however, Osler's dream strikes us as a moment of revelation, crystallized but not consciously realized. It expresses the most awful paradox of the war: that all the progress of western "civilization" had done no more than equip the "primitive" which remained at its heart with modern industrial weapons. In this dream, the attempts of western explorers to colonize the natural resources of "darkest Africa" proved an invasion too far. The deadly gas they liberated flowed forth and crushed all before it with the irresistible force of a natural disaster. The accumulated rationality and learning of all the potentates of the University of Oxford, for educated Britons one of the most powerful symbols of "civilization", could not save them. The gas spilled out even from the grotesque world of the nightmare, and Osler awoke fighting for breath. His own psyche had conspired to choke him. The dream represented the suicidal reality of the war, the unexpected eruption of primal instincts in the midst of everyday "civilized" life, played out on the individual mind.

Osler's dream not only exposes fears which dominated the medical imagination in wartime, but also ways of looking at the world which shaped medical responses to psychological breakdown in soldiers. In the early twentieth century, evolutionary theories of human development governed medical approaches to mind, nerves, and brain: radical

---

[3] Osler, 'Address on Science and War', 798, 801.

antitheses of "primitive" and "civilized" structured the scientific world-view of doctors who treated "shell-shocked" men. The contents of Osler's dream reveal a mode of understanding which permeated medical mentalities beyond the somnolent fantasies of one individual, as evidenced in the later elaboration of diagnostic categories and treatments for "shell-shock" which were saturated with evolutionary assumptions. His narration of the dream also makes a different gesture, perceptible only in hindsight, towards newer perspectives on human nature which extended their reach over the course of the war. Osler did no more than outline his dream, and it is unlikely that his audience made any further attempts at interpretation. In 1915, this did not seem like a lack; in 1919, it would have been an aberration. In the immediate aftermath of the war, most likely even the sternest critics of psychoanalysis would have noticed Osler's failure to delve into the unconscious, and assumed it was a deliberate decision; this dream-sketch would have triggered an entirely different chain of associations in listeners' minds. This book asks what changed in this short space of time, and why.

So: what did change? In simple terms, it might be said that "shell-shock" formed a bridge between Darwinian and Freudian understandings of human mind and behaviour. In the first decades of the twentieth century, British psychological medicine was dominated by evolutionary modes of thought. These evolutionary foundations were gradually overlaid by forms of psychological understanding which wittingly and unwittingly drew on concepts such as the unconscious, repression, and drives. In these decades, a distinctive set of concepts emerged within psychological medicine which, albeit in modified forms, continue to shape the way that most people in the western world explain their own behaviour to themselves and others today. This book assesses the role of the First World War as a catalyst for these changes in medical understandings of human mind and behaviour in Britain. It argues that although psychodynamic theories and therapies infiltrated medical culture through the conduit of "shell-shock", this did not involve fundamental revision of existing modes of explanation. In early twentieth-century psychological medicine, evolutionary and psychoanalytical theories and practices were not opposed, or even based within separate paradigms. Newer forms of psychological knowledge aligned with existing evolutionary modes of understanding, and were often expressed in quite conventional terms. Psychoanalytically informed approaches infused British medical culture because they melded with its native traditions, not because they nullified or overturned them.

This book explores the influence of evolutionary modes of understanding on the formation and operation of the diagnosis of "shell-shock".

This involves looking at "shell-shock" from a different angle to most histories. Often, historians approach "shell-shock" by reading backwards from a position of assumed psychological knowledge and depict psychological and physical approaches to the disorder as inherently opposed. Here, I try to read forwards from an understanding of the assumptions and knowledges which doctors brought to their work with "shell-shocked" men, as detailed in the first and second chapters. This perspective, which emphasizes doctors' shared commitment to evolutionary modes of explanation, challenges several elements of the conventional story of twentieth-century psychological medicine. It reveals pre-war medical culture as more variegated and open to "psychological" approaches than usually realized; draws out continuities between pre-war, wartime, and post-war psychological medicine; underlines similarities between different scientific approaches to "shell-shock" (such as the neurological, psychological, and physiological); and locates "shell-shock" itself within the mainstream of medical culture rather than as an object of expertise for either military psychiatry or the civilian "psy" disciplines. Crucially, it shows that although the experience of war contributed to important reorientations of theory and practice within psychological medicine, these changes developed out of established modes of knowledge formation and negotiation between different approaches to the problems of understanding human nature. The experience of "shell-shock" sparked a revolution in British psychological medicine, but this occurred through evolution rather than rupture.

This argument raises questions about how we understand the war itself as an historical event which (potentially) caused specific shifts within medical culture. As a diagnostic category, "shell-shock" was a product of war, but it was also formed out of the knowledges of civilian medicine. Awareness of this dual heritage is integral to understanding its origins, contents, and afterlife in medical culture. "Shell-shock" doctors also pondered the exact relation of the disorder to war as they repeatedly returned to the question of why some men broke down while others did not. In wartime, this question most often led into debates over the relative influence of heredity, life experience, or exposure to horrific events as causative factors in "shell-shock". Furthermore, doctors' own patriotic or ambivalent emotions about the pursuit of war also affected medical theorizations of "shell-shock". The wartime context was not merely background to medical discourse on "shell-shock", but also shaped that discourse in powerful and ill-understood ways. The fact of war undoubtedly provoked radical questions about the limits of endurance, the relative influence of nature and nurture on behaviour, and the relation of mind to body. However, while the war was ongoing, it also limited and contained the potential radicalism of the answers to these questions. Most doctors accepted it as self-evident that war exposed men to severe and unusual horrors which could lead to breakdown. This meant that as long as war lasted, doctors could explain "shell-shock" as an understandable response to exceptional circumstances and so were not forced to fundamentally revise their explanatory frameworks. Perversely, "shell-shock" had most real influence on psychological medicine in the post-war period.

"Shell-Shock", War, and Social Change

Since the 1960s, debates on war and social change have dominated social and cultural histories of the First World War.[4] In histories of medicine and psychiatry, a counterpart of these debates asks whether the experience of "shell-shock" stimulated sweeping changes in psychological medicine. In 1985, Martin Stone put forward the influential argument that the wartime episode of "shell-shock" redefined 'the boundary of the pathological ... at all its constitutive levels' and 'brought the neuroses into the mainstream of mental medicine and economic life'.[5] Stone contended that British doctors showed little interest in medical psychology before 1914, but received practical introductions to psychodynamic approaches (including psychoanalysis) when forced into professional contact with "shell-shocked" men in wartime. By the end of the war, hundreds of doctors had developed considerable expertise in the diagnosis and treatment of nervous disorders, and in the 1920s, these effects rippled out across psychological medicine: in books and articles on psychopathology and psychotherapy, in new associations set up to promote research in medical psychology, and in the creation of facilities for the treatment of psychiatric disorders outside the asylum system. Because "shell-shock" proved that any man could break down under sufficient stress, it severely dented psychiatric orthodoxies such as belief

[4] Important contributions to these debates include A. Marwick, *The Deluge: British Society and the First World War* (Harmondsworth: Penguin, 1965); A. Marwick, *War and Social Change in the Twentieth Century: A Comparative Study of Britain, France, Germany, Russia, and the United States* (Basingstoke: Palgrave Macmillan, 1974); P. Fussell, *The Great War and Modern Memory* (London, Oxford, and New York: Oxford University Press, 1975); J.M. Winter, *The Great War and the British People*, 2nd edn (Basingstoke and New York: Palgrave Macmillan, 2003) [1986].
[5] M. Stone, 'Shellshock and the Psychologists', in W.F. Bynum, R. Porter, and M. Shepherd (eds.), *The Anatomy of Madness: Essays in the History of Psychiatry. Volume 1: People and Ideas* (London and New York: Tavistock, 1985), p. 266. An important precursor to this essay is E. Leed, *No Man's Land: Combat and Identity in World War One* (Cambridge: Cambridge University Press, 1979), pp. 169–80.

in hereditary degeneration. Stone concluded that radical changes to psychiatric practice such as those enabled by the Mental Treatment Act (1930), which made treatment without certification available to 'rate-aided patients', should therefore be seen as a direct outcome of the wartime experience of "shell-shock".

For the next decade, most scholarship on "shell-shock" and early twentieth-century psychological medicine endorsed this interpretation, which chimed with the prevalent emphasis on rupture and change in histories of the First World War.[6] In the early 2000s, around the same time as the first full-length monographs on "shell-shock" were published, it began to be subjected to serious and sustained challenges. Historians pointed out that medical engagement with psychoanalytic theory was evident even before 1914 while the doctrine of hereditary degeneration survived into the post-war decades and beyond.[7] Nor did psychoanalytic therapies gain much purchase in the wartime treatment of "shell-shock": only a handful of wartime doctors employed radical "analytic" therapies, with most continuing to espouse conventional treatments such as rest, warm baths, and bromides.[8] In wartime, resources were diverted from mentally ill civilians to soldiers, so civilian patients did not benefit from advances in military psychiatry.[9] War did not overturn the public stigma attached to mental illness, as many "shell-shocked" veterans faced a lack of sympathy and ongoing battles to prove their right to pensions.[10] In all, "shell-shock" had almost no influence on the army's practices over the interwar period and few concrete effects on civilian psychological medicine. The majority of doctors never endorsed Freudian psychoanalytic theories, and before

---

[6] T. Bogacz, 'War Neurosis and Cultural Change in England, 1914–22: The Work of the War Office Committee of Enquiry into "Shell-Shock"', *Journal of Contemporary History*, 24 (1989), 227–56; M. Pines, 'The Development of the Psychodynamic Movement', in G.E. Berrios and H. Freeman (eds.), *150 Years of British Psychiatry, 1841–1991* (London: Gaskell, 1991), pp. 213–15; C. Feudtner, '"Minds the Dead Have Ravished": Shell Shock, History, and the Ecology of Disease Systems', *History of Science*, 31 (1993), 377–420.

[7] M. Thomson, *Psychological Subjects: Identity, Culture, and Health in Twentieth-Century Britain* (Oxford and New York: Oxford University Press, 2006), pp. 182–6.

[8] P. Leese, '"Why Are They Not Cured?" British Shellshock Treatment During the Great War', in M. Micale and P. Lerner (eds.), *Traumatic Pasts: History, Psychiatry and Trauma in the Modern Age, 1870–1930* (Cambridge: Cambridge University Press, 2001); P. Leese, *Shell Shock: Traumatic Neurosis and the British Soldiers of the First World War* (Basingstoke: Palgrave, 2002), pp. 68–84.

[9] M. Thomson, 'Status, Manpower and Mental Fitness: Mental Deficiency in the First World War', in R. Cooter, M. Harrison, and S. Sturdy (eds.), *War, Medicine and Modernity* (Stroud: Sutton, 1998), pp. 149—66.

[10] Leese, *Shell Shock*, pp. 123–58; P. Barham, *Forgotten Lunatics of the Great War* (New Haven, CT, and London: Yale University Press, 2004).

1930 there were few outpatient clinics in Britain.[11] Cumulatively, this research emphasized continuities in the ideas, practices, and institutions of pre- and post-war psychological medicine.

Each of these revisionist claims is backed by substantial evidence. On an individual basis, each claim convinces. Nevertheless, this scholarship fails to prove that the war did not critically and permanently alter British psychological medicine.[12] The determinist undercurrent of some revisionist scholarship on war and social change is troubling, as it seems to assume that specific developments would have happened despite the war.[13] This does no more than flip on their head earlier narratives of psychiatric enlightenment via wartime "lessons learned". Both interpretations are equally teleological: no matter what happened, we were always going to end up where we are now. I find this difficult to accept, and so resist describing the consequences of "shell-shock" for psychological medicine in the bare idiom of continuity or change. The effects of an event as complex as the First World War cannot be reduced to the choice between complete rupture or mere ripples on the calm surface of medical culture. Instead, this book examines how existing approaches to disorders of mind, nerves, and brain were adapted, exploited, and stretched in wartime to accommodate newer modes of thought, and how these processes ultimately encouraged acceptance of the novel and transfigured established ideas and practices. This interpretation contributes to those cultural histories of the First World War which complicate the relation between "tradition" and "modernity" (and therefore continuity and change). These explorations show how older forms and practices could take on new meanings in different contexts, and how contemporaries self-consciously negotiated understandings of the "traditional" and the "modern" as they sought to make sense of the war as a defining moment in their own lives and the life of the nation.[14]

---

[11] B. Shephard, *A War of Nerves: Soldiers and Psychiatrists, 1914–1994* (London: Pimlico, 2002), pp. 133–68; E. Jones and S. Wessely, *Shell Shock to PTSD: Military Psychiatry from 1900 to the Gulf War* (Hove, East Sussex and New York: Psychology Press, 2005).

[12] My own views on this question have changed since the publication of T. Loughran, 'Shell-Shock and Psychological Medicine in First World War Britain', *Social History of Medicine*, 22:1 (2009), 79–95.

[13] M. Harrison, 'The Medicalization of War – The Militarization of Medicine', *Social History of Medicine*, 9:2 (1996), 270.

[14] J. Winter, *Sites of Memory, Sites of Mourning: The Great War in European Cultural History* (Cambridge, New York, and Melbourne: Cambridge University Press, 1995); A. Light, *Forever England: Femininity, Literature and Conservatism between the Wars* (London and New York: Routledge, 1991); S. Goebel, *The Great War and Medieval Memory: War, Remembrance and Medievalism in Britain and Germany* (Cambridge and New York: Cambridge University Press, 2006); Carden-Coyne, *Reconstructing the Body*. See also

In the early decades of the twentieth century, acceptance of psycho-analytic theories and practices depended on the "translation" of these ideas into the established vernacular of mainstream psychological medicine. This acceptance was always actively negotiated, often partial, and conditional on a more extensive process of "translation" than the mere removal of allegedly "offensive" aspects of Freudian theory. Psychoanalytic concepts infiltrated medical culture through three main processes: "translation", consisting of assimilation into more familiar modes of explanation, and/or denial of their fundamental novelty; their modification or adaptation to suit existing modes of interpretation, such as emphasizing social rather than sexual instincts and impulses; and their incorporation into eclectic systems of diagnosis and treatment. These processes of "translation", modification, and eclecticism were used before, during, and after the war. However, the post-war period wit-nessed the proliferation of psychological debates in mainstream medical culture as well as important shifts within the conventional explanatory mechanisms of psychological medicine. Yet while confrontation with "shell-shock" forced doctors to consider new approaches to nervous and mental disorders, these established processes of incorporation made incremental revolution seem like the continuation of established trad-ition. Often, protestations of psychiatric orthodoxy reveal not the absence of change, but how it manifested: claims about "tradition" cloaked the introduction of novel elements into psychological medicine and eased their acceptance.

I use the term "translation" to describe the process through which newer forms of psychological knowledge were partially assimilated through being (re-)presented as consonant with established aspects of British medical culture, even when dealing with concepts initially expressed in English, because transposition into different contexts was always accompanied by shifts in meaning. As a result, many words and concepts in common use within British psychological medicine were not clearly defined or always used in exactly the same way. Often, the same words and concepts were disputed, in flux, or even kept deliberately imprecise. Indeed, "shell-shock" is perhaps the paradigmatic example of a word/concept at the same time serviceably vague, fiercely contested, and constantly mutable: similarly fluid descriptive terms include "psychic", "functional", and "analytic". These forms and uses of lan-guage both reflected and shaped how doctors understood and responded to the symptoms of "shell-shock".

M. Francis, 'Attending to Ghosts: Some Reflections on the Disavowals of British Great War Historiography', *Twentieth Century British History*, 25:3 (2014), 355–6.

The indeterminacy of the language of early twentieth-century psychological medicine raises all kinds of problems for the historian. How is it
possible to research and write about words of indefinite meaning, or past
forms of understanding articulated in vocabularies that have since shifted
meaning or fallen out of use? I argue that it is necessary not only to
interrogate the meaning of ill-defined words and concepts but also
to adopt the specific language of wartime medical texts. In some cases,
only a word no longer used can adequately convey past modes of
understanding. For example, in the period covered here, the term
"psychic" described symptoms which were not (or not primarily) somatic, but it did not usually incorporate any sophisticated model of psychological processes. The existence of such a word, which describes a
gap between the physical and what we now think of as the psychological,
explains much about medical mentalities, as does the gradual abandon-
ment and reconfiguration of this term in the post-war decades. Such
words and concepts cannot be fully translated into today's idiom; the full
extent of their past meanings is unreachable and unassimilable. For this
reason, I use double quotation marks around terms or concepts which
contemporaries contested (such as "shell-shock"), those involving
value judgements essential to conveying past mentalities (such as "civilized" or "primitive"), and those for which current uses do not adequately
reflect past meaning (such as "psychic" and, in some contexts,
"psychological").[15]

This use of double quotation marks is intended to jar: it illustrates the
awkwardness of these concepts, including "shell-shock" itself. It is a
visual reminder not to take meaning for granted, a combination of the
familiar and the strange which echoes the admixture of the habitual and
the incongruous in post-war psychological medicine. The experience of
war fostered dramatic reorientation of conceptual and, to a lesser extent,
therapeutic approaches to the psychological within mainstream medical
culture. However, dramatic changes in the character and extent of psychological debate in medical culture, which stemmed directly from the
war, coexisted with apparent continuities in older ways of understanding
human nature and the world. Continuities went hand in hand with
fundamental changes in the status and contents of psychological understanding in post-war medical culture. Revolutions do not always consist
of sudden and radical paradigm shifts: sometimes a revolution takes
place when, as a result of clearly identified events, there is an accelerated

---

[15] For similar reasons, I use indeterminate male pronouns wherever contemporary authors
did so: this communicates the gendered construction of certain terrains, which was an
important part of their mental worlds.

movement of marginal tendencies into the mainstream, where this constellation of changes constitutes something 'innovative and novel'.[16] After the war, the landscape of British psychological medicine had an appreciably different appearance from that of 1914. The most likely explanation for this difference is that the experience of "shell-shock" deepened and accelerated existing trends towards the adoption of psychodynamic approaches. This form of revolution via evolution cannot be easily broken into the basic blocks of continuity/change, "traditional"/"modern", or radical/conservative. These kinds of binary divisions encourage simplistic narratives of linear progress towards psychological understanding, such as those told in histories which claim a straightforward journey from "shell-shock" to post-traumatic stress disorder (PTSD). The propagation of such stories has important consequences for how we think about the existence of war and trauma in our own societies.

"Shell-Shock", Trauma, and PTSD

The historical narrative which takes us from "shell-shock" to PTSD is contested, but still powerful. Although there is a definite historical relationship between the diagnostic constructions and experiences of "shell-shock" and PTSD, the two syndromes are not direct equivalents or the same condition under different names. The subject of this history is "shell-shock", not PTSD: they are not the same thing. It is important to make this absolutely clear because, as the history of "shell-shock" demonstrates, processes of naming affect abstract conceptualizations of illness, medical practices, and historical understanding. Even in wartime, "shell-shock" was a controversial label, lambasted for its misleading inference that symptoms resulted from physical injury to the central nervous system and rejected by many doctors, yet retaining resonance in spite of widespread disfavour. "Shell-shock" was coined early in the war, and was in use among soldiers before it was first committed to print in February 1915 by the academic psychologist Charles Myers (1873–1946). In an influential article, Myers described the symptoms of "shell-shock", but remained non-committal as to their cause. These symptoms appeared after exposure to shell blasts, but were also similar to hysteria.[17] Although cases of nervous and mental breakdown in soldiers

---

[16] G. Weisz, 'Reconstructing Paris Medicine', *Bulletin of the History of Medicine*, 75:1 (2001), 108.

[17] C.S. Myers, 'A Contribution to the Study of Shell Shock: Being an Account of Three Cases of Loss of Memory, Vision, Smell, and Taste, Admitted into the Duchess of

had been reported in the medical press months before the publication of Myers' article, and despite his caution, "shell-shock" now took on a life of its own. The act of naming transformed disparate symptoms into a syndrome which could be researched, debated, or rejected, but not wished away. With the naming of "shell-shock", a distinct diagnosis was created. The description of symptoms under this label made available new forms of identification, understanding, and behaviour.[18] The public act of naming had real and important effects on medical approaches to what was now perceived as a definite disorder and on the lives of men now known as "shell-shocked". Names are not neutral. Names matter.

The aetiological ambiguities Myers noted have never been fully resolved. In wartime, definitional problems attached to "shell-shock" affected both the treatment of individual soldiers and their entitlement to pensions for war-related injury. The term "shell-shock" was soon appropriated by the army, who did not know quite what to do with it. Until late in 1915, men presenting with nervous and mental symptoms were classified under a variety of headings.[19] The Army Council then issued a writ commanding that cases be labelled either wounded ('shell-shock W') or sick ('shell-shock S') depending on whether or not symptoms resulted from 'enemy action'. Only 'shell-shock W' cases were entitled to wound stripes and military pensions.[20] With this ruling, the military officially recognized 'a grey area between cowardice and madness' for the first time, but also maintained its traditional distinction between 'battle-casualties' and 'sickness' in relation to "shell-shock".[21] Regimental Medical Officers (RMOs) found it difficult to classify cases using this scheme. In practice, they often mislabelled soldiers caught in shell blasts as 'shell-shock S' and vice versa, or failed to modify the label "shell-shock" with the appropriate letter, meaning that many eligible men were not deemed to be battle casualties.[22]

Westminster's War Hospital, Le Touquet', *Lancet*, 13 February 1915, 316–20; C.S. Myers, *Shell Shock in France 1914–1918: Based on a War Diary* (Cambridge: Cambridge University Press, 1940), p. 11.

[18] This interpretation is influenced by Ian Hacking's theories of 'dynamic nominalism' and 'the looping effects of human kinds'. See I. Hacking, 'Making Up People', in T.C. Heller *et al.* (eds.), *Reconstructing Individualism: Autonomy, Individuality and the Self in Western Thought* (Stanford, CA: Stanford University Press, 1986); I. Hacking, 'The Looping Effects of Human Kinds', in D. Sperber, D. Premack, and A.J. Premack (eds.), *Causal Cognition: A Multidisciplinary Approach* (Oxford: Clarendon Press, 1994).

[19] Leese, *Shell Shock*, p. 53.   [20] Myers, *Shell Shock in France*, pp. 93–5.

[21] Shephard, *War of Nerves*, pp. 28–9.

[22] Myers, *Shell Shock in France*, p. 94. For a detailed analysis of the use of these classifications at one neurological centre, see Jones and Wessely, *Shell Shock to PTSD*, p. 30.

In June 1917, the army introduced a new classification procedure which created almost as many problems as the old one. When new specialist units for the rapid treatment of nervous and mental cases were established close to the fighting lines, it was decided to initially label men sent to these centres 'NYDN (Not Yet Diagnosed Nervous)' and determine via enquiries to their units whether they should ultimately be classified 'shell-shock W' or 'shell-shock S'. As the War Office Committee of Enquiry into "Shell-Shock" concluded in 1922, this procedure was 'unfair and unworkable in practice'. In September 1918, the classification 'shell-shock W' was finally abolished in treatment centres in France, and used only for cases of serious disabilities which warranted transfer to the United Kingdom, where neurological boards at special centres recommended their classification as battle casualties (or not).[23]

Although the military eventually developed more effective procedures for managing the influx of "shell-shock" cases at home and abroad, it never satisfactorily dealt with the classificatory and definitional problems "shell-shock" posed. This failure had immediate consequences for soldiers wrangling with the Ministry of Pensions over just compensation for war-related conditions, but it also affects historians. At the most basic level, problems around naming affected the compilation of reliable statistics on "shell-shock". When the official history of the First World War medical services was published in 1923, full statistics were not available, and the compilers worked mainly from data relating to the number of reported casualties in particular units over specific periods.[24] To calculate the incidence of "shell-shock", compilers used Ministry of Pensions statistics for the total number of cases of "shell-shock" reported as battle casualties in France up to the end of 1917, doubled these to include those reported as 'sick', added an allowance to cover the period until the end of 1918, and arrived at the figure of 80,000.[25] This method of calculation did not account for variations in the incidence of "shell-shock" over different phases of fighting, the likely possibility of unequal numbers of 'sick' and 'wounded', or that cases of relapse might have been counted several times over.

---

[23] *Report of the War Office Committee of Enquiry into "Shell-Shock"* (*RWOCESS*) (London: Imperial War Museum, 2004) [1922], p. 119.

[24] T.J. Mitchell and G.M. Smith, *History of the Great War Based on Official Documents. Medical Services: Casualties and Medical Statistics of the Great War* (London: HMSO, 1931), pp. x–xiii.

[25] W.G. Macpherson, W.P. Herringham, T.R. Elliott, and A. Balfour (eds.), *History of the Great War Based on Official Documents. Medical Services: Diseases of the War*, 2 vols. (London: HMSO, 1923), vol. 2, pp. 1–7.

These statistics, unreliable at face level, disintegrate entirely when the problematic relation between diagnostic label and symptom is taken into account. Pressure on time and resources meant that sometimes doctors could offer little more than cursory examination before shuttling soldiers along to another point in the medical system. Adolphe Abrahams (1883–1967), medical officer in charge of the Connaught Hospital at Aldershot during the war, claimed that he often received patients bearing wildly inappropriate diagnoses, including 'a case of aneurysm sent up as myalgia' and 'a case of oesophagal carcinoma labelled "This man is always complaining"'.[26] These kinds of problems were magnified when dealing with a disorder as ill-defined as "shell-shock". Apart from anything else, there was considerable disagreement among doctors about what actually counted as "shell-shock". One doctor might treat cardiac irregularities and fits as somatic conditions while another viewed the same symptoms as evidence of psychological disturbance; other physicians might label certain kinds of head injury as "shell-shock", applying the term more literally than most; some sympathetic doctors categorized "mentally deficient" men as "shell-shocked" to remove them from active service; and sometimes, doctors even tried to avoid any kind of official diagnosis for fear of stigmatizing the patient.[27] It is impossible not only to know how many soldiers were officially diagnosed with "shell-shock" and related disorders, but also what symptoms actually sheltered under official headings – and this is before we even start to consider those who were haunted for decades by their wartime experiences, but never came under medical attention.[28]

There are all kinds of practical reasons why acts of naming mattered to soldiers and continue to matter to historians of "shell-shock". But names also matter to historians because they often involve claims about identity: that X in the past *was the same as* (or was identical to) Y in the present.[29] Most historians are alert to the possibility that in different cultural and historical settings, the same word does not always describe the same

[26] A. Abrahams, 'The Medical Officer in Charge of a Division', *Journal of the RAMC*, 33:1 (July 1919), 83–5.
[27] Leese, *Shell Shock*, p. 53; M. Culpin, 'The Early Stage of Hysteria', *British Medical Journal (BMJ)*, 13 April 1918, 225.
[28] On invisible emotional responses to war, see J. Winter, *Remembering War: The Great War between Memory and History in the Twentieth Century* (New Haven, CT, and London: Yale University Press, 2006), p. 62.
[29] A. Cunningham, 'Transforming Plague: The Laboratory and the Identity of Infectious Disease', in A. Cunningham and P. Williams (eds.), *The Laboratory Revolution in Medicine* (Cambridge: Cambridge University Press, 1992), p. 210.

concept.[30] In relation to "shell-shock", the reverse is often assumed: that different names – "shell-shock", trauma, PTSD – describe the same concept. In many contexts, "shell-shock" is portrayed as merely an older name for PTSD, a present-day psychiatric syndrome which develops from exposure to an 'extreme traumatic stressor'. However, the diagnostic criteria for "shell-shock" and PTSD are not exact equivalents.[31] In contrast to the clearly delimited clinical syndrome of PTSD, for contemporaries "shell-shock" described a range of afflictions which incorporated physical, physiological, and psychological factors, including hysterical paralyses, severe depression, and persistent headaches and amnesia. Although many recorded cases of "shell-shock" from the First World War would meet the criteria for a diagnosis of PTSD, many more would not. By a comparison of symptoms and diagnostic criteria, the two syndromes do not match up: "shell-shock" is not PTSD.[32]

Why does this matter? "Shell-shock" should not be conflated with PTSD because this stance involves a number of other positions that are rarely explicitly articulated, but that are frighteningly far-reaching: that no matter what contemporaries believed, in reality, "shell-shock" is only one name for a psychological reaction to warfare which has existed in roughly the same form in several different historical cultures; that today's psychiatric establishment has succeeded where previous medical systems failed in accurately identifying the core elements of this psychological syndrome; and that during the First World War, when they described cases as "shell-shock", doctors often perceived, reported, emphasized, or interpreted symptoms wrongly. Assumptions of uncomplicated equivalence between "shell-shock" and PTSD involve the implicit claim that "we" now know better. This is an unintentional collapse into an unarticulated moral position. The disorders which soldiers suffered were painful and real. At the same time, any history which positions itself as telling the story of the gradual realization of the truth about "shell-shock", the story of the recognition of a transhistorical psychological illness now properly understood and correctly identified under the banner of PTSD, is inevitably teleological. Such histories cut off the

---

[30] On 'word history' and 'concept history', see T. Dixon, *The Invention of Altruism: Making Moral Meanings in Modern Britain* (Oxford and New York: Oxford University Press, 2008), pp. 28–39.

[31] T. Loughran, 'Shell Shock, Trauma, and the First World War: The Making of a Diagnosis and Its Histories', *Journal of the History of Medicine and Allied Sciences*, 67:1 (January 2012).

[32] For an extensive discussion of this view, see A. Young, *The Harmony of Illusions: Inventing Post-Traumatic Stress Disorder* (Princeton, NJ: Princeton University Press, 1995).

possibility of alternative histories of "shell-shock", which are not about psychological recognition, but the manifold possible trajectories of a disorder with protean symptoms.[33]

In this book, I define "shell-shock" as the constellation of symptoms and conditions which wartime doctors identified as a related set of psychiatric, psychological, and physiological responses to war.[34] This is a messy definition, but there are no neat resolutions to the problems raised by a nebulous, disputed, and endlessly elastic diagnostic category. In some respects, this approach echoes wartime usage. Often, doctors expressed severe misgivings about the designation "shell-shock" but used it as a last resort, either with the aim of being immediately understood or to make non-prescriptive aetiological and descriptive statements about the nervous and mental disorders of war. The term "shell-shock" became an unavoidable form of shorthand for war-related nervous and mental disorders, and it is used in this spirit here. This definition shifts the object of study from the history of psychological trauma to the historical reconstruction of the now-discarded diagnosis of "shell-shock". It is an approach which tries to preserve the pastness of the past, to keep potential future histories open, and to understand the disorder on its own fluctuating and contested ground.[35] Because it does not characterize "shell-shock" as a coherent, bounded, and essentially knowable entity, this definition generates a history which shifts focus to the production of knowledge about "shell-shock" rather than knowledge of the disorder itself. In turn, this means thinking about the diagnosis of "shell-shock" as produced by historically specific medical communities and through historically specific and discrete mechanisms.

"Shell-Shock" and Medical Culture

This book examines the construction of the diagnosis of "shell-shock" and the medical mentalities underpinning this act of construction.

---

[33] On other possible trajectories for histories of "shell-shock", see Loughran, 'Shell Shock, Trauma, and the First World War'.

[34] I have not included within this definition symptoms and syndromes most often studied and treated separately to "shell-shock", such as functional cardiac disorders, even though by the end of the war, many cardiologists and "shell-shock" doctors believed that similar mechanisms were at work in the production of war neurosis and functional cardiac disorders. I have also excluded discussions of malingering; although military doctors necessarily tried to separate malingerers from the genuinely ill, and conscious simulation of illness from "shell-shock", most accepted that there was a genuine difference.

[35] On the avoidance of present-day perspectives and the importance of allowing for contingency in the history of psychology, see R. Smith, 'Does the History of Psychology Have a Subject?', *History of the Human Sciences*, 1:2 (1988), 147–77.

An understanding of medical approaches to "shell-shock" is integral to understanding the disorder in its fullest dimensions. As both medical professionals and representatives of the state, "shell-shock" doctors held an unusual degree of power over vulnerable patients. They decreed diagnostic labels, length of stay in hospital, types of treatment, the soldier's future part in the war (discharge, light duty, or return to combat), and the size of his pension. What doctors said and did influenced how patients suffered, their possibilities for agency or resistance, and the physical, emotional, and financial resources of their future lives. This book explores the intellectual resources available to medical men as they took these life-changing decisions; how knowledge was produced, organized, and deployed in encounters between doctors and patients; and how newer forms of psychological knowledge were assimilated into earlier schemes of explanation. This is achieved through a research method which combines analysis of the structure and contents of publicly circulating forms of medical knowledge with attention to the producers of this knowledge, including their professional interests, sites of practice, and networks.

The main evidence base is a comprehensive survey of published wartime medical discourse on "shell-shock" and related disorders, incorporating generalist civilian and military medical journals; specialist publications on neurology, psychiatry, and psychology; and textbooks authored by "shell-shock" doctors or dealing with relevant topics.[36] These publications provide information about specific formulations of "shell-shock" as well as the contexts which shaped these understandings. In histories of "shell-shock", the status of published medical discourse as a form of evidence is ambiguous. As the most extensive and easily accessible unified body of evidence about "shell-shock", it is cited more often than any other type of source. At the same time, the value of this type of evidence is rarely explicitly assessed. It is sometimes implied that unpublished sources, such as the diaries of frontline medical officers, or hospital case notes, provide greater insight into the construction and operation of the diagnosis at ground level.[37] Yet while unpublished

---

[36] This includes a complete review of the following publications for the period 1914–19: *British Medical Journal (BMJ)*, *Lancet*, *Edinburgh Medical Journal*, *Practitioner*, *The Medical World*, *Proceedings of the Royal Society of Medicine*, *Journal of the Royal Army Medical Corps*, *Brain*, *Journal of Mental Science*, and the *British Journal of Psychology*.

[37] Leese, *Shell Shock*, pp. 73–4; S.C. Linden and E. Jones, '"Shell Shock" Revisited: An Examination of the Case Records of the National Hospital in London', *Medical History*, 58:4 (2014), 2–3. For examples of histories drawing extensively on unpublished material, see B. Shephard, '"The Early Treatment of Mental Disorders": R.G. Rows and Maghull 1914–1918', in H. Freeman and G.E. Berrios (eds.), *150 Years of British Psychiatry. Volume 2: The Aftermath* (London: Athlone, 1996), pp. 434–64; Leese, '"Why

records illuminate aspects of clinical practice and the day-to-day operation of institutions which are not evident in published medical discourse, they are not repositories of deeper truths about medical
practice. Published and unpublished sources reveal different kinds and
layers of knowledge, and published texts are valuable sources in their
own right.

Knowledge about "shell-shock" was created in different ways and at
several locations. Clinical encounters between doctors and patients
formed the most important route to such knowledge. However, these
encounters were mediated through shared knowledge about "shell-
shock" and related disorders circulating in medical culture. This culture
was partially constituted through the medical press, which provided a
medium for the exchange and flow of ideas and information, performed
the social function of reporting on a communal world, and enabled
physicians to locate their own professional lives within local, national,
and international activities. If we think of the medical press as the
primary site for the construction of public professional knowledge about
"shell-shock", it becomes clear that published medical texts did not
simply smooth over the "real" work of knowledge production performed
in face-to-face encounters between doctors and patients. There was no
disjuncture between published medical discourse and on-the-ground
clinical practice: these texts were an active vehicle for knowledge formation and comprised a form of practice.

Medical journals were public productions which reflected the views of
their contributors and engaged the attention of their readers. The medical press represented the activities of on-the-ground communities and
organizations, but in presenting these activities to different audiences and
in different contexts, it reshaped their meaning. It was a site for debates
which expressed conflict between different stances, but it also helped to
determine the nature of these positions and provided a public expression
of viewpoints which others could identify with or against.[38] The journals
used here catered to diverse medical constituencies and made vital
contributions to the exchange and flow of ideas and information.

Are They Not Cured?'"; E. Jones, 'Shell Shock at Maghull and the Maudsley: Models of
Psychological Medicine in the UK', *Journal of the History of Medicine and Allied Sciences*,
65:3 (2010), 368–95; M. Humphries and K. Kurchinski, 'Rest, Relax and Get Well:
A Re-Conceptualisation of Great War Shell Shock Treatment', *War & Society*
[University of New South Wales], 27:2 (2008), 89–110.
[38] For example, see letters under the heading 'Correspondence: Psycho-Analysis', *BMJ*, 6,
13, 20, and 27 January 1917, 32–3, 64–5, 102–4, 138–9; those marked 'Hypnotism',
Times, 22, 23, and 25 April 1919; and those headed 'Hypnotism, Suggestion, and
Dissociation', *BMJ*, 26 April, 10, 17, and 31 May 1919, 561, 592–3, 624–5, 693.

Wartime articles should not be read as complete statements on "shell-shock", but as part of a thriving discourse in continual flux and evolution. In drawing on the wartime medical press, this book does not delineate a genealogy of pure ideas, but deals with the mess and confusion, as well as the unexpected convergences and contrasts, which accompanied the construction of "shell-shock" in real time and space.

To fully understand the status, contents, and influence of published medical discourse on "shell-shock", it is also essential to consider its producers, and above all, the relation of these authors to "shell-shocked" men. The authors of these wartime medical texts generated knowledge of "shell-shock" and related disorders which publicly circulated and influenced understandings of the disorder within medical culture and beyond. If we think of these authors as an identifiable cohort of "shell-shock" doctors, it is possible to generalize about their backgrounds, wartime activities, and post-war careers in ways which help us to understand both the diagnostic construction of "shell-shock" and the legacies of the disorder in post-war medical culture. This approach shifts the focus from a handful of influential or notorious physicians to the location of both familiar and now-forgotten doctors, concepts, practices, and debates within wider medical culture.[39] Of course, this cohort is not representative of all those who worked with "shell-shocked" men. The desire and ability to publish demonstrated unusual commitment to active theoretical articulation or knowledge formation and often indicated elevated actual or potential professional achievement. As a cohort, published "shell-shock" doctors collected many honours – including peerages, parliamentary seats, and prestigious professional prizes – and were extremely active in international, national, regional, and local medical and scientific associations. Many held posts in universities and medical schools.[40] These doctors exerted great influence on medical culture through their publications, professional achievements, and high

---

[39] Excellent biographical studies include R. Leys, 'Traumatic Cures: Shell Shock, Janet, and the Question of Memory', *Critical Inquiry*, 20 (Summer 1994), 623–62; A. Young, 'W.H.R. Rivers and the War Neuroses', *Journal of the History of the Behavioral Sciences*, 35:4 (1999), 359–78; D. Cantor, 'Between Galen, Geddes, and the Gael: Arthur Brock, Modernity, and Medical Humanism in Early-Twentieth-Century Scotland', *Journal of the History of Medicine and Allied Sciences*, 60:1 (2005), 1–41; J. Forrester, 'The English Freud: W.H.R. Rivers, Dreaming, and the Making of the Early Twentieth-Century Human Sciences', in S. Alexander and B. Taylor (eds.), *History and Psyche: Culture, Psychoanalysis, and the Past* (Basingstoke and New York: Palgrave Macmillan, 2012), pp. 71–104.

[40] For the detailed biographical information on this cohort of "shell-shock" doctors on which the subsequent discussion is based, see T. Loughran, 'Shell-Shock in First World War Britain: An Intellectual and Medical History, c. 1860–c. 1920', unpublished PhD thesis, University of London (2006), pp. 240–89.

levels of involvement in associational life. Precisely because they were not typical, they were able to shape medical discourse at different levels and from many different sites.

A quasi-prosopographical approach yields two critical insights into the diagnostic construction of the disorder. First, publicly circulating forms of medical knowledge on "shell-shock" were produced by civilian doctors who had either joined up for the duration, or not at all. Second, these doctors were drawn from a range of medical specialisms, not just the disciplines of mind, nerves, and brain. In wartime, "shell-shock" was located within the mainstream of medical culture rather than the confines of either military psychiatry or the civilian "psy" disciplines. This raises questions about the kinds of knowledge about mind, brain, and nerves which doctors brought to their encounters with "shell-shocked" men, illuminates specific elements of the wartime construction of the diagnosis, and helps to explain the pervasive influence of "shell-shock" on post-war medical culture.

All the doctors in this cohort worked with "shell-shocked" men in different capacities and at different locations within the extensive military medical network.[41] In wartime medical discourse, "shell-shock" was usually conceptualized as a disorder arising from conditions on the western front, and it was a diagnosis produced for the most part by doctors who served on the home front.[42] At home, published "shell-shock" doctors worked in military or civilian hospitals, Ministry of Pensions clinics, Homes of Recovery, and private practice. Overseas, they served in advanced neurological centres, general and voluntary hospitals, field ambulances, and Casualty Clearing Stations, and as consulting physicians to different commands. Although one of the most well-known accounts of war strain in 1914–18, Lord Moran's *Anatomy of Courage* (1945), was written by a former Regimental Medical Officer, this cohort includes no RMOs, perhaps because they generally spent little time with "shell-shocked" men (their role was to send them down the line for treatment), or perhaps because their duties provided little time for reflection and publication. While it is sometimes assumed that doctors with experience of overseas service were 'better placed to give an opinion on the effects of battle on soldiers' minds', home-front doctors did have

---

[41] On wartime treatment networks, see The Long, Long Trail, 'The Royal Army Medical Corps of 1914–1918', http://www.1914–1918.net/ramc.htm, accessed 6 January 2017, F. Reid, *Broken Men: Shell Shock, Treatment and Recovery in Britain 1914–1930* (London and New York: Continuum, 2010), pp. 29–34.

[42] Only one-third of published "shell-shock" doctors are known to have served overseas (mainly in France, but also in Italy, Malta, Salonika, Egypt, India, and Russia).

close contact with "shell-shocked" men.[43] A doctor with experience gained entirely in home front hospitals would have found it near impossible to achieve the return-to-duty rates of front-line doctors, but the latter would have found their methods equally ill-adapted for patients first diagnosed months or years previously. These should be seen as different orders of professional experience, rather than ranked as superior or inferior.[44]

The nature of their military service undoubtedly influenced individual doctors' views of "shell-shock". However, the wartime relation of medicine to the military establishment played an even more important role in determining approaches to the disorder among the cohort as a whole. The massive expansion of the Royal Army Medical Corps (RAMC) meant that civilians in uniform vastly outnumbered regular members, and in the opinion of one high-ranking physician with a temporary commission, this resulted in a 'fusing of the two branches' of civilian and military medicine.[45] Awareness of the interplay between the civilian and military medical establishments helps us to place "shell-shock" in a different perspective. For good reason, the disorder is often written about as part of the history of military psychiatry: "shell-shock" was suffered by soldiers, dealt with primarily by the military authorities, and, in the first instance at least, framed by many doctors as a military problem. Yet although the urgent war situation stimulated prolific and creative debates on "shell-shock", the civilian heritage of doctors determined the precise contents of these debates.

The most striking fact in support of this contention is that although more than two-thirds of the cohort held temporary commissions, none had chosen military medicine as a career.[46] As an institution, the regular RAMC did not trouble itself much with mental illness. It provided no

---

[43] E. Jones, 'The Psychology of Killing: The Combat Experience of British Soldiers during the First World War', *Journal of Contemporary History*, 41:2 (2006), 235.

[44] For accounts of the differences in patients and treatment methods at various points in the treatment network, see J.S. Fraser, 'War Injuries of the Ear: A Résumé of Recent Literature', *Edinburgh Medical Journal (EMJ)*, 18 (January–June 1917), 107; F. Dillon, 'Neuroses among Combatant Troops in the Great War', *BMJ*, 8 July 1939, 66; I. Whitehead, 'The British Medical Officer on the Western Front: The Training of Doctors for War', in R. Cooter, M. Harrison, and S. Sturdy (eds.), *Medicine and Modern Warfare* (Amsterdam: Rodopi, 1999), p. 176.

[45] W.P. Herringham, *A Physician in France* (London: Edward Arnold, 1919), p. 56. By the end of the war, nearly 13,000 doctors had been recruited into the army's medical services. R.L. Atenstaedt, 'The Organisation of the RAMC during the Great War', *Journal of the RAMC*, 152 (2006), 83; I. Whitehead, *Doctors in the Great War* (Barnsley, South Yorkshire: Leo Cooper, 1999), pp. 60–1.

[46] The number holding temporary commissions may have been even higher, but this is difficult to discover because the service records of temporary officers were destroyed after 1920.

instruction at all in military psychiatry until 1917, when a voluntary three-month training programme for medical officers was established at Maghull Military Hospital, and quickly shed these limited requirements for psychiatric expertise after 1918.[47] Although they served the needs of the military, "shell-shock" doctors continued to publish in the civilian medical press and to attend meetings of civilian medical societies. "Shell-shock" was formally defined and treated under the purview of military medicine, but medical discourse on the disorder was a product of the civilian as well as the military spheres. Doctors based their knowledge of the disorder on the cases they treated, but viewed these cases through the lens of pre-war civilian medical culture.

How did this lens shape responses to "shell-shock"? Quite unexpectedly, psychiatrists, psychologists, and neurologists make up only just over half of the cohort of published "shell-shock" doctors. Doctors from miscellaneous specialisms, including general hospitalmedicine, ophthalmology, surgery, gastroenterology, physiology, pathology, radiology, speech therapy, otolaryngology, and anatomy, make up the remainder.[48] The hotchpotch composition of the cohort resulted from the uncertain aetiological mechanism and varied symptomatology of "shell-shock" as well as inconsistencies in the overburdened wartime treatment network. Blind soldiers might be sent to psychiatrists, neurologists, or ophthalmologists; officers with uncontrollable vomiting might be seen by gastroenterologists or psychologists; paralysed soldiers might be examined by surgical specialists before being diagnosed as functional cases. But it is also true that some specialisms chose not to assert sovereignty over "shell-shock". The psychiatric *Journal of Mental Science* published several articles on "shell-shock", but the neurological journal *Brain* and the *British Journal of Psychology* printed only one article each on the disorder over the entire course of the war. Although neurologists and psychologists treated "shell-shocked" men, they published on the disorder in non-specialist forums. Indeed, the overwhelming majority of wartime discussions of "shell-shock" were published in generalist medical journals.

[47] Shephard, "'Early Treatment of Mental Disorders'", 447; E. Jones and S. Wessely, 'The Impact of Total War on the Practice of British Psychiatry', in R. Chickering and S. Förster (eds.), *The Shadows of Total War: Europe, East Asia, and the United States, 1919–1939* (Cambridge: Cambridge University Press, 2003), p. 139.

[48] Contemporaries occasionally noted and celebrated the heterogeneity of "shell-shock" doctors as likely to have beneficial effects on post-war psychological medicine. See Anon., 'The Effect of the War upon Psychiatry in England', *Lancet*, 1 September 1917, 352; Anon., 'Review: G. Elliot Smith and T.H. Pear, Shell-Shock and Its Lessons', *EMJ*, 19 (July–December 1917), 272.

The fact that most "shell-shock" doctors chose to publish in general medical journals rather than specialist forums tells us much about how they conceptualized the disorder, including their belief that knowledge of "shell-shock" was important and of interest to non-specialist medical audiences. The disorder was not colonized by specialists, but shaped by the knowledge and expertise on mind, brain, and nerves diffused throughout the medical world. The diagnosis was deeply embedded within medical culture. This is essential to understanding the construction, wartime evolution, and post-war influence of the diagnosis. "Shell-shock" was a product of medical culture in its fullest dimensions, not its specialist branches. To understand its origins and afterlife, this is where it must be located.

"Shell-Shock" and National Memories of the First World War

This is a history of "shell-shock" in British medical culture. Although "shell-shock" was undoubtedly a 'transnational condition', experienced by soldiers of all combatant nations, there were definite limits to transnational interchange in wartime.[49] While British medical journals reported on developments in all combatant nations, it was much easier to access material on military allies, especially France. Before 1920, the only translations of full-length foreign-language monographs to appear in Britain were French works published in the same series.[50] When doctors did manage to consult German authorities on war neurosis, this was sufficiently unusual for reviewers to point it out.[51] Practical obstacles to the exchange of ideas were sometimes compounded by the knee-jerk xenophobia unleashed by the war, as when opponents condemned the 'moral leprosy' of Germans and Austrians.[52] Only after the war had ended were most doctors able to acquaint themselves with medical literature from all combatant nations. Even in 1919, E.E. Southard's

---

[49] J. Winter, 'Shell Shock', in J. Winter (ed.), *The Cambridge History of the First World War. Volume III: Civil Society* (Cambridge and New York: Cambridge University Press, 2013), p. 321.

[50] J. Babinski and J. Froment, *Hysteria or Pithiatism and Reflex Nervous Disorders in the Neurology of War* (London: University of London Press, 1918); G. Roussy and J. Lhermitte, *The Psychoneuroses of War* (London and Paris: University of London Press/Masson et Cie, 1918); J. Lépine, *Mental Disorders of War* (London and Paris: University of London Press/Masson et Cie, 1919); A. Léri, *Shell Shock: Commotional and Emotional Aspects* (London: University of London Press, 1919).

[51] Anon., 'Review: G. Elliot Smith and T.H. Pear, Shell-Shock and Its Lessons', 273.

[52] D.G. Thomson, 'Correspondence: Psycho-Analysis', *BMJ*, 6 January 1917, 32.

extensive compilation of case histories drawn from all belligerent nations acknowledged difficulties obtaining German and Austrian material.[53]

There has been scarcely more international interchange among historians: "shell-shock" still attracts much more attention from historians of Britain than other nations, and relatively few English-language works on European experiences of war neurosis have been published.[54] Nevertheless, it is clear that recurrent themes – such as debates over the physical or psychological origins of soldiers' symptoms or the struggles of veterans with pensions systems – played out quite differently according to existing traditions of medical knowledge. Perversely, this makes more explicit some of the national dimensions of "shell-shock" and most of all the ways in which European ideas were altered by their transposition to the context of British psychological medicine. I refer to this process as "translation" because it involves both literal translation and less obvious shifts in meaning which can only be inferred from context. The identification of this process of "translation" as one of the major mechanisms by which psychological ideas infiltrated mainstream medical culture is one of the most important insights of this book. Although this remains a national history, it is attentive to the porousness of borders and to the extensive transnational intellectual crossings which were a major feature of early twentieth-century medical culture.

Today, "shell-shock" occupies radically different places within the mental landscapes of different nations. The role of "shell-shock" in myths and memories of the war is intimately related to the relative importance of the war in different national traditions, as well as to how each nation "remembers" its own part in the conflict. As social and political contexts change, different facets of war experience assume prominence or fade into the background of cultural memory. Within Britain, the First World War is popularly viewed as the foundational

---

[53] E.E. Southard, *Shell-Shock and Other Neuropsychiatric Problems, Presented in Five Hundred and Eighty-Nine Case Histories from the War Literature, 1914–1918* (Boston, MA: W.M. Leonard, 1919), Preface.

[54] J. Winter, 'Shell-Shock and the Cultural History of the Great War', *Journal of Contemporary History*, 35:1 (2000), 7–11; *Journal of Contemporary History*, 35:1 (2000), Special Issue: Shell-Shock; H. Binneveld, *From Shell Shock to Combat Stress: A Comparative History of Military Psychiatry* (Amsterdam: Amsterdam University Press, 1997); M. Micale and P. Lerner (eds.), *Traumatic Pasts: History, Psychiatry and Trauma in the Modern Age, 1870–1930* (Cambridge: Cambridge University Press, 2001); P. Lerner, *Hysterical Men: War, Psychiatry and the Politics of Trauma in Germany, 1890–1930* (Ithaca, NY and London: Cornell University Press, 2003); J. Crouthamel, *The Great War and German Memory: Society, Politics and Psychological Trauma, 1914–1945* (Exeter: University of Exeter Press, 2009); G. M. Thomas, *Treating the Trauma of the Great War: Soldiers, Civilians, and Psychiatry in France, 1914–1940* (Baton Rouge, LA: Louisiana State University Press, 2009).

moment of the twentieth century and the most important native catastrophe in modern history. In this context, "shell-shock" is an attractive symbol of collective trauma and victimhood and is easily assimilated into wider historical narratives of the war as a pivotal moment in the nation's history.

Unlike most European nations, Britain has no official national day which commemorates a significant event or symbolic moment in the nation's history. Arguably, in recent years, Remembrance Sunday, which commemorates the efforts of British and Commonwealth service personnel in the two world wars and in subsequent conflicts, has played a similar part in the national calendar. Rituals around Remembrance Sunday have now attained quasi-religious status, and public figures who refuse to participate in conventional forms of commemoration face questioning of their motives or even outright condemnation from some sections of the population.[55] In this context, trauma has gradually claimed a central place within the cultural memory of the First World War, and the repetition of reassuring narratives of psychological progress helps to forge new national myths. I think we tell and retell these stories of eventual knowledge and understanding because they are comforting and because they help us not to face certain truths: that war still causes trauma, that we do not know how to avoid this, and that we do not know how to fix broken soldiers. These myths help us to live with war, and with our own complicity in its making.

This book tries to explain the effects of "shell-shock" on British psychological medicine. It argues that war created conditions under which certain forms of understanding, already nascent within pre-war psychological medicine, emerged as distinctive ways of thinking about human mind and behaviour. This is the story of a quiet revolution, but it does not reinscribe comforting narratives of progress. New forms of understanding were assimilated into existing modes of explanation and presented as novel restatements of known facts. "Shell-shock" did not shatter the explanatory paradigms of pre-war psychological medicine but stretched and remade them. Nevertheless, the war matters in this narrative because we cannot assume that the changes it wrought would have happened anyway. "Shell-shock" should not be co-opted into linear narratives of the triumph of psychological approaches: its alternative

---

[55] Witness, for example, the press furore around newsreaders not wearing remembrance poppies on air: BBC News, 'TV's Jon Snow Rejects "Poppy Fascism"', 10 November 2006: news.bbc.co.uk/1/hi/uk/6134906.stm, accessed 6 January 2017 J. Denham, 'Charlene White Hits Back after Racist Abuse for Not Wearing a Poppy', *Independent*, 13 November 2013: www.independent.co.uk/incoming/charlene-white-hits-back-after-racist-abuse-for-not-wearing-a-poppy-8937123.html, accessed 6 January 2017.

potential histories must remain open. These potential histories matter to our reflexive understanding of the human condition here and now. War and trauma are crucial parts of the stories we tell ourselves about ourselves, about who we are, who we have been, and who we should be. It is important to get these stories as right as possible. If the history presented here achieves this, then it shows that understandings of ourselves as psychologically aware creatures, as people who learnt lessons from the bloodshed of twentieth-century warfare, are at least partly founded on a series of misunderstandings, elisions, and forgettings.

1   Frameworks of Understanding
Reconstructing the Human from Darwin to the First World War

In early 1915, as the war turned from awful novelty to the backdrop of life, Sigmund Freud (1856–1939) reflected on how the conflict had led to disillusionment about the achievements of modern "civilization". Europeans, seduced by their own myths of unstoppable progress had been hit hard by the shock of war, he claimed. Their pre-war innocence demonstrated fundamental misunderstanding of human nature and "civilization". No matter how "civilized", imperishable "primitive" instincts and drives persisted within each person and fought for control of the mind. Yet "civilization" was built on the renunciation of instinctual satisfaction. All "civilized" peoples and societies, embroiled in the constant act of repression, existed in a state of perpetual tension between instinct and the higher self. This tension could not be dissolved, and the maintenance of "civilization" could never be assured. In retrospect, the outbreak of war was inevitable: it made manifest instincts and impulses simmering beneath the surface of "civilized" life even at outwardly peaceful times.[1] Freud's 'piece of topical chit-chat', written to satisfy the publisher, caught the prevalent mood of anxious contemplation on the consequences of war for "civilization".[2]

The broad sweep of Freud's argument was not alien to British intellectual and scientific culture, which had long incorporated views of "civilization" as built on the conquest of individual, anti-social desires.[3] In the recent past, these ideas had been reworked along psychobiological lines in Darwin's

---

[1] S. Freud, 'Thoughts for the Times on War and Death' [1915], in *The Standard Edition of the Complete Works of Sigmund Freud* [*SE*], translated from the German under the General Editorship of James Strachey in collaboration with Anna Freud, assisted by Alix Strachey and Alison Tyson, vol. 14, pp. 282–6.

[2] D. Pick, *War Machine: The Rationalisation of Slaughter in the Modern Age* (New Haven, CT and London: Yale University Press, 1993), quotation p. 218; S. Hynes, *A War Imagined: The First World War and English Culture* (New York: Atheneum, 1991), pp. 3–24; P. Crook, *Darwinism, War and History: The Debate over the Biology of War from the Origin of Species to the First World War* (Cambridge and New York: Cambridge University Press, 1994), pp. 130–52.

[3] J. Reed, *Victorian Will* (Athens, OH: Ohio University Press, 1989), pp. 18–19, 65–7.

reconstitution of man as a creature driven by the foundational, unconscious, and ineradicable force of animal instinct.[4] For many of those who followed Darwin, his vision of instinct as at the centre of human nature trampled over meliorating dreams of "progress".[5] The animal within could only be policed, never destroyed. It was a necessary constituent of human identity, but one which must be constantly rejected in order to maintain the human and "civilization" itself. For late Victorians, 'living self-consciously in an age of evolutionary belief', the doubts and anxieties provoked by evolutionary theory were live matters.[6] Men of science raised in the fervent atmosphere of the Darwinian revolution, including older "shell-shock" doctors, transmitted to younger generations both their absolute confidence in the evolutionary framework of understanding and the insecurities about "man's place in nature" which it stimulated. The ideas about mind, nerves, and brain which doctors took into the war were formulated within this evolutionary framework of understanding, and replicated the latent pessimism and uncertainties of earlier debates on evolution and human nature.

This chapter examines forms and sites of "psychological" knowledge within pre-war medical culture, arguing that these extended far beyond specialist disciplines and institutions. In the late nineteenth and early twentieth centuries, an evolutionary framework of understanding underpinned medical approaches to mind, nerves, and brain. The evolutionary model of mind was structured by dichotomies of "high" and "low" (human/animal, mind/body, civilized/primitive), but the emphasis within evolutionism on transition simultaneously undermined these hierarchies. Because psychological medicine was infused with evolutionary assumptions, it reflected and contributed to debates about human identity and "modern civilization" which ranged across and drew together many disciplines.[7] As a unified system underlying various models of mind, the evolutionary framework of understanding also bridged some of the main concepts of late nineteenth-century psychological medicine and later psychodynamic approaches. Awareness of the pervasive influence of evolutionism helps us to understand how British doctors responded to psychoanalysis during and after the war, and the series of transitions between

---

[4] C. Darwin, *The Descent of Man, and Selection in Relation to Sex*, 2nd edn (London: Penguin, 2004) [1879], especially pp. 127–37; Crook, *Darwinism, War and History*, p. 21.

[5] For alternative reactions to Darwinian theories of instinct, see Dixon, *Invention of Altruism*, pp. 136–40.

[6] R. Smith, *Free Will and the Human Sciences in Britain, 1870–1910* (London and Brookfield, VT: Pickering and Chatto, 2013), pp. 14, 169–70.

[7] Dixon, *Invention of Altruism*, pp. 152, 314.

Darwin and Freud in British psychological medicine. The evolutionary model of mind carried over into theories of "shell-shock", which can be seen as part of the longer attempt to work out the human and animal attributes of "civilized" persons. Up to and beyond the First World War, the medical imagination was haunted by visions of the animal and the "primitive" at the heart of the human and of "civilization".

Understanding Mind, Nerves, and Brain in Pre-War Medical Culture

If many of the doctors who treated "shell-shock" were not specialists in mind, nerves, or brain, what knowledge of these entities did they bring to their encounters with "shell-shocked" men? There were two main paths to such knowledge: practical professional experience of treating nervous and mental disorders and education (formal and informal). The most obvious location for professional practical experience was the asylum, the site of the development of the psychiatric profession in Britain. Around half of the published "shell-shock" doctors had some background in asylum psychiatry. In the absence of public provision for non-custodial treatment, the asylum remained the main site for the care of those with severe or chronic mental health problems. The period spanning the late nineteenth and early twentieth centuries is often seen as the nadir of psychiatric provision in Britain, with most asylums overcrowded and understaffed, and the overall system inflexible and insufficient to cope with the full range of mental illnesses.[8] However, before 1914, many asylum psychiatrists vocally supported proposals for the early and non-custodial treatment of mental disorders and actively worked towards the 'hospitalization of the asylum'.[9] The most visible manifestation of this movement was the foundation in 1907 of the Maudsley Hospital,

[8] A. Scull, *The Most Solitary of Afflictions: Madness and Society in Britain, 1700–1900* (New Haven, CT, and London: Yale University Press, 1993).

[9] Quotation G.M. Robertson, 'The Employment of Female Nurses in the Male Wards of Mental Hospitals in Scotland', *EMJ*, 16 (January–June 1916), 203. See also Shephard, '"Early Treatment of Mental Disorders"'; T.S. Clouston, 'The Possibility of Providing Suitable Means of Treatment for Incipient and Transient Mental Diseases in Our Great General Hospitals', *Journal of Mental Science (JMS)*, 48:203 (October 1902), 697–709; E.W. White, 'Psychological Medicine in Relation to the Medical Practitioner', *King's College Hospital Reports (KCHR)*, 1 (1893–4), 49–54; D.G. Thomson, 'Teaching of Psychiatry', *JMS*, 54:226 (July 1908), 553; R.G. Rows, 'The Development of Psychiatric Science as a Branch of Public Health', *JMS*, 58:240 (January 1912), 26; G.M. Robertson, 'The Teaching of Mental Diseases in Edinburgh', *EMJ*, 21 (July–December 1918), 230; J. Mackenzie, 'The Aim of Medical Education', *EMJ*, 20 (January–June 1918), 35; G.L. Gulland, 'The Teaching of Medicine', *EMJ*, 21 (July–December 1918), 23.

intended for the 'care and treatment of acute recoverable cases of mental disease' – although the fact that the hospital did not open at all until January 1916, and was not open for civilian use until 1923, also points to the difficulties faced by reformers.[10] While "shell-shock" undoubtedly provided an urgent impetus towards reform of the asylum system, powerful currents of change existed before the war.

Outside the asylum, doctors observed and treated temporary or less severe psychological or "nervous" afflictions at several sites. Minor nervous illnesses, such as hypochondriasis and neurasthenia, were often perceived as the responsibility of hospital physicians and neurologists. Cases of these disorders were encountered in hospitals on general wards, observation wards, and specialist wards for the treatment of 'alcoholism, poisoning, and mental derangement'.[11] In addition, before 1914, outpatient departments for psychiatric and nervous illnesses had been founded at several institutions, including four London teaching hospitals.[12] Although these sites provided no opportunities for systematic study of mental disorders and their treatment, it was widely recognized among the medical profession that non-specialists had to deal with minor nervous and mental illnesses as part of their daily work. Reformers emphasized that an ideal medical curriculum would provide instruction in the diagnosis and treatment of these illnesses, not least to enable recognition and preventative treatment at an early stage of mental disorder.[13] Medical students learnt and plied their trade in general hospitals and their attached outpatient clinics, and non-specialists among the published "shell-shock" doctors had almost certainly encountered different forms of nervous and mental disorders at these sites.

[10] P. Allderidge, 'The Foundation of the Maudsley Hospital', in G.E. Berrios and H. Freeman (eds.), *150 Years of British Psychiatry, 1841–1991* (London: Gaskell, 1991), p. 83; A. Walk, 'Medico-Psychologists, Maudsley and the Maudsley', *British Journal of Psychiatry*, 128 (1976), 19–30.

[11] Clouston, 'Possibility of Providing Suitable Means of Treatment', 703; 'Discussion: The Training of the Student of Medicine, XLII–XLVII', *EMJ*, 21 (July–December 1918), 246; E. Matthew, 'The Teaching of Medicine', *EMJ*, 21 (July–December 1918), 29.

[12] R. Mayou, 'The History of General Hospital Psychiatry', *British Journal of Psychiatry*, 155 (1989), 764–76; White, 'Psychological Medicine in Relation to the Medical Practitioner', 52; T.S. Clouston, 'The Position of Psychiatry and the Role of General Hospitals in Its Improvement', *JMS*, 61:252 (January 1915), 1–17.

[13] Clouston, 'Possibility of Providing Suitable Means of Treatment', 703; Clouston, 'Position of Psychiatry', 3; Rows, 'Development of Psychiatric Science', 32; R.D. Clarkson, 'The Teaching of Psychology to Medical Undergraduates', *EMJ*, 21 (July–December 1918), 243; B. Hart, 'Psychology and the Medical Curriculum', *EMJ*, 21 (July–December 1918), 215; E. Bramwell, 'The Teaching of Neurology', *EMJ*, 21 (July–December 1918), 211.

This period also saw increased medical specialization. In the half century or so before 1914, new journals and societies focusing on the problems of mind, nerves, and brain proliferated.[14] Although these forums promoted different disciplinary stances, practitioners in each field were also aware of connections between the specialisms. In its early years, presidents of the neurological section of the Royal Society of Medicine (RSM) were chosen by rotation to represent different faces of the topic: 'one year special neurology, another general medicine, another surgery, another psychology, another physiology, each with special bearing upon the subject of the nervous system'.[15] When the *British Journal of Psychology* was struggling to get off the ground, the *Journal of Mental Science* called for financial and moral support for the venture, portraying the aims of the new journal as inextricably tied to those of its own subscribers.[16] Specialization did not preclude interest in adjacent fields. The Medico-Psychological Association (M-PA) was "officially" the organization of asylum psychiatrists, but several psychologists and neurologists among the published "shell-shock" doctors were members or attended its meetings.[17] Likewise, the British Neurological Society welcomed asylum doctors and physiologists, and the British Psychological Society held joint meetings with the psychiatric section of the RSM, the Aristotelian Society, and the Mind Association.[18] Neurologists played an important part in the foundation of the section of psychiatry of the RSM in 1912.[19] The personnel, subject matter, and activities of specialist organizations often overlapped. In the late nineteenth and early twentieth centuries, the boundaries between psychology, psychiatry, and neurology were porous.

In the early stages of differentiation between these disciplines, when fewer specialist forums existed, individuals congregated at any event which pursued knowledge of mind, nerves, and brain. For example, the annual meeting of the M-PA in 1900 hosted representatives of the psychiatric old guard such as the alienists Charles Mercier (1851–1919) and Robert Armstrong-Jones (1857–1943) as well as future leaders of

---

[14] M. Shepherd, 'Psychiatric Journals and the Evolution of Psychological Knowledge', in W.F. Bynum, S. Lock, and R. Porter (eds.), *Medical Journals and Medical Knowledge: Historical Essays* (London and New York: Routledge, 1992), pp. 196, 201.

[15] P. Hunting, *The History of the Royal Society of Medicine* (London: Royal Society of Medicine Press, 2002), p. 264.

[16] Anon., 'A New Journal', *JMS*, 49:206 (July 1903), 523–4.

[17] John Collie, David Eder, Edward Fearnsides, Charles Myers, and W.H.R. Rivers were members of the M-PA; Harry Campbell, Howard Tooth, and James Purves Stewart attended meetings.

[18] See lists of meetings in the *British Journal of Psychology*, 1914–19.

[19] Hunting, *History of the Royal Society of Medicine*, p. 323.

British psychology including Alexander Shand (1858–1936) and W.H.R. Rivers (1864–1922).[20] Associations such as the M-PA played an important in part in building professional networks and fostering interaction between individuals with different outlooks and interests. Shand and Rivers helped to establish the *British Journal of Psychology*. Another founder member of this journal was Charles Myers. He and Rivers were both members of the 1898 Cambridge anthropological expedition to the Torres Straits and worked alongside each other at the Cambridge experimental psychology laboratory. Both were also alumni of St Bartholomew's medical school. Myers' election to membership of the M-PA in 1909 was proposed by Rivers, the early proponent of psychodynamic psychology W.H.B. Stoddart (1868–1950), and Robert Armstrong-Jones, an asylum superintendent strongly attached to hereditary theories of mental illness. The only apparent link between Armstrong-Jones and the more sophisticated psychologists is that he was also a Barts man, roughly contemporaneous with Rivers. Rivers and Myers rarely attended the M-PA, but when its quarterly meeting was held at Cambridge in February 1909, they gave a demonstration of equipment in the psychological laboratory. Armstrong-Jones and Charles Mercier were again present.[21] These connections between leading asylum psychiatrists and the foremost figures in academic psychology, spanning two decades, demonstrate the fluidity of relations within the fields of psychological medicine and research.

The flipside of fluidity was insecurity: free exchange of ideas and personnel was necessary while these disciplines were ill-established. Yet the differentiation and refinement of approaches to mind, nerves, and brain also point to deep engagement with these issues within parts of medical culture. Pre-war psychological medicine is often characterized as reactive or stagnant, but the inertia of the formal structures of mental health provision coexisted with supra-structural flux as new disciplines were established and sought to work out their relations to each other. Psychiatrists, psychologists, and neurologists had not yet defined their remits: sometimes, they were not even sure how to describe what they were doing. When 'psychiatry' was touted as a name for the new section of the RSM, there was confusion over how to pronounce the word until a lexicographer declared that if the society planned to adopt the term, it

---

[20] For a full list of those present at this meeting, see Anon., 'Medico-Psychological Association of Great Britain and Ireland: General Meeting', *JMS*, 46:194 (July 1900), 601.

[21] Anon., 'Notes and News: The Medico-Psychological Association of Great Britain and Ireland', *JMS*, 55:229 (April 1919), 391–3.

could settle the pronunciation itself.[22] The generalist medical press regularly printed lectures and reviewed books on psychiatry and psychology, with commentators testifying to the 'real living interest' in such topics.[23] Although doctors disagreed on the best way forward, the extent of debate – even the volume of complaints about the asylum system – shows that this was a moment of change within psychological medicine. These shifts arose out of dissatisfaction and despair with aspects of existing mental health care provision, but also generated much excitement and activity.

Psychology, Psychiatry, and Medical Education

Apart from practical professional experience of patients suffering from mental or nervous illnesses, doctors were most likely to have gained some knowledge of mind, nerves, and brain from their medical education and training. A fairly standardized medical curriculum had emerged by the 1890s.[24] This included a compulsory course in psychological medicine, and some teaching hospitals and medical schools began offering such courses as early as the 1860s.[25] These courses usually consisted of attendance at a series of lectures, and at clinical demonstrations held at a public asylum near the hospital.[26] By 1900, most newly qualified doctors had received some training in psychological medicine, but reformers argued for more extensive changes still. They complained that the fundamentals of psychological medicine could not be fully taught in

[22] Hunting, *History of the Royal Society of Medicine*, p. 324.
[23] Anon., 'Review: Modern Problems in Psychiatry', *EMJ*, 12 (January–June 1914). For example, W.H.B. Stoddart's Morison lectures on 'the new psychiatry' were delivered to the Royal College of Physicians and printed in the *Edinburgh Medical Journal* and the *Lancet* before being published in book form. W.H.B. Stoddart, 'The New Psychiatry. Lecture I', *EMJ*, 14 (January–June 1915), 244–60; W.H.B. Stoddart, 'The Morison Lectures on the New Psychiatry', *Lancet*, 20 and 27 March 1915; W.H.B. Stoddart, *The New Psychiatry* (London: Baillière, Tindall and Cox, 1916).
[24] A. Digby, *The Evolution of British General Practice 1850–1948* (Oxford: Oxford University Press, 1999), pp. 54–7; K. Waddington, *Medical Education at St Bartholomew's Hospital 1123–1995* (Woodbridge, Suffolk: Boydell Press, 2003), pp. 116–17.
[25] White, 'Psychological Medicine in Relation to the Medical Practitioner', 51; J.L. Crammer, 'Training and Education in British Psychiatry 1770–1970', in H. Freeman and G.E. Berrios (eds.), *150 Years of British Psychiatry. Volume 2: The Aftermath* (London: Athlone, 1996), pp. 217–18.
[26] For descriptions of typical courses, see White, 'Psychological Medicine in Relation to the Medical Practitioner'; St Bartholomew's Hospital Archive (SBHA): MS 20, *St Bartholomew's Hospital and College Sessions 1875–1876*, p. 41; *St Bartholomew's Hospital and College Sessions 1892–1893*, pp. 52, 68; *St Bartholomew's Hospital and College Sessions 1894–1895*, p. 61; King's College Hospital and Medical School Archive (KCHMSA): KH/SYL1/2: *King's College Hospital Medical School 1911–1912 Abridged Syllabus*, p. 18; KH/SYL1/1: *The Medical School of King's College Hospital 1910–1911*, p. 54.

the time available, that the advanced cases of insanity students saw in asylums bore little relation to the 'borderland and incipient cases' more often found in general practice, and that examining bodies did not consistently and rigorously enforce assessment in psychological medicine.[27] Yet psychological medicine did make solid gains within medical education in the decades before the war. In 1885, the M-PA set up a certificate of efficiency in psychological medicine. Although this certificate never really took off among medical students, in London and the four Scottish universities those studying for the degree of doctor of medicine could specialize in psychiatry if they wished. By 1914, it was also possible to take a postgraduate diploma in psychiatry at the universities of Durham, Edinburgh, Manchester, Leeds, and Cambridge.[28] As courses proliferated, universities set up lectureships and chairs in psychiatry and related disciplines.[29] Although only highly committed students opted for specialist courses, these decades nevertheless saw solid increases in provision for education in psychological medicine.

Even medical students who did not pursue specialist training or pay close attention to compulsory lectures and demonstrations would have found it difficult to avoid acquiring some "psychological" knowledge in the course of their studies. Because psychiatry shared territory with many other branches of medicine, instruction in mind, brain, and nerves was scattered throughout the curriculum.[30] At Barts in the 1880s, the course on 'principles and practice of medicine' dealt with diseases of the brain and spinal cord, as well as chorea, epilepsy, hysteria, and delirium tremens. Over the decade, the content of this course gradually expanded to encompass everything from headache to sleep problems, stammering, and writers' cramp.[31] In lectures on anatomy and physiology, students were introduced to the structure and functions of the nervous system, and to 'the Physiology of the MIND'.[32]

---

[27] Thomson, 'Teaching of Psychiatry', 552; Clouston, 'Position of Psychiatry', 8–9; Clarkson, 'Teaching of Psychology', 241; Robertson, 'Teaching of Mental Diseases', 227; G. Newman, *Recent Advances in Medical Education in England: A Memorandum Addressed to the Minister of Health* (London: HMSO, 1923), pp. 139, 141; Matthew, 'Teaching of Medicine', 25.

[28] Clouston, 'Position of Psychiatry', 7–8; Crammer, 'Training and Education in British Psychiatry', pp. 220–3; Digby, *Evolution of British General Practice*, p. 61.

[29] S.T. Anning and W.K.J. Walls, *A History of the Leeds School of Medicine: One and a Half Centuries, 1831–1981* (Leeds: Leeds University Press, 1982), p. 109; Robertson, 'Teaching of Mental Diseases', 225.

[30] Crammer, 'Training and Education in British Psychiatry', 213.

[31] SBHA: MS 20, *St Bartholomew's Hospital and College Sessions 1878–1879*, p. 30; *St Bartholomew's Hospital and College Sessions 1881–1882*, p. 33; *St Bartholomew's Hospital and College Sessions 1887–1888*, p. 33.

[32] SBHA: MS 20, *St Bartholomew's Hospital and College Sessions 1876–76*, pp. 32, 44.

This included instruction on the relations of physiology to psychology and body to mind, 'functions associated with mind' such as 'consciousness, perception, and will', and even 'unconscious cerebration'.[33] Meanwhile, courses on forensic medicine and medical jurisprudence routinely dealt with insanity, malingering, and the relation of unsound states of mind to criminal acts.[34] Medical students did not have to be committed to a career in psychiatry to acquire a passing acquaintance with some of its key concepts, diagnostic practices, and treatments.

For students actively interested in psychological medicine, there were several less formal avenues to knowledge within their teaching institutions. Hospital medical societies fostered cross-generational links and served as potential conduits for the vertical transmission of knowledge. The cohort of "shell-shock" doctors mostly took an active part in the associational life of their educational institutions, whether as students or teachers, and their paths sometimes crossed at pre-war meetings of student medical societies.[35] The records of student medical societies and in-house journals suggest a growing appetite for papers on "psychological" subjects in the late nineteenth and early twentieth centuries. The St Barts' Abernethian Society and *Hospital Reports* often hosted discussions of functional and neurotic disorders, including hysteria and neurasthenia, and of matters such as 'mental disturbance after operations' or 'medicine and the mind'.[36] When the Abernethian Society put on papers on 'manifestations of hysteria' or 'the psychology of dreams', respectable numbers attended (respectively, twenty-four and sixty-five listeners). But when the speaker was well known, such as the neurologist Henry Head (1861–1940) or Robert Armstrong-Jones, the number of attendees could climb to more than 200.[37]

---

[33] P.H. Pye-Smith, *Syllabus of a Course of Lectures on Physiology Delivered at Guy's Hospital* (London: J. & A. Churchill, 1885), pp. 2, 43, 47.

[34] SBHA: MS 20, *St Bartholomew's Hospital and College Sessions 1875–1876*, p. 38 and *St Bartholomew's Hospital and College Sessions 1886–1887*, p. 40. KCHMSA: KH/SYL1/1: *The Medical School of King's College Hospital 1910–1911*, p. 54. Guy's Hospital Medical School Archive (GHMSA): G/PUB/6/1: Guy's Hospital Examination Papers 1889–1890.

[35] For example, between 1884 and 1914, seven doctors from the cohort published in the *St Bartholomew's Hospital Reports* or gave papers to the Abernethian Society (Howard Tooth, W.H.R. Rivers, Harry Campbell, Charles Myers, Robert Armstrong-Jones, Adolphe Abrahams, and Anthony Feiling); seven more published in the *Guy's Hospital Reports* or gave papers to the Pupil's Physical Society (Harry Campbell, E.A. Peters, A. W. Ormond, Arthur Hurst, George Savage, J.L.M. Symns, and Laughton Scott).

[36] W.P. Herringham, 'Cases of Mental Disturbance After Operations', *SBHR*, 21 (1885), 165–7; S. West, 'Five Cases of Functional Nervous Disorder', *SBHR*, 21 (1885); F.A. Bainbridge, 'Some Neuroses of Children', *SBHR*, 37 (1901). See also lists of proceedings of the Abernethian Society, *SBHR*, 27 (1891), 285; *SBHR*, 29 (1893), 350; *SBHR*, 39 (1903), 239; *SBHR*, 44 (1908), 217.

[37] See lists of proceedings of the Abernethian Society, *SBHR*, 48 (1912), 167; *SBHR*, 49 (1913), 111; and *SBHR*, 50:2 (1914), 176.

The associational life of other teaching hospitals in the thirty years or so before the war shows similar patterns. The Medical (later Listerian) Society of King's College Hospital heard papers on insanity,[38] malingering,[39] functional nervous disorders (including hysteria and neurasthenia),[40] and Freud.[41] At Guy's, the Pupil's Physical Society, the Physiological Society, and the *Guy's Hospital Reports* covered topics including insanity and related disorders,[42] the nature of mind (in its conscious and unconscious aspects, its material and other manifestations, and normal and abnormal psychology),[43] and sleep and dreams.[44] There was a notable increase in the number of papers on hypnotism and suggestion, perennial favourites of student medical societies, from around 1900. These usually attracted higher than average audiences.[45] In a record for the Medical Society, eighty-six people

[38] KCHMSA: KHU/C1/M7, Mr Distin, 'Medical Experiences in a Lunatic Asylum' (3 February 1893); KHU/C1/M8, Dr White, 'Epilepsy Associated with Insanity' (27 January 1899); R.P. Williams, 'Insanity and Crime' (19 March 1901).

[39] KCHMSA: KHU/C1/M7, Mr Birch, 'Malingering' (27 January 1887); KHU/C1/M8, A.H. Cheatle, 'Malingering in Ear Disease' (4 March 1910).

[40] KCHMSA: KHU/C1/M7, Dr Dent, 'Hysterical Dysponea with Some Remarks on [Ospahectomy?]' (3 December 1885); KHU/C1/M8; F.W. Mott, 'On the Causation of Nervous Diseases' (16 February 1900); Mr Whittington, 'A Case of Traumatic Neurasthenia' (21 January 1910); unnamed speaker, 'A Case of Functional Paraplegia' (27 October 1911).

[41] KCHMSA: KHU/C1/M8, W. Brown, 'Freud's Theory and Its Uses in Diagnosis' (21 January 1913).

[42] GHMSA: G/S7/55, W.A. Slater, 'The Medico-Legal Aspects of Insanity' (7 October 1882); G/S7/1, printed card advertising Pupil's Physical Society session 1889–90, E. Goodall, 'Mental Diseases'; G/S6/7, A.H. Gool, 'The Physiological Aspects of Lunacy' (undated, 1907–8); G.H. Savage, 'Suicide as a Symptom of Mental and Nervous Disorder', *Guy's Hospital Reports*, 50 (1893).

[43] GHMSA: G/S6/3, H.O. Brookhouse, 'Unconscious Mentality – Its Existence and Value' (4 December 1902); G/S6/5, S.S. Brook, 'The Force of Mind (undated, 1904–5); G/S6/6, J.L. Atkinson, 'The Ignorance of Science, Especially as Regards the Physical Basis of Mind' (12 March 1906); G/S6/10, G.S. Miller, 'Volition and Will' (undated, 1909–10); G/S6/12, W.W. Payne, 'Abnormal Psychology' (undated, 1912–14).

[44] GHMSA: G/S7/1, printed card advertising Pupil's Physical Society session 1910–11, J.L.M. Symns, 'Night Terrors' (29 January 1913); G/S6/6, G.H. Haycraft, 'Dreams and Delusions' (undated, 1905–6); G/S6/4, L. Mandel, 'Sleep' (27 January1904); G/S6/7, A. Neville-Cox, 'Sleep' (undated, 1906–7); G/S6/9, W.S. George, 'Sleep' (30 November 1908); G/S6/11, F.V. Bevan, 'Sleep' (undated, 1910–1911); G/S6/13, T.L. Heath, 'The Physiology of Sleep' (9 February 1914).

[45] KCHMSA: KHU/C1/M8, Dr Milne Bramwell, 'Hypnotism' (31 January 1902); GHMSA: G/S7/1, printed card advertising Pupil's Physical Society session 1907–8, Douglas Bryan, 'Hypnotism' (27 November 1907); H.D. Rolleston, 'Treatment by Hypnotic Suggestion', *SBHR*, 25 (1889), 115–26; G/PUB 1/1/1/2, G.L. Scott, 'Ten Consecutive Cases Treated by Hypnotism', *Guy's Hospital Neurological Studies*, 67 (1913), 114–19; see also lists of the proceedings of the Abernethian Society, *SBHR*, 34 (1898), 328; *SBHR*, 48 (1912), 169; *SBHR*, 51 (1915), 56.

attended one such lecture at King's.[46] The opportunity for showman-
ship formed part of the appeal of hypnotism, with more than one set of
minutes recording the excitement of practical demonstrations.[47] However, hypnotism also afforded students the chance to explore topics
covered only sketchily on the formal curriculum: dreaming, memory,
the existence of the unconscious, the influence of the mind on the
body, the role of the doctor's personality in healing, the fine lines
separating normal and abnormal psychological processes, and the
limits of free will and individual autonomy.[48] Little wonder, then, that
such papers often stoked lively discussions.[49]

The formal and informal structures of medical education offered many
opportunities to find out about psychological matters. Diligent scholars,
or those heavily involved in the associational life of colleges and hospitals,
would undoubtedly have acquired some such knowledge, albeit in an
unorganized and piecemeal fashion. In this way, non-specialists could
obtain some basic knowledge of nervous and mental disorders. Perhaps
more importantly, the evolutionary framework which shaped specialist
understandings of mind, nerves, and brain also formed the foundation of
approaches to mind and body within medical education. Via the influence of evolutionary forms of understanding, specialists and non-
specialists had access to some similar kinds of psychological knowledge,
although these were elaborated more explicitly and in greater detail
within specialist disciplines. This evolutionary model of mind was carried
over into constructions of the diagnosis of "shell-shock", and is crucial to
understanding commonalities between apparently different conceptualizations of the disorder.

The Evolutionary Model of Mind in Pre-War
Psychological Medicine

By the end of the nineteenth century, evolutionary frameworks of understanding dominated British intellectual and scientific culture. The author
of the essay on 'Evolution' in the 1911 edition of the *Encyclopaedia*

---

[46] KCHMSA: KHU/C1/M8, Dr Bramwell, 'Hypnotism and Treatment by Suggestion' (15
October 1909).
[47] KCHMSA: KHU/C1/M8, J. Woods, 'Treatment by Suggestion with and without
Hypnosis' (25 March 1908); Anon., 'The Medical Society', *KCHR*, 5 (1897–8), 237.
[48] See, for example, GHMSA: G/S6/4, C.A.L. Meyer, 'Animal Magnetism' (undated,
1903–4); G/S6/5, S.S. Brook, 'The Force of Mind' (undated, 1904–5); G/S6/11,
J. Stevenson, 'Hypnotism' (undated, 1910–11).
[49] See comments on H. Wingfield's paper on 'The Nature and Phenomena of Hypnotism'
in lists of proceedings of the Abernethian Society, *SBHR*, 27 (1891), 284.

Britannica commented that in the space of only two editions, since Huxley's exposition of the topic in 1878, 'the doctrine of evolution has outgrown the trammels of controversy and has been accepted as a fundamental principle'.[50] In the half-century leading up to the First World War, when "shell-shock" doctors undertook their professional training, evolution gradually permeated the preclinical medical curriculum. Most topics invited an evolutionary standpoint or required some engagement with evolutionary theory. The examination questions at St Barts on comparative anatomy, biology, morphology, embryology, physiology, and botany demonstrate that by the 1880s at the latest, evolution was firmly entrenched in the mainstream of medical education.[51] In the same decades, evolutionary principles structured the course of physiology lectures at Guy's, which began with 'distinctions between man and the lower animals', and then provided evolutionary-infused overviews of comparative anatomy, morphology, and individual and racial development.[52] In 1918, when the Edinburgh Pathological Club hosted an extensive enquiry into the ideal training of medical students, many different specialists still emphasized the role of evolutionary theory in their subjects, including botany, zoology, anatomy, and general medicine.[53] The evolutionary framework of understanding underpinned most aspects of formal medical education in the opening decades of the twentieth century.

The less formal elements of medical education also immersed students in evolutionary thought. In the two decades before the war, several of the papers delivered to the Guy's Hospital Physiological Society that tackled mind or related topics explicitly referred to Darwin or alternative theories of evolution.[54] The evolutionary account of mind in one paper on

[50] P.C. Mitchell, 'Evolution', *Encyclopaedia Britannica*, 11th edn, 29 vols. (Cambridge: Cambridge University Press, 1910), vol. 10, p. 34.
[51] See SBHA: MS 20, *St Bartholomew's Hospital and College Sessions* for *1878–1879* and *1897–1880*. Compare the annual *St Bartholomew's Hospital and College Sessions* from 1875–95 for further examples of questions employing an evolutionary framework.
[52] Pye-Smith, *Syllabus of a Course of Lectures*, pp. 2, 5, 44–5.
[53] B. Balfour, 'Botany in Medical Education', *EMJ*, 20 (January–June 1918), 115; J.C. Ewart, 'The Connection of Zoology with Medicine', *EMJ*, 20 (January–June 1918), 118, 121; D. Waterson, 'The Teaching of Anatomy', *EMJ*, 20 (January–June 1918), 184; Prof. Robinson, 'The Place of Anatomy in the Medical Curriculum', *EMJ*, 20 (January–June 1919), 185; D.E. Dickinson, 'The Training of Medical Students for General Practice: Recollections and Reflections', *EMJ*, 21 (July–December 1918), 364.
[54] GHMSA: G/S6/3, Russell, 'Origin of Life' (undated, 1902–3); G/S6/5, E.M. Lobb, 'Temperament' (October 1904), 10; G/S6/6, W.L. Hibbert, 'Crime and the Criminal' (October 1905), 4, 13; H.W. Heasman, 'The Cerebro-Spinal Nervous System' (27 November 1905), 7; G/S6/9, J.A. Bullbrook, 'Instinct and Reason' (2 November 1908), 7, 13–15, 19; G/S6/11, R.O.H. Jones, 'The Physiology of the Child' (undated, 1910–11); W.E. James, 'The Biological Aspect of Socialism' (13 March 1911); G/S6/12,

'Consciousness' stressed racial hierarchy, with the speaker claiming that 'the difference between the consciousness of the dogs, apes, etc., and between that of the lowest races of mankind such as the Aztecs, the Veddahs, and the Polynesians, is a great deal less than the corresponding difference between these uncivilised races, and the higher specimens of thoughtful genius in man, such as Shakespeare, Darwin, Goethe, Milton, and Pope'.[55] This explicit statement on the evolutionary hierarchy of mind articulated and systematized the implicit assumptions scattered throughout other student papers.

At every stage in their training, doctors were taught to conceptualize the human body and mind as shaped by a long process of evolution. When the circumstances of war forced doctors who were not specialists in mind, brain, or nerves to take responsibility for treating "shell-shocked" men, they fell back on the knowledge of mind and its workings gleaned from their medical education. When doctors reflected on the development of psychology in Britain, they usually credited Darwin with originating a truly scientific (by which they meant biological) approach to the subject. In the words of one "shell-shock" doctor, Darwin had 'rescu[ed] psychology from the thraldom of medieval thought' and shown 'its true ancestry, coeval with animal life'.[56] The way of seeing fostered by the evolutionary framework of understanding united surgeons, ophthalmologists, gastroenterologists, medical psychologists, psychiatrists, and neurologists. Although there were many distinctions between practitioners from different disciplines and traditions, this shared mode of thought makes it possible to set out some general features of an evolutionary model of mind common to psychiatrists, psychologists, and neurologists as well as doctors from other specialisms.

The doctrine of psycho-physical parallelism, sometimes identified as the most popular medical view of mind–body relations, formed an important common ground in mainstream approaches within neurology, psychiatry, and psychology.[57] As employed by doctors in this period, psycho-physical parallelism meant that mental and physical processes were viewed as occurring in tandem with each other and as in some

P.G. McEvedy, 'The Origin of Life' (24 January 1913); G/S6/13, Anon., 'The Origin of Life' (undated, 1914–16); Anon., 'Vitalism and Mechanism' (undated, 1914–16); G/S6/14, R.S. Ralph, 'The Vertebrate Character of Man' (undated, 1917–19).

[55] GHMSA: G/S6/2, G.W. Rontley, 'Consciousness' (undated, 1901–2), 6–7.

[56] J.H. Parsons, *Mind and the Nation* (London: Bale, Sons and Danielsson, 1918), p. 4.

[57] T.C. Shaw, *Ex Cathedra: Essays on Insanity* (London: Adlard and Son, 1904), p. 113; M. Craig, *Psychological Medicine: A Manual on Mental Diseases for Practitioners and Students*, 3rd edn (London: J. & A. Churchill, 1917), p. 1; J.R. Lord, 'Psychology the Science of Mind', *JMS*, 73:314 (July 1930), 544.

way connected, but the nature of the causal relation was not specified.[58] Psycho-physical parallelism allowed psychiatrists to identify their relatively insecure discipline with more established and scientifically reputable neurological and physiological approaches.[59] It also meant that doctors could justify focusing on mind *or* body without denying the importance of either. Joseph Ormerod (1848–1925), a specialist in nervous disorders with a particular interest in hysteria, compared physiologists and psychologists to men looking at a coin from opposite sides and arguing whether it was heads or tails: 'the two sides are indissolubly connected, just as there is some unknown but certain connection between mind and matter'.[60] The psychologist William Brown, meanwhile, argued that as doctors knew more about mental processes than corresponding brain activities, it made sense to explain mental disturbances in terms of 'memory, ideas, imaginations, desires, and wishes' rather than through reference to 'hypothetical nerve cells and nerve fibres'.[61] The disciplines of mind, nerves, and brain were therefore linked by the doctrine of psycho-physical parallelism, uses of which both reflected the incomplete separation of these fields and glossed the differences between them. As will be seen in the next chapter, the use of ambiguous concepts and strategies to justify particular stances or to forge practical working theories was central to the practice of pre-war British psychological medicine.

Although the doctrine of psycho-physical parallelism was not universally accepted, it was widely believed that the evolution of mind and nervous system proceeded hand in hand. The foremost British neurologist of the nineteenth century, John Hughlings Jackson (1835–1911), argued that the nervous system consisted of 'levels' laid down at different evolutionary moments which corresponded to functions rather than anatomical structures. The functions performed at the most ancient levels were simple, highly organized, and automatic. At the higher levels,

---

[58] This departs from current standard use, which denies a causal relation. See the definitions in E.J. Foley, 'Consciousness and Sensation', in G. Rhodes (ed.), *The Mind at Work: A Handbook of Applied Psychology* (London: Thomas Murby, 1914), pp. 58–66, 64–5; Craig, *Psychological Medicine*, 3rd edn, pp. 1–2.

[59] M.J. Clark, 'The Rejection of Psychological Approaches to Mental Disorder in Late Nineteenth-Century British Psychiatry', in A. Scull (ed.), *Madhouses, Mad-Doctors and Madmen: The Social History of Psychiatry in the Victorian Era* (Philadelphia, PA: University of Pennsylvania Press, 1981), pp. 283–4.

[60] J.A. Ormerod, 'The Lumleian Lectures on Some Modern Theories Concerning Hysteria. I', *Lancet*, 25 April 1914, 1164.

[61] W. Brown, 'Freud's Theory of Dreams', *Lancet*, 19 April 1913, 1115. See also W.A. White and S.E. Jelliffe, 'Preface', in W.A White and S.E. Jelliffe (eds.), *The Modern Treatment of Nervous and Mental Diseases, by American and British Authors* (London: Henry Kimpton, 1913), p. v.

which provided the basis for consciousness, activity was less organized, more complex, and more voluntary. The higher levels controlled the lower levels. Any impairment of the higher levels released the lower levels from this control and resulted in the development of pathological conditions such as aphasia (a partial or total loss of the ability to produce or to comprehend language). Jackson named this process 'dissolution' and believed that as disease or injury stripped back the higher levels of the nervous system, behaviour characteristic of an earlier stage in the evolution of the species could be viewed. The 'pathological' symptoms and behaviours released by dissolution represented what was once the highest level of phylogenetic development.[62]

Jackson's influence was felt across the other disciplines of mind, nerves, and brain. The psychologist William McDougall (1871–1938) described 'each step of mental evolution' as 'the effect or expression of a corresponding step of nervous evolution'.[63] For the physiologist Edward Schäfer (1850–1935; later Sharpey-Schafer), all human mental achievement resulted from 'the acquisition by a few cells in a remote ancestor of a slightly greater tendency to react to an external stimulus'.[64] Robert Cole (1866–1926), a specialist in mental diseases and author of a well-received textbook of psychiatry, concluded that mind was best regarded from 'the Evolutionary standpoint' because study of the animal kingdom demonstrated 'the gradual development of Mind *pari passu* with the evolution of the Brain'.[65] On the eve of the First World War, Cole's statement described the outlook of most medical men on the origins and evolution of the mind and nervous system.

The Faculties of Mind: Thought, Emotion, and Will

The evolutionary model prevalent within the pre-war disciplines of mind, nerves, and brain depicted mind as a unified and integrated structure consisting of three basic faculties: emotion, thought, and volition.[66]

[62] Young, 'W.H.R. Rivers and the War Neuroses', 363.
[63] W. McDougall, *Psychology: The Study of Behaviour* (London: Williams and Norgate, 1914), pp. 73–4, 140–1.
[64] E. Schäfer, 'Presidential Address on the Nature, Origin, and Maintenance of Life', *Lancet*, 7 September 1912, 676, 682.
[65] R.H. Cole, *Mental Diseases: A Text-Book of Psychiatry for Medical Students and Practitioners* (London: University of London Press, 1913), pp. 14–15.
[66] A. Bain, *The Emotions and the Will* (London: John W. Parker and Son, 1859), p. 3; G. Rhodes, 'Introduction', in Rhodes (ed.), *Mind at Work*, pp. 1–13; W.C. Coupland, 'Philosophy of Mind', in D.H. Tuke (ed.), *A Dictionary of Psychological Medicine*, 2 vols. (London: J. & A. Churchill, 1892), vol. 1, pp. 27–49; Cole, *Mental Diseases* [1913], p. 14; McDougall, *Psychology*, p. 63.

Healthy mental functioning was conceived as a matter of balance between these faculties: their interdependence meant that disorder in any part affected all the other aspects of mind. These faculties of mind were also aligned with nervous processes and incorporated into a hierarchical model of nervous evolution.[67] Authors of works on psychological medicine continually calibrated the degree to which each faculty of mind was animal or human, "primitive" or "civilized", and dependent on nature or nurture. Within this model of mind, individuals and races were deemed more or less "civilized" to the extent that their behaviour was dominated by the "higher" faculties of reason or will, or the "lower" faculty of emotion. However, the animal and the "primitive" were constituent parts of even the most "civilized" human and could rise to the surface at any time. Although the "civilized" was defined through its opposition to the "primitive", and these conditions marked different ends of the evolutionary spectrum, because the same scale instituted a series of transitional steps between the two positions, evolutionism underlined the precariousness of "civilization" and even the human itself.

The instability of established understandings of human nature in the post-Darwinian world is evident in late nineteenth-century psychological accounts of reason and instinct. Conventionally, reason had been viewed as a unique attribute which separated human behaviour from the instinct-driven actions of animals. The Liberal philosopher L.T. Hobhouse (1864–1929), born in the middle of the decade separating *Origin of Species* from *The Descent of Man*, dimly recalled being taught as a child 'that man had reason, while animals had instinct'. By the time he reached adulthood, this conception had broken down. Instead, Hobhouse recounted, it was now known that 'no impassable gulf' separated instinct from intelligence and that intelligence actually evolved out of instinct. All human behaviour, including reason, was based in heredity and instinct. Although man benefitted from 'the guidance of experience and reflection', it was impossible to completely separate out instinct from intelligence. Man was 'no more regulated by pure reason than animals by pure instinct'.[68] The British psychologist Conwy Lloyd Morgan (1852–1936) confirmed this view of intelligence as little more than modified instinct: instinct was 'inherited adaptation', while intelligence was an 'inherited power' which permitted reasoned adaptation within the lifetime of the individual.[69] Another psychologist, James Sully (1842–1923), marvelled

---

[67] Cole, *Mental Diseases* [1913], pp. 69–70.
[68] L.T. Hobhouse, *Mind in Evolution* (London: Macmillan, 1901), pp. 46–7.
[69] C.L. Morgan, 'Instinct', *Encyclopaedia Britannica*, 11th edn, 29 vols. (Cambridge: Cambridge University Press, 1910), vol. 14, p. 650.

that the development of 'the most ordinary child' revealed 'the points of contact of man's proud reason with the lowly intelligence of the brutes' and demonstrated 'the great cosmic action, the laborious emergence of intelligence out of its shell of animal sense and appetite'.[70]

In the evolutionary model of mind, the position of reason as the most "human" mental attribute was determined by its relation to other elements. Volition, or reasoned will, stood at the apex of human mind, and the inherited racial attribute of emotion at its base. The hereditary, biologically inscribed attribute of emotion was closely aligned with instinct, and sometimes even portrayed as little more than a basic nervous reflex.[71] Commentators contrasted emotion with the acquired (and therefore more *human*) characters of reason and will, as in Darwin's claim that the main emotions were 'innate or inherited', and therefore beyond 'the will of the individual'.[72] Other authors portrayed emotion as the direct opposite of volition.[73] The American psychologist William James (1842–1910) went so far as to deny any separation of emotion from the body. In 'What is an emotion?' (1884), James argued that bodily changes do not take place as a consequence of emotion: rather, the perception of bodily change *is* the emotion. He stated that a 'purely disembodied human emotion' was inconceivable: if a strong emotion was analysed and its 'characteristic bodily symptoms' abstracted, there was 'nothing left behind, no "mind-stuff" out of which the emotion can be constituted'. A 'cold and neutral state of intellectual perception is all that remains'.[74] Although James' theory was far from universally accepted, it was seen to prove 'the capital importance of physiological factors in emotion'.[75]

[70] J. Sully, 'Introduction', in B. Perez, *The First Three Years of Childhood* (London: Swan Sönnenschein, 1889), pp. vi–vii.

[71] For definitions of instinct and reflex, see G. Romanes, 'Instinct', in Tuke (ed.), *Dictionary of Psychological Medicine*, vol. 2, p. 704; E.J. Foley, 'Cognition and Ideation', in Rhodes (ed.), *Mind at Work*, p. 156; Anon., 'The Science and Philosophy of Instinct', *Nature*, 92 (September 1913–February 1914), 627. For the alignment of instinct with emotion, see T. Ribot, *The Psychology of the Emotions*, 2nd edn (New York and Melbourne: Walter Scott Publishing, 1911), pp. vii–viii; A.F. Shand, *The Foundations of Character: Being a Study of the Tendencies of the Emotions and Sentiments* (London: Macmillan, 1914), pp. 188–92; Cole, *Mental Diseases* [1913], pp. 55, 59.

[72] C. Darwin, *The Expression of the Emotions in Man and Animals*, 2nd edn (London: Fontana Press, 1999) [1889], pp. 348–9; see also Coupland, 'Philosophy of Mind', pp. 39–40.

[73] See, for example, T.C. Shaw, 'Suicide and Sanity', *Lancet*, 20 April 1907, 1067.

[74] W. James, 'What Is an Emotion?', *Mind*, 9 (1884), 188–93.

[75] Ribot, *Psychology of the Emotions*, pp. 93–97; Cole, *Mental Diseases* [1913], pp. 49–50; S.S. Colvin, 'Education', in White and Jelliffe (eds.), *Modern Treatment of Nervous and Mental Diseases*, p. 89.

This association of emotion with the body demonstrates its status as a "primitive" faculty of mind. The psychiatrist W.H.B. Stoddart claimed that emotion always operated in essentially the same way, whether it expressed the 'sensations of a cat when she sees a mouse' or the 'sensations of a lover who sees his sweetheart walking with another man'.[76] Emotion was characterized as a product of the earliest stages of human evolution, and individuals or groups apparently ruled by emotion were perceived as "backward" or "uncivilized". To observe emotion in its purest, unmediated state, Darwin studied four main groups: 'the commoner animals', 'savage' races, the insane, and infants.[77] Along similar lines, medical commentators described emotion as a prominent feature of the mental life of women and the working classes.[78] The social and racial prejudices of these assessments of 'emotionality' depended on circular reasoning: the behaviour of these groups was dominated by emotion and instinct, and so they must be located at a lower point on the evolutionary scale; because they were less highly evolved, the actions of these groups must be governed by emotion and instinct, rather than reason and volition.

As a manifestation of the lower levels of mind, emotion required strict control by the higher faculties. Uncontrolled or overabundant emotion was undesirable, and actions based on unmediated emotion were seen as uncritical, impulsive, and driven by "primitive" suggestion and belief rather than reasoned volition.[79] There was no substantial difference between the actions of a person in a state of uncontrolled emotion and those of a lunatic.[80] While doctors acknowledged emotion as a necessary element of life, which imbued the world with 'warmth' and 'human value', they also insisted that it was valuable only in proportion to intelligence.[81] Authors constructed elaborate hierarchies of affective states organized by the degree to which cognition and volition entered into their constitution. The lowest level was feeling, a reflex reaction to simple

[76] W.H.B. Stoddart, *Mind and Its Disorders: A Text-Book for Students and Practitioners*, 2nd edn (London: H.K. Lewis, 1912), p. 69.
[77] Darwin, *Expression of the Emotions*, pp. 20–4. See also Bain, *Emotions and the Will*, pp. 4–6.
[78] Cole, *Mental Diseases* [1913], pp. 50, 53, 71; Stoddart, *Mind and Its Disorders* [1912], p. 103.
[79] McDougall, *Psychology*, p. 239; R.C. Temple, 'Administrative Value of Anthropology', *Nature*, 92 (September 1913–February 1914), 208; Cole, *Mental Diseases* [1913], p. 122.
[80] T.C. Shaw, 'A Lecture on the Mental Processes in Sanity and Insanity', *Lancet*, 27 January 1912, 213.
[81] Colvin, 'Education', p. 87; H. Campbell, 'The Feelings', *JMS*, 46:193 (April 1900), 226; T.C. Shaw, 'A Lecture on the Special Psychology of Women', *Lancet*, 2 May 1908, 1265.

corporeal pleasure or pain; then came emotion, still 'reflexly and involuntarily aroused', but provoked by 'a perception or idea' rather than mere sensation; finally, in the highest affective level of sentiment, voluntary attention was directed to ideas. In the 'intellectualised emotions' of sentiments, such as truth, justice, duty, conscience, and aesthetic taste, feeling was attached 'to an object of pure intellect'.[82] As emotion was incrementally augmented by reason and volition, it was gradually "civilized". The ideal development of emotion was therefore a movement further and further away from reflex and the body, until the animal was entirely written out of its definition.

In contrast to emotion, the perfectly directed will represented the apex of human mental achievement. Evolutionists' veneration of free will might be seen as logically inconsistent with determinist views of the human mind as the outcome of material processes, and as subject to the same laws which determined the motions of all other physical matter.[83] If will were a natural phenomenon like any other, then there could be 'no such thing as liberty of will even in man: man is simply the slave and the obedient slave of his nerve cells'. Indeed, the human will had 'no more freedom than that of the higher animals', from which it differed 'only in degree – not in kind'.[84] The removal of will from the mystical realm of the soul, and of man from his status as divinely appointed lord and master of all creation, was a dangerous assault on comforting fictions of human power.[85] A thoroughgoing determinism should have levelled all the faculties of mind and retained no special place for will. In practice, however, doctors went to some lengths to retain the higher status of will, even while recasting its power in naturalistic terms.[86] Medical psychologists continued to insist that volition was the highest product of evolution, even while elaborating rejections of metaphysical notions of will which ran to several hundred pages.[87] This feat was achieved through the construction of evolutionary scales of development tracing the growth of will from the instinct of 'the simplest microscopic animalcule' up to 'the most truly purposive actions of man,

---

[82] Cole, *Mental Diseases* [1913], pp. 47–8, 53–4; Coupland, 'Philosophy of Mind', pp. 39–40; Stoddart, *Mind and Its Disorders* [1912], pp. 59, 93.

[83] Dixon, *Invention of Altruism*, p. 179.

[84] GHMSA: G/S6/2, G.W. Rontley, 'Consciousness' (undated, 1901–2), 10–11.

[85] M. Wiener, *Reconstructing the Criminal: Culture, Law and Policy in England, 1830–1914* (Cambridge: Cambridge University Press, 1990), pp. 159–71, 184; Smith, *Free Will and the Human Sciences*, pp. 7–8.

[86] L.J. Daston, 'The Theory of Will versus the Science of Mind', in W.R. Woodward and M.G. Ash (eds.), *The Problematic Science: Psychology in Nineteenth-Century Thought* (New York: Praeger, 1982), p. 111; Smith, *Free Will and the Human Sciences*, pp. 43–4, 138–9.

[87] H. Maudsley, *Body and Will* (London: Kegan Paul, Trench, 1883), p. 295.

actions sustained and renewed through long years by a firm self-conscious resolution to achieve some clearly conceived end'.[88] The evolutionary narratives created by psychologists, psychiatrists, and neurologists used the language of natural science but tenaciously clung to the possibility of free and inviolate will.[89]

In some ways, fears within medical culture about the pernicious effects of theories and practices which seemed to undermine the will were tiresomely repetitive: responses to Darwin echoed earlier disquiet around mesmerism and anticipated the uneasiness provoked by psychoanalysis.[90] Nevertheless, the encounter with Darwinism did alter concepts of will. As doctors and other theorists emphasized the animal origins of will, they simultaneously undermined the potential of its reach and underlined the potency of the forces it had to contain. Like thought and emotion, will was simultaneously linked to and divided from instinct. It developed out of instinct, but existed to police and contain lower forms of activity.[91] The crucial mediator between instinct and volition, as between emotion and sentiment, was intelligence: the French psychologist Theodule Ribot (1839–1916) described the relation between will and intelligence as 'the robust blind man carrying on his shoulders the paralytic who sees clearly'.[92] The perfect direction of will depended on harnessing intelligence to determine the right end of action, and suppressing emotion which might interfere with judgement or the execution of an action. The precise deployment of will, on which "civilized" human identity hinged, involved forbearance as well as positive action, and could even be defined as the power *not* to act.[93] Because human development depended on the suppression of instinct and emotion, the capacity for repression proved the measure of man.[94]

[88] McDougall, *Psychology*, pp. 152–3; see also Stoddart, *Mind and Its Disorders* [1912], p. 70; Cole, *Mental Diseases* [1913], p. 55; Coupland, 'Philosophy of Mind', pp. 41–2.

[89] L.S. Jacyna, 'Somatic Theories of Mind and the Interests of Medicine in Britain, 1850–1879', *Medical History*, 26 (1982), 240, 244; Clark, 'Rejection of Psychological Approaches', pp. 275–7; L.J. Ray, 'Models of Madness in Victorian Asylum Practice', *Archives Européenes de Sociologie*, 22 (1981), 243, 251–2.

[90] D. Pick, 'Maladies of the Will: Freedom, Fetters and the Fear of Freud', in R. Bivins and J.V. Pickstone (eds.), *Medicine, Madness and Social History: Essays in Honour of Roy Porter* (Basingstoke: Palgrave Macmillan, 2007).

[91] Colvin, 'Education', p. 96; Stoddart, *Mind and Its Disorders* [1912], p. 70; Coupland, 'Philosophy of Mind', pp. 41–2; Cole, *Mental Diseases* [1913], pp. 61–2; McDougall, *Psychology*, p. 154.

[92] Ribot, *Psychology of the Emotions*, p. 440.

[93] T. Ribot, 'Will, Disorders of', in Tuke (ed.), *Dictionary of Psychological Medicine*, vol. 2, p. 1367; Stoddart, *Mind and Its Disorders* [1912], p. 71; Reed, *Victorian Will*, p. ix.

[94] Bain, *Emotions and the Will*, pp. 404, 407–8.

The heightened emphasis on will as perhaps the most important aspect of human identity is even perversely reflected in the late nineteenth-century creation of aboulia, a disorder defined as the absence of will (and deemed to be more common in women than men).[95] The will shaped by 'education and experience' was the cornerstone of character and the most distinctively "human" of all mental faculties.[96] As the 'force in Nature in which consciousness reaches its acme', humans achieved 'the dignity of personality' and dominion over the earthly universe through the exercise of will.[97] Yet if the special character of man was that 'racially and personally he has grown into the habit of inhibiting himself from brutishness', this only underscored that he had '*much*, complex and various, *to inhibit*'.[98] Reformulations of will enabled man to cling to a distinctively human status, but only by the skin of his recognizably canine teeth. Will both defined human identity and performed an essential social function: it restrained individual desire, prevented anarchy, and formed the foundation of "civilization" itself.[99] Without will, there could be no duty and responsibility, only the selfish indulgence of individual desire.[100] The dark shadow of impairment of will was the precarious status of all human achievement.

Mind and Its Disorders

The incorporation of mind in the evolutionary scale of development meant that any disorder of its faculties could be construed as a perilous return to "primitive" origins. Although disorder might originate in any of the three faculties of mind, its existence always demonstrated the slackening of 'the vigilant control of the will', the highest coordinating faculty of mind.[101] All disorders of mind were therefore also disorders of will. As one of the most recent acquirements of the human mind, any

[95] Ribot, 'Will, Disorders of', 1366–7; G. Van Ness Dearborn, 'Kinesthesia and the Intelligent Will', *American Journal of Psychology*, 24:2 (April 1913), 227.
[96] Stoddart, *Mind and Its Disorders* [1912], p. 71; G.H. Savage, 'An Address on Mental Disorders', *Lancet*, 26 October 1912, 1134–7; Coupland, 'Philosophy of Mind', p. 42; Rhodes, 'Mechanism of the Will', pp. 188, 191; Bain, *Emotions and the Will*, p. 340; Cole, *Mental Diseases*, pp. 55–7.
[97] Cole, *Mental Diseases* [1913], pp. 56, 61–2; Colvin, 'Education', p. 99; E.J. Foley, 'Modes of Consciousness', in Rhodes (ed.), *Mind at Work*, p. 90; Reed, *Victorian Will*, p. 130.
[98] Van Ness Dearborn, 'Kinesthesia and the Intelligent Will', 235–6 [emphasis in the original].
[99] E. Buttar, 'Physiology of the Brain and Nervous System', in Rhodes (ed.), *Mind at Work*, pp. 31–2.
[100] Smith, *Free Will and the Human Sciences*, p. 3.
[101] Coupland, 'Philosophy of Mind', p. 29; A.J. Brock, 'Habit as a Pathological Factor', *EMJ*, 13 (July–December 1914), 142.

impairment of will constituted a regression; because it harnessed and directed all the "lower" faculties of mind, loss of will unleashed primal traits and testified to the animal origins of man. In the 1870s, psychiatrist Henry Maudsley (1835–1918) interpreted the 'brute-like characteristics' of the insane as reminders that every man had 'the brute nature within him'.[102] Forty years later, Robert Armstrong-Jones reaffirmed this view. As 'a vertebrate animal with the instincts of the animal', man attained the 'veneer of civilization' only through the 'the power of inhibition' and 'the influence of his environment'. In insanity, all the accoutrements of "civilization" were shed 'in inverse order of their acquirement', 'until at last a man is left a wreck barely above the level of the animal'.[103] For both alienists, madness meant reversion to mental states characteristic of earlier stages in individual development and racial evolution.

Thomas Claye Shaw (1841–1927), whose professional career spanned most of these forty years, put forward a similar view of insanity. From the early 1870s until his retirement in 1911, Claye Shaw was superintendent of Banstead Asylum and lecturer in psychological medicine at St Bartholomew's Hospital.[104] He described madness in Jacksonian terms as 'dissolution' or 'devolution' from 'the highest state of the individual'.[105] Volition, a recently acquired and highly elaborate aspect of mind, was shed first in mental illness.[106] In turn, 'intellectual comprehension' shrank, emotion ran riot, and 'the type of early, undeveloped life' dominated: hence, the insane resembled 'uncivilized persons', 'savages', 'islanders', 'primitive races', children, and even 'the brute creation'.[107] As dissolution showed, man's original nature was still that of 'a wild beast, impulsive and liable to explode'. Indeed, the 'readiness with which civilized man reverts to the savage type shows simply that the original ferocity is only tamed, not changed'. Although modern societies were built on 'the cultivation of inhibition', at the current stage of evolution, this could only ever be an 'artificial restraint'.[108] For Claye Shaw, the

---

[102] H. Maudsley, *Body and Mind: An Inquiry into Their Connection and Mutual Influence, Specially in Reference to Mental Disorders* (New York: D. Appleton, 1871), p. 51.

[103] R. [Armstrong-]Jones, 'An Address on Temperaments: Is There a Neurotic One?' *Lancet*, 1 July 1911, 5–6; R. [Armstrong-]Jones, 'Para-Myo-Clonus Multiples and Insanity', *SBHR*, 46 (1910), 28–9.

[104] R. Armstrong-Jones, 'In Memoriam: Thomas Claye Shaw', *SBHR*, 60 (1927), 1.

[105] Shaw, *Ex Cathedra*, p. 94.

[106] Shaw, 'A Lecture on the Special Psychology of Women', 1266; Shaw, 'Suicide and Sanity', 1068.

[107] T.C. Shaw, 'On Degradation of Type in the Insane', *SBHR*, 20 (1884), 169, 170–3, 177.

[108] T.C. Shaw, 'A Contribution to the Analysis of the Mental Process in Criminal Acts', *Lancet*, 9 November 1907, 1307; T.C. Shaw, 'On the Forecast of Destructive Impulses in the Insane', *SBHR*, 21 (1885), 11.

extent of mental instability in modern life demonstrated the inevitable appearance of 'throw-backs or reversions, failures and impossibilities'.[109] Moreover, in practice, mankind could not be divided into the definitively mad and the absolutely sane. Individuals perpetually seesawed above and below an average level of sanity, and any 'phonographic repetition of the day's sayings and a cinematographic representation of the day's doings would show many ups and downs in the levels of development'.[110] Ultimately, the evolutionary framework of understanding undermined the boundaries between animal and human, "primitive" and "civilized", insane and sane.

This construction of mental disorder as regression, a slippage down the evolutionary scale of development, carried over into conceptions of war neurosis. "Shell-shock" doctors imbibed these ideas from the culture around them, but more specifically from their formal and informal education. These influences were direct and indirect. Although he published extensively on insanity, belonged to many medical societies, and merited obituaries in leading medical journals, Claye Shaw was not a great psychological theorist or even one of the leading psychiatrists of his day. Yet he was deeply immersed in the institutional and associational life of one of the great teaching hospitals: an 'attractive' lecturer with 'well-attended' classes, who favoured rising juniors at the Abernethian Society with his patronage and contributed an article to almost every volume of the *St Bartholomew's Hospital Reports* published between the mid-1870s and 1900.[111] As such, Claye Shaw's influence on psychological medicine extended over several decades. During his tenure as lecturer in psychological medicine at Barts, several "shell-shock" doctors passed through the school, including Armstrong-Jones, Charles Myers, and W.H.R. Rivers, the three doctors to publish most extensively on the disorder.[112] We cannot know how, or even if, Claye Shaw influenced the intellectual development of these students. However, the concept of mental illness as regression recurs in different ways in the work of all three physicians.[113] The constellation of future "shell-shock" doctors at Barts offers an intriguing insight into potential mechanisms for the

[109] Shaw, 'Contribution to the Analysis of the Mental Process', 1307.
[110] Shaw, *Ex Cathedra*, p. 110.
[111] Anon., 'Obituary: Thomas Claye Shaw', *BMJ*, 22 January 1927; Armstrong-Jones, 'In Memoriam: Thomas Claye Shaw', 3. See lists of proceedings of Abernethian Society, *SBHR*, 32 (1896); *SBHR*, 33 (1897), 231; *SBHR*, 40 (1904), 157; *SBHR*, 46 (1910), 199. For his articles, mainly on insanity, see *SBHR*, 1874–1900.
[112] The others are Adolphe Abrahams, Harry Campbell, Alfred Carver, Anthony Feiling, Robert Hotchkis, John Herbert Parsons, Howard Tooth, and William Aldren Turner.
[113] On ideas of the "primitive" and "civilized" in the work of Rivers and Myers, see M. Thomson, '"Savage Civilisation": Race, Culture and Mind in Britain,

transmission of knowledge within medical schools, and the influence of medical education on the later careers of students, in a period when evolutionary frameworks of understanding shaped many aspects of the medical curriculum.

Conclusion

In the final decades of the nineteenth century, British doctors, like their contemporaries in other fields, revised their visions of human nature in the wake of the Darwinian revolution. This involved the reconfiguration, rather than erasure and reinvention, of earlier ideas of mind, brain, and nerves. After Darwin, the traditional boundaries of high and low which governed western thought were reconstituted as gateways between the categories they delineated. The evolutionary framework of understanding came to dominate medical education. During their training, doctors were exposed to a model of mind in which human mental faculties were perceived as repositories of earlier stages of evolutionary development, overlaid by the fragile acquisitions of "civilization". Volition was the cornerstone of human identity and the controlling mechanism of the mind, but it also grew out of instinct and attested to man's animal origins. As an insecure attainment, will was liable to waver in the course of everyday life, but under extreme strain it could even break down completely, unleashing the "primitive" forces it contained. When doctors trained in this tradition tried to explain "shell-shock", they fell back on this conception of mind, and depicted the nervous and mental disorders of war as painful failures of will.

In its barest outlines, this evolutionary model had much in common with Freud's representation of mind in his 1915 paper on war and death. Freud argued that "civilization" was superficial: scratch the surface of the "civilized" mind, and an ineradicable mass of primitive drives and instincts pulsates beneath. "Civilization" demanded the repeated renunciation of instinctual satisfaction from each of its members, and so survived on the shakiest of foundations. Freud's paper recapitulated the dominant themes of late nineteenth-century intellectual and scientific culture. Indeed, in the view of ophthalmologist John Herbert Parsons (1868–1957), the Freudian-derived "'New Psychology" [had] its origin in the "Origin of Species"'.[114] The evolutionary framework of understanding instituted points of

1898–1939', in W. Ernst and B. Harris (eds.), *Race, Science and Medicine, 1700–1960* (London and New York: Routledge, 1999), pp. 235–58.
[114] Parsons, *Mind and the Nation*, p. 8.

exchange for ideas about human mind, body, and culture across medicine and the human, social, and natural sciences.

Across several domains of thought, individuals raw with the abrasions of the post-Darwinian universe niggled away at the dangerous proximity of the human to the animal. Anthropological expeditions which set out to confirm 'biologically based otherness and inequality' ended by revealing 'the "savage" and "primitive" basis of the "civilized" mind'.[115] Psychological investigations attempted to establish what made a coherent and rational person, but instead tore open the unstable borderlines between consciousness and the 'obscure recesses' of the mind.[116] In this way, the conceptual gateways that evolutionary theory instituted between "high" and "low" also constituted a different, historical point of exchange, between the psychological medicine of the late nineteenth-century and the psychodynamic approaches to mind which gained medical and scientific purchase in Britain in the interwar period. The Freudian theory of the unconscious drew on 'well-known theories of the pervasive influence of unconscious mental processes', but it also transformed them.[117] The concept of organic memory – the transmission of thoughts, memories, and cultural achievements across generations – permeated Freudian psychoanalysis. Only the belief that ontogeny recapitulates phylogeny (that individual development repeats racial development) allowed Freud to 'view human history through the child and through the neurotic as well as through the unconscious of the "normal" individual'.[118] The same concepts of evolution, inheritance, and "civilization" that saturated psychological culture in Britain also formed the backdrop of psychoanalytic theory, against which Freud formulated his more radical ideas.

These interfaces demonstrate the existence of shared questions and concerns about the fundamental make-up of human nature, although the answers were very different. Freudian psychoanalysis is often viewed as the main intellectual resource of psychodynamic medical psychologists in the years around the First World War, but it was not the only form of knowledge that forced reappraisal of established certainties. The evolutionary framework of understanding which pervaded intellectual and

[115] Thomson, '"Savage Civilisation"', p. 236; M. Thomson, 'Psychology and the "Consciousness of Modernity" in Early Twentieth-Century Britain', in M. Daunton and B. Rieger (eds.), *Meanings of Modernity: Britain from the Late-Victorian Era to World War Two* (Oxford and New York: Berg, 2001), pp. 100–5.

[116] J.B. Taylor, 'Obscure Recesses: Locating the Victorian Unconscious', in J.B. Bullen (ed.), *Writing and Victorianism* (London and New York: Longman, 1997), pp. 143, 157.

[117] Ibid., p. 140.

[118] L. Otis, 'Organic Memory and Psychoanalysis', *History of Psychiatry*, 4 (1993), 372; L. Otis, *Organic Memory: History and the Body in the Late Nineteenth and Early Twentieth Centuries* (Lincoln, NE and London: University of Nebraska Press, 1994), pp. 1–49.

scientific culture in the early twentieth century also encouraged reassessment of the constituents of human identity and workings of mind. This
framework of understanding shaped medical approaches to the bodies
and minds of "shell-shocked" soldiers. As will be seen, concepts of
emotion, will, and animal inheritance dominated understandings of the
disorder until the end of the war and beyond. The evolutionary model of
mind remained integral to medical understandings of mental breakdown.
But in the decades before the war, as the disciplines of mind, nerves, and
brain gradually separated and defined their own territories, attempts to
understand the relations between animal and human, body and mind,
and the individual and the social also led to flux and mutation within
medical culture.

2   Languages of Diagnosis
Hysteria, Neurasthenia, and Changing Pre-War Psychological Medicine

A medical diagnosis identifies the symptoms which make up an illness. It groups together the symptoms combined in each condition and allows doctors to distinguish between different disorders which include similar symptoms. It involves assessments of the possible causes of these symptoms and predictions of their likely effects, and implies further judgements about the most effective forms of treatment. A diagnostic label is convenient shorthand for this knowledge, which eases communication among doctors and between doctors and patients. However, the assurance of understanding implied in this ability to name a condition is deceptive. A medical diagnosis almost always involves some uncertainties. Is it definitely this condition and not another? What is the ultimate cause? Which form of treatment is best in this particular case? Doctors are usually aware of the ambivalence contained within diagnostic terms, even if patients are not. It is less often realized that diagnostic labels conceal consensus as well as disagreement. A medical diagnosis is never a purely objective statement of what happens in the body. It also necessarily rests on shared assumptions, mostly unarticulated, about what constitutes body, mind, and environment; what is most important about each for understanding the individual's illness; how these domains might interact; and what counts as a pathological form or response. A diagnosis is a way of organizing knowledge about the world. As the contents and boundaries of a diagnosis shift, this knowledge is reorganized. Flux within diagnostic categories demonstrates the instability of knowledge about the world and represents the attempt to classify and conquer what remains indeterminate.

"Shell-shock" was an unstable diagnosis made up of other unstable diagnoses. Most doctors disliked the designation and used it, if at all, as an umbrella term for all the conditions seen as forming part of the nervous and mental disorders of war: hysteria, neurasthenia, traumatic neurosis, concussion, "commotional shock", exhaustion, physiological malfunction, "soldier's heart", epilepsy, insanity, and sometimes forms of psychosis. This diagnostic messiness reflected the broad symptomatology and unclear aetiology of "shell-shock", and had important and immediate practical implications. Without clear understanding of causes and symptoms, effective treatment was a matter of guesswork. However, this level of diagnostic chaos also reveals more fundamental ambiguities, not only about the nature of "shell-shock", but also around all those elements which might or might not affect the development of the disorder. Medical efforts to understand "shell-shock" therefore also involved attempts to work out the relations between mind and body, the relative influence of nature and nurture in individual cases of "shell-shock", and the potential physical, social, and emotional causes and consequences of the disorder. These were not new problems. Difficulties in determining the contents and boundaries of "shell-shock" arose not only from questions thrown up by the war, such as the possible effects of modern industrial weapons on the human organism, but also from ambivalences and tensions within existing conceptions of similar disorders.

In 1914, understandings of the relations of mind, body, and environment were in flux. As doctors tried to organize knowledge about "shell-shock" into manageable and useful categories, they drew on pre-existing diagnostic classifications. Many symptoms of "shell-shock" corresponded to those found in other disorders such as hysteria, neurasthenia, and traumatic neurosis. However, the fact that doctors recognized some of what they saw did not resolve anything. There is no safety in falling back on shifting ground. Medical understanding of these conditions was characterized by profound divisions over causation, contents, and treatment. In pre-war psychological medicine, these conditions occupied a no-man's land between physical and "psychological" illness. Within this space, doctors could either attempt to work out the relations of psyche and soma or shelve the fundamental problem of mind–body relations to concentrate on the immediate and practical issue of cure. Both approaches enabled engagement with psychological theorizing within the predominantly somatic paradigm of British psychological medicine. Before 1914, this engagement took the form of efforts to get to grips with European theories developed to explain functional disorders, especially hysteria.

The classificatory categories and language used to describe these conditions reveal medical uncertainty about what they were, and how best to treat them. Hysteria, neurasthenia, traumatic neurosis, and, later on, "shell-shock", were all usually categorized as functional diseases or disorders. Often, doctors used the term "psychic" to describe either these disorders or medical approaches to them. Although useful working terms, the designations "functional" and "psychic" cloaked fundamental conceptual ambiguities. Functional disorders were characterized by disturbances or changes in the functions of an organ not attributable to any discernible organic disease.[1] Classification of an illness as functional meant that it occupied the hinterland between mind and body. As will be seen, it was through the category of functional disorder that "psychological" forms of thought first infiltrated British psychological medicine. "Psychic" described symptoms or approaches which were not primarily somatic, but the term did not usually incorporate more sophisticated comprehension of psychological processes. The term implied that an illness was not physical, and that symptoms could be attributed to the mind, but its use did not rest on a fully worked out or coherent understanding of mental operations or the relation of mind to body. One of the central arguments of this chapter is that before 1914, British medical culture did not possess any fully developed psychological mode of understanding, although in retrospect, we can trace a series of shifts through which such ways of thinking had started to come into being.

Within pre-war psychological medicine, one important trend was an incremental shift towards greater openness to "psychological" thinking. However, this coincided with another critical movement: the resurgence of biological modes of explanation for mental illness. This is most evident in the rise of the eugenics movement, but even doctors who were not committed eugenicists debated the roles of heredity and environment in individual cases of health and illness, and often stated their belief in the ultimate power of nature over nurture. Logically, this biological turn might seem to pull against psychological theorizing, but both tendencies coexisted quite happily in the thought of most doctors. Again, the ambivalent status of functional disorders explains this apparent contradiction. Because these disorders were defined by the lack of solid knowledge about their origins, attempts at medical explanation were predicated on non-commitment to known first causes. This meant that doctors could simultaneously posit hereditary weakness among the first causes of such disorders *and* develop explanations concentrating on the interaction of heredity with environment. An example of such thinking is the late nineteenth-century medical identification of a degenerate urban "residuum". Belief in an inherently biologically flawed underclass did not prevent attempts to tackle the problem of degeneration through public health measures, as well as eugenically influenced proposals.[2] In practice, sufferers were still condemned as biological failures, but a

---

[1] D.H. Tuke (ed.), *A Dictionary of Psychological Medicine*, 2 vols. (London: J. & A. Churchill, 1892), vol. 1, p. 518.

[2] G.S. Jones, *Outcast London: A Study in the Relationship between Classes in Victorian Society* (Harmondsworth: Penguin, 1984), pp. 281–314; D. Porter, '"Enemies of the Race": Biologism, Environmentalism, and Public Health in Edwardian England', *Victorian Studies*, 34 (1991), 159–78.

theoretical space existed which allowed for the potential influence of the environment. Because the category of functional disorder enabled doctors to elaborate practical knowledge of symptoms and treatments without fully articulating beliefs about causes, and therefore to avoid denial or endorsement of particular positions, "psychological" and biological modes of thought did not clash.

This chapter uses the diagnoses of hysteria and neurasthenia as case studies to demonstrate the flux and tension within pre-war British psychological medicine.[3] These 'elusive and protean' disorders open up debates on body and mind, nature and nurture, and the social and political ramifications of illness.[4] Because hysteria and neurasthenia later formed component parts of the diagnosis of "shell-shock", they are particularly helpful for understanding the knowledges and uncertainties doctors took into their encounters with "shell-shocked" patients, and exactly how the war reshaped medical approaches to disorders of mind, nerves, and brain. As doctors related the sufferings of soldiers to civilian maladies, they imbued the diagnosis of "shell-shock" with the values and assumptions of pre-war psychological medicine, and became locked into intractable questions about the nature of human identity, "modernity", and "civilization". However, if the experience of "shell-shock" further destabilized knowledge of these domains, it also propelled the refashioning of ideas about the individual and social, body and mind, and the "primitive" and "civilized". All that was new about "shell-shock" was refracted through the prism of existing modes of understanding, but this did not alter the fundamental unknowability and awful novelty of war itself.

Hysteria and Neurasthenia in Pre-War Medical Discourse

Languages of diagnosis can be slippery. In the pre-war period, the same diagnostic term could describe different symptom sets and shoulder different ideological burdens over a relatively short space of time. Different meanings did not simply replace one another, but were used simultaneously in separate contexts, and gradually overlapped with and infused one another. It follows that languages of diagnosis were diffuse, but also highly particular and context-specific. The contents and

---

[3] See my earlier discussion in T. Loughran, 'Hysteria and Neurasthenia in Pre-1914 British Medical Discourse and in Histories of Shell-Shock', *History of Psychiatry*, 19:1 (March 2008), especially 26–7.

[4] Quotation, M. Micale, 'Hysteria and Its Historiography: The Future Perspective', *History of Psychiatry*, 1 (1990), 45–6. Micale refers to hysteria, but his description fits neurasthenia equally well.

meanings of diagnostic terms only partially crossed the boundaries between different specialties or nations: doctors drew on the medical literatures of many traditions, but "translation" into the native idiom always constituted a change in the signified as well as the signifier. This "translation" was not always literal.[5] Ideas transformed as they were taken up and used in different contexts, even if doctors were apparently speaking the same language. These "translations" reflected attitudes and assumptions ingrained in the new context, but also determined the extent to which understanding was possible across boundaries, and shaped the future uses of particular ideas. What first seem like misunderstandings or misappropriations can be viewed as practical attempts to mesh new ideas with existing traditions. The coexistence of apparently contradictory positions could represent attempts to find workable means of coping with illness in the absence of concrete knowledge.

This is evident in relation to hysteria and neurasthenia. Although both diagnoses crossed national borders, their uses within British psychological medicine reflected the particular concerns of this national tradition. Both were perceived as older forms of illness now more prevalent under the stresses and strains of modern life. Medical accounts readily acknowledged the ancient lineage of hysteria, but British doctors also insisted that neurasthenia, a term popularized from the 1860s, described a familiar condition under a new name.[6] Both disorders also incorporated extensive lists of symptoms, which were distinctively inflected in different national contexts. The *grande hysterie* or hysterical fit, archetypal symptom of the disease in French literature, was rarely observed in Britain.[7] However, as hysteria was characterized by its mimicry of organic disease, it could manifest in virtually any imaginable way: in disorders of sensation, movement, and circulation as well as in the capricious behaviours and emotional outbursts associated with the hysteric

---

[5] But sometimes it was: comparisons of English translations of German psychoanalytic texts suggest that these translations 'differ considerably in register from those originals'. English psychoanalytic terminology was more technical in character and, even more importantly, shifted the emphasis of discussions from 'process' to 'structure'. See G. Richards, 'Britain on the Couch: The Popularization of Psychoanalysis in Britain 1918–1940', *Science in Context*, 13:2 (June 2000), 218.

[6] R. Arndt, 'Neurasthenia', in Tuke (ed.), *Dictionary of Psychological Medicine*, vol. 2, p. 843; R. Porter, 'Nervousness, Eighteenth and Nineteenth Century Style: From Luxury to Labour', in M. Gijswijt-Hofstra and R. Porter (eds.), *Cultures of Neurasthenia: From Beard to the First World War* (Amsterdam and New York: Rodophi, 2001), pp. 40–1; J. Oppenheim, *"Shattered Nerves": Doctors, Patients, and Depression in Victorian England* (Oxford and New York: Oxford University Press, 1991), p. 95.

[7] J.A. Ormerod, 'Hysteria', in T.C. Allbutt (ed.), *A System of Medicine*, 8 vols. (London and New York: Macmillan, 1898), vol. 8, pp. 96–7.

personality.[8] The diagnosis of neurasthenia was similarly capacious and open to interpretation, comprising a range of somatic and "psychic" symptoms: nervous exhaustion and fatigue, constant tiredness, general aches and pains affecting any or several bodily functions (circulation, digestion, sexual activity), inability to concentrate, headache, insomnia, depression, excitability, irritability, introspection, and excessive emotion. Although the "psychological" elements of the disorder were emphasized in some countries, in Britain neurasthenia was most often perceived as a condition of nervous weakness or exhaustion with attached "psychic" symptoms.[9]

The British tradition of thought on both hysteria and neurasthenia emphasized bodily and mental elements, and refused to definitively allocate either disorder to one realm over another. By 1914, it was widely acknowledged that the 'gallant attempts' of British theorists to find a physical basis for hysteria had failed, but lack of convincing physical explanations did not lead to the production of sophisticated psychological theories.[10] Doctors instead emphasized the interaction of bodily and mental processes in hysteria, and suggested that the disorder was produced by some combination of hereditary weakness, exhaustion, poor education, suggestion, and/or emotional shock.[11] They explained neurasthenia as the outcome of a similar blend of physical and "psychic" factors.[12] Medical textbooks listed possible somatic causes including

[8] J. Paget, 'Clinical Lectures on the Nervous Mimicry of Organic Diseases. Lecture I', *Lancet*, 11 October 1873, 511–13; Tuke (ed.), *Dictionary of Psychological Medicine*, vol. 1, pp. 641–2; W.H.B. Stoddart, *Mind and Its Disorders: A Text-Book for Students and Practitioners* (London: H.K. Lewis, 1908), pp. 370–3.

[9] J.D. Nagel, *Nervous and Mental Diseases: A Manual for Students and Practitioners* (London: Hodder and Stoughton, 1905), pp. 171–2; C.S. Potts, *Nervous and Mental Diseases for Students and Practitioners*, 2nd edn (London: Henry Kimpton, 1908), pp. 405–7; T.A. Ross, 'The Nature and Treatment of Neurasthenia', *EMJ*, 12 (January–June 1914), 297. Stoddart's inventory of neurasthenic symptoms in *Mind and Its Disorders* [1908] ran to nearly three pages: see pp. 362–4.

[10] J.A. Ormerod, 'Two Theories of Hysteria', *Brain*, 33:3 (January 1911), 270. For physiological theories of hysteria, see H.C. Bastian, *Various Forms of Hysterical or Functional Paralysis* (London: H.K. Lewis, 1893); T.D. Savill, *Lectures on Hysteria and Allied Vaso-Motor Conditions* (London: Henry J. Glaister, 1909).

[11] Stoddart, *Mind and Its Disorders* [1908], pp. 368–70; Cole, *Mental Diseases* [1913], pp. 216–17; Potts, *Nervous and Mental Diseases*, pp. 411–12.

[12] The aetiological accounts of most doctors blended physical and mental factors or acknowledged the possibility of different causes in different cases (including the potential for apparently neurasthenic symptoms to mask more serious organic disorders). See C. Oldfield, 'Some Pelvic Disorders in Relation to Neurasthenia', *Practitioner*, 91:3 (September 1913), 335; I.G. Cobb, 'Neurasthenia – Its Causes and Treatment', *Practitioner*, 95 (July–December 1915), 229; Anon., 'Review: The Conquest of Nerves by J.W. Courtney', *Lancet*, 27 July 1912; J.S.R. Russell, 'The Treatment of Neurasthenia', *Lancet*, 22 November 1913, 1453; F.W. Mott, 'Neurasthenia and Some Associated Conditions', *Practitioner*, 86:1 (January 1911), 1–10; H. Head and E.G. Fearnsides,

hereditary weakness, nervous incapacity or irritability, chemical imbalance, bacterial infection, or auto-intoxication. The nervous weakness of neurasthenia might be inborn (the result of heredity) or acquired (the result of environmental factors such as shock, illness, or an undesirable mode of life), but this was not sufficient to determine the development of the illness. Instead, doctors portrayed the final descent into neurasthenia as triggered by behavioural factors such as overwork, poor diet, lack of exercise, sexual excess, or emotional strain.[13]

Because doctors perceived nervous weakness as a stepping stone between physical and "psychic" illnesses, hysteria and neurasthenia were borderland diagnoses in which body and mind were both implicated. The treatment most often recommended for both conditions was a modified version of the rest cure devised by the American physician Silas Weir Mitchell (1829–1914), which combined physical and psychological elements.[14] The treatment consisted of seclusion (removal from the patient's usual surroundings and severe restrictions on visitors), lengthy and complete bed rest combined with massage to prevent muscle wastage, and a regime of 'over-feeding' to build up the patient and prevent physical fatigue.[15] British doctors emphasized the "psychological" elements of this treatment. Mitchell stressed the need to attain complete 'moral influence' over the patient and to alter his or her poisonous 'moral environment'.[16] The Weir Mitchell treatment therefore tackled the moral weaknesses of hysterical and neurasthenic patients as well as potential physical conditions, and this is why physicians with quite different views about the causes and nature of hysteria and neurasthenia endorsed it. The rest cure was a perfect treatment for functional disorders because it dealt with body and mind, and it allowed either aspect to be emphasized in treatment. The popularity of the Weir Mitchell treatment perhaps also reflects the resurgence of medical holism in the

'The Clinical Effects of Syphilis of the Nervous System in the Light of the Wassermann Reaction and Treatment with Neosalvarsan', *Brain*, 37:1 (September 1914), 9.

[13] T.C. Allbutt, 'Neurasthenia', in T.C. Allbutt (ed.), *A System of Medicine*, 8 vols. (London and New York: Macmillan, 1898), vol. 8, pp. 150–2; Ross, 'Nature and Treatment of Neurasthenia', 296; Stoddart, *Mind and Its Disorders* [1908], p. 362; Cole, *Mental Diseases* [1913], pp. 220–1; J. Ritchie, 'Neurasthenia', *EMJ*, 12 (January–June 1914), 115.

[14] Ormerod, 'Hysteria', 121–3; Ritchie, 'Neurasthenia', 118–9; Stoddart, *Mind and Its Disorders* [1908], pp. 366, 377; Cole, *Mental Diseases* [1913], pp. 219–20, 222; Ross, 'Nature and Treatment of Neurasthenia', 297.

[15] H. Marland, '"Uterine Mischief": W.S. Playfair and His Neurasthenic Patients', in Gijswijt-Hofstra and Porter (eds.), *Cultures of Neurasthenia*.

[16] Oppenheim, *"Shattered Nerves"*, p. 214; T. Lutz, 'Varieties of Medical Experience: Doctors and Patients, Psyche and Soma in America', in Gijswijt-Hofstra and Porter (eds.), *Cultures of Neurasthenia*, p. 55.

early twentieth century in response to the fragmentation of medicine into ever-smaller specialties. Medical holists saw diagnostic labels as useful for classifying knowledge, but warned that they should not be confused with 'the actual manifestation of illness in the individual patient', which could not be 'reduced to the action of a microbe on the body or a failing in one body system'.[17] The ideal treatment dealt with the whole patient, rather than individual symptoms.

Hysteria, Neurasthenia, and Functional Disease

The ambiguities within medical discourse on hysteria and neurasthenia did not result from ignorance alone, but also from flux within understandings of the role of body and mind in the production of nervous and mental disorders. Although late nineteenth- and early twentieth-century British psychological medicine is often perceived as rigidly somatic, the empirical bent of this tradition allowed more space for alternative approaches than the explicit statements of doctors might seem to allow. Symptoms mattered more than causes. To take one example: the core symptom of neurasthenia was nervous exhaustion, but the effects of emotions such as anxiety and dread were still important parts of the clinical picture of the condition. In some cases, doctors argued that the patient's anxiety about minor physical ailments set up a vicious circle which resulted in total nervous exhaustion.[18] Doctors who remained formally committed to somatic explanations nevertheless drew up models of causation which implicated body and mind. This approach might seem contradictory and hopelessly confused, and some doctors did try to turn neurasthenia into a more coherent diagnosis. One method was to divide the symptoms of neurasthenia into different subcategories according to whether they were physical, "psychic", or a mixture of both.[19] Another tactic, which increased in popularity in the years leading up to the war, was redistribution of the "psychic" symptoms into new diagnoses, thereby stripping the old one down to its pure core of nervous exhaustion, a primarily somatic category.[20] But for the most part, doctors

---

[17] D. Cantor, 'The Diseased Body', in R. Cooter and J. Pickstone (eds.), *Companion to Medicine in the Twentieth Century* (London and New York: Routledge, 2003), p. 351; C. Lawrence, 'Incommunicable Knowledge: Science, Technology and the Clinical Art in Britain, 1850–1914', *Journal of Contemporary History*, 20 (1985), 503–20.

[18] Ross, 'Nature and Treatment of Neurasthenia'.

[19] Russell, 'Treatment of Neurasthenia', 1453.

[20] Anon., 'Medical Societies: Nottingham Medico-Chirurgical Society', *Lancet*, 11 November 1911, 1338; J.M. Clarke, *Hysteria and Neurasthenia* (London and New York: John Lane, 1905), p. 191. See Loughran, 'Hysteria and Neurasthenia', 35–6, on the relation between neurasthenia and anxiety neurosis.

continued to diagnose patients with neurasthenia and to remain fairly confident that other physicians would know, at least more or less, what they meant when they used the term. They complained all the time that neurasthenia was too wide-ranging to be a meaningful diagnosis, but continued to publish articles about neurasthenia and to diagnose it in their own patients; if it was not meaningful, neither was it redundant. In practice, doctors exploited the elasticity of neurasthenia in order to deal with symptoms they could not otherwise explain.

The ambivalent characterization of hysteria and neurasthenia therefore demonstrates lack of knowledge about causes, but it also reflects a distinctively British mode of conceptualizing functional disorders in which coherence mattered less than practical application. As physician Clifford Allbutt (1836–1925) explained,

In England we cling to concrete experience; we look for friction, unexpected turns, compromises, chances; we have little belief in systems of thought and dialectics, and in medicine, as in political and social affairs, have trusted to experiment, to touch; we find safety not in ideal revolutions, nor in rigid organization, but in broadening down, in criticism, and in the fertility of intuitive action.[21]

British doctors were self-consciously proud of the empiricism of their medical tradition, and contrasted it to the perceived French and German taste for abstract theorization.[22] However, medical recourse to the category of functional disorder eventually opened up space for explicit psychological theorization within the dominant somatic paradigm of British psychological medicine.

The concept of functional disease originated as a convenient designation for disorders for which no organic cause could be found. It therefore described effects without ascribing first causes, and this fundamental ambiguity enabled it to become a storehouse for all that appeared temporarily unexplainable within physical terms.[23] As already seen in

---

[21] T.C. Allbutt, 'President's Address on the Universities in Medical Research and Practice', *BMJ*, 3 July 1920, 7.

[22] Xenophobic distaste for abstract thought is evident in the exacting specifications accompanying provision for the endowment of a chair of Rational Logic and Scientific Method at the University of London in psychiatrist Charles Mercier's will: 'The professor is to be chosen for his ability to think and reason and to teach, and not for his acquaintance with books on logic, or with the opinions of logicians or philosophers. Acquaintance with the Greek and German tongues is not to be an actual disqualification for the professorship, but in case the merits of the candidates appear in other respects approximately equal, preference is to be given first to him who knows neither Greek nor German; next, to him who knows Greek but not German; next to him who knows German but not Greek; and last of all, to a candidate who knows both Greek and German'. Anon., 'Notes and News: The Late Dr. C.A. Mercier', *JMS*, 67:145 (January 1921), 146.

[23] Bastian, *Various Forms of Hysterical or Functional Paralysis*, p. 2.

relation to hysteria, lack of physical explanation did not immediately lead to the creation of psychological theories. In the late nineteenth and early twentieth centuries, British psychiatry lacked a purely psychological paradigm, and so what remained when organic change had been excluded was not automatically referred to the mind. Rather, as older ways of understanding certain illnesses proved barren, and certain kinds of symptoms seemed to manifest more often, doctors reconsidered what they thought they knew. The concept of functional disease gradually stretched to accommodate new ways of thinking about psyche, soma, and their relations. Functional disorders such as hysteria and neurasthenia were gradually redefined to include psychological elements in another manifestation of the same process by which the concept of trauma, originally denoting a cut or wound, was transposed from the physical to the psychological sphere during the late nineteenth century.[24] The category of functional disorder, originally created in the expectation that organic explanations would be found for the symptoms it housed, eased these movements of redefinition and reconceptualization.

Before 1914, no convincing physical explanation could be found for disorders described as functional, but there was no other fully developed mode of understanding illness. Although approaches to hysteria and neurasthenia found a place for the potential "psychic" causes of illness, these cannot be described as fully "psychological" explanations because this implies a way of conceptualizing mind and its disorders which was still embryonic within British psychological medicine. In retrospect, it seems that we can trace a transition to recognizably "modern" understandings of the psyche from around the mid-nineteenth century, and that this movement gathered speed from around 1900. But doctors at the time did not know what would happen next, and they did not see their explanatory options as simply divided into the physical or the psychological. Instead, because British psychological medicine operated within a somatic paradigm, the first point of reference within the concept of functional disorder was the body. The concept of functional disorder was predicated on the notion of an organic non-event, not on the possibility of a psychological event. This non-event, the absence of traceable organic change, operated as the only positive and universal defining feature of

---

[24] M. Micale and P. Lerner, 'Trauma, Psychiatry, and History: A Conceptual and Historiographical Introduction', in M. Micale and P. Lerner (eds.), *Traumatic Pasts: History, Psychiatry, and Trauma in the Modern Age, 1870–1930* (Cambridge: Cambridge University Press, 2001) pp. 1–27; I. Hacking, 'Memory Sciences, Memory Politics', in P. Antze and M. Lambek (eds.), *Tense Past: Cultural Essays in Trauma and Memory* (New York and London: Routledge, 1996), pp. 75–6; M. Neve, 'Public Views of Neurasthenia: Britain, 1880–1930', in Gijswit-Hofstra and Porter (eds.), *Cultures of Neurasthenia*, p. 141.

functional diseases. The body was not merely the first, but the only point of reference within definitions of functional disorder.

This somatic frame of reference is evident in the lists of functional diseases in early twentieth-century textbooks of nervous and mental diseases: these typically featured epilepsy, chorea, tetanus, aphasia, muscular spasm, writers' cramp, facial hemiatrophy, exophthalmic goitre, and various kinds of paralysis.[25] Today, these seem entirely different orders of experience to hysteria and neurasthenia, but their inclusion makes sense against the somatic paradigm of pre-war psychological medicine. Through the category of functional disease, disorders which did not fit the somatic paradigm could be understood via reference to it. This is demonstrated in the work of Joseph Ormerod, who wrote extensively on European theories of hysteria.[26] In order to introduce and make plausible the notion of disruption of psychological function, Ormerod reiterated the physiological meaning of function, explaining that 'by "function" we generally mean a combination of bodily events, so that they work harmoniously together towards some given physiological end ... for the due performance of a function an organisation, comparable to this bodily organisation, must have been made in the mind'.[27] For British medical audiences, psychological concepts became comprehensible only when filtered through the lens of physiological – and thus concrete, knowable, and scientifically palatable – processes.

Another demonstration of the dominance of the somatic paradigm in concepts of functional disorder is the stated allegiance of British commentators to an as-yet undiscovered organic basis for hysteria, the archetypal functional disease. For decades before 1914, most British doctors focused on "psychic" factors in their writings about the causes and symptoms of hysteria. However, they framed this decision as resulting from lack of knowledge about the physical processes involved in the production of hysteria rather than as a positive statement about its psychological basis. In the 1890s, it was still possible to suppose that 'the light of improved knowledge and experience' would reveal the organic origin of many symptoms of hysteria.[28] This optimism faded slightly in subsequent years, but doctors still insisted hysteria was 'as real as smallpox or cancer, and that it has a

---

[25] Nagel, *Nervous and Mental Diseases*, pp. 138–90; Potts, *Nervous and Mental Diseases*, pp. 385–437.

[26] H.D. Rolleston, 'In Memoriam Joseph Arderne Ormerod', *SBHR*, 59 (1926), 3.

[27] J.A. Ormerod, 'The Lumleian Lectures on Some Modern Theories Concerning Hysteria. II', *Lancet*, 2 May 1914, 1238–9; Ormerod, 'Two Theories of Hysteria', 275. See also Brock, 'Habit as a Pathological Factor', 142.

[28] T. Buzzard, 'Simulation of Hysteria by Organic Disease of the Nervous System', in Tuke (ed.), *Dictionary of Psychological Medicine*, vol. 1, p. 1163.

physical basis', and therefore "psychological" theories could prove a useful stopgap measure until this organic foundation was discovered.[29] In fact, when improved diagnostic techniques revealed that some symptoms traditionally associated with hysteria did have an organic basis, a process which began just before 1900 and continued throughout the first few decades of the twentieth century, this caused the contraction of the disorder rather than the provision of a physical explanation for it.[30] But by the time this occurred, alternative ways of understanding non-physical illnesses had developed, and it made more sense to explain hysteria along these lines. This development could not have been foreseen by doctors in the late nineteenth century, although in the years immediately before the war, some had started to acknowledge this possibility, albeit in a halting and inchoate fashion.

So far, this account of functional disorders might suggest that before 1914, British psychological medicine remained stubbornly, even dogmatically, wedded to somatic explanations. But the example of Ormerod's rhetorical strategy hints at an apparently paradoxical fact: the very strength of the somatic paradigm enabled psychological ideas to infiltrate mainstream medical discourse. In the opening decades of the twentieth century, British doctors readily acknowledged that their compatriots had produced 'comparatively little of an authoritative character' on hysteria.[31] In the late nineteenth century, the recognized European experts on hysteria were French physicians, above all Jean-Martin Charcot (1825–93).[32] In the years immediately before the war, accounts of hysteria in the British medical press most often took the form of expositions of Continental theorists such as Joseph Babinski (1857–1932), Pierre Janet (1859–1947), and Sigmund Freud.[33] These theorists had 'to a great extent superseded the doctrines of Charcot, though … none of them has passed into the region of accepted fact'.[34] New theories of

[29] J.P. Stewart, *The Diagnosis of Nervous Diseases* (London: Edward Arnold, 1906), p. 307; S.A.K. Wilson, 'Some Modern French Conceptions of Hysteria', *Brain*, 33:3 (January 1911), 336–7; Ormerod, 'Lumleian Lectures. I', 1169.

[30] M. Micale, 'On the "Disappearance" of Hysteria: A Study in the Clinical Deconstruction of a Diagnosis', *Isis*, 84 (1993), 504–10.

[31] Anon., 'Modern Views of Hysteria', *Lancet*, 8 April 1911, 951.

[32] See for example Tuke (ed.), *Dictionary of Psychological Medicine*, vol. 1, p. 618.

[33] J.S. Fowler, 'Recent Literature: Critical Summaries and Abstracts. Medicine: Modern Theories of Hysteria – Babinski, Janet, and Freud', *EMJ*, 6 (January–June 1911), 443–8; B. Hart, 'Freud's Conception of Hysteria', *Brain*, 33:3 (January 1911), 339–66; Wilson, 'Some Modern French Conceptions of Hysteria'; Anon., 'Freud's Theory of Dreams', *Lancet*, 10 May 1913, 1327; Brown, 'Freud's Theory of Dreams'; T.R. Glynn, 'Abstract of the Bradshaw Lecture on Hysteria in Some of Its Aspects', *Lancet*, 8 November 1913, 1303; Ormerod, 'Lumleian Lectures'.

[34] Anon., 'Freud's Theory of Hysteria and Other Psychoneuroses', *Lancet*, 21 May 1910, 1424.

hysteria were extensively discussed in the British medical press, in many different formats, including reports of papers delivered to regional medical societies, which demonstrate ground-level interest in this research.[35] Although these theories were often rejected, significantly modified, or unwittingly altered in "translation" as British doctors sought to accommodate some of their insights, they contributed to shifting the boundaries of the somatic paradigm.

Most British medical commentators (re-)presented the theories of Babinski, Janet, and Freud via reference to the somatic paradigm, in the process normalizing them. Undoubtedly, this approach resulted partly from the inability to comprehend psychological theorization. One doctor alluded to Babinski during a meeting of the Liverpool Medical Institution, but confessed himself unable to 'fully follow this distinguished French physician'; he probably articulated the secret sentiments of many.[36] However, precisely because they were unable to think far outside the somatic paradigm, some doctors did not reject psychological theories outright. A common policy of sceptical engagement can be seen in discussions of Freud. The British medical establishment was not, as is sometimes alleged, uniformly hostile to Freud before the First World War.[37] Despite some famous examples of antagonistic responses, such as the silent exodus of the entire audience from a psychoanalytic paper presented by Montague David Eder (1865–1936), many members of the medical community were extremely interested in Freud's theories, if not entirely convinced by them.[38] In the pre-war medical press, Freud was most often viewed as one of many thinkers who had contributed to the study of hysteria. Like these others, his theories did not have to be swallowed whole.[39] For

---

[35] Anon., 'Medical Societies: Liverpool Medical Institution', *Lancet*, 9 April 1910, 1001–2; Anon., 'Medical Societies: Nottingham Medico-Chirurgical Society'; Anon., 'Sheffield Medico-Chirurgical Society: Some Recent Conceptions of Hysteria', *Lancet*, 12 April 1913, 1024–5.

[36] Anon., 'Medical Societies: Liverpool Medical Institution', 1001.

[37] Stone, 'Shellshock and the Psychologists', p. 243; E. Showalter, *The Female Malady: Women, Madness and English Culture, 1830–1980* (London: Virago, 1987), p. 189. For an alternative view, see S. Raitt, 'Early British Psychoanalysis and the Medico-Psychological Clinic', *History Workshop Journal*, 58 (Autumn 2004), 67–8, 77.

[38] See E. Glover, 'Eder as Psycho-Analyst', in J.B. Hobman (ed.), *David Eder: Memoirs of a Modern Pioneer* (London: Victor Gollancz, 1945), p. 89. The mixture of support and criticism in responses to a paper on Freudian psychoanalysis given in 1913 more accurately reflects the variety and temper of medical opinion. KCHMSA: KHU/C1/ M8, W. Brown, 'Freud's Theory and Its Uses in Diagnosis' (21 January 1913).

[39] W.H.B. Stoddart, 'The New Psychiatry. II', *EMJ*, 14 (January–June 1915), 343. Graham Richards suggests that the appeal of psychoanalytic doctrine lay 'precisely in the fact that it provided a menu of ideas from which readers could selectively pick and choose while many of its propositions and concepts were open to quite varied interpretations'. Richards, 'Britain on the Couch', 186, 219.

example, Ormerod could not stomach the inductive basis of Freud's theories – 'very unsubstantial, and literally such stuff as dreams are made of' – but he valued some psychoanalytical insights, such as the belief that expression of repressed emotion helped to relieve symptoms.[40]

This magpie approach was typical of British medical authors.[41] They picked and chose apparently useful aspects of particular theories, and in doing so re-inflected and tamed the whole. Perversely, this limited openness to new ideas was only possible because medical allegiance to the somatic paradigm was so strong. As long as doctors believed hysteria had an organic basis not yet discovered, they could view psychological theories simply as expedient adjuncts to this supposed foundation. The outcomes of this process – perhaps more accurately described as welding than assimilation – can seem incongruous to modern readers. In his well-received 1913 textbook, Robert Cole, a specialist in mental diseases, incorporated new psychological theories into his account of hysteria. He referenced Babinski, Janet, and Freud, and initially defined hysteria as 'a disorder of the subconscious mind; it is a peculiar mental state in which the psychical and physical symptoms are largely due to auto-suggestion'. However, only a few pages later, Cole proposed possible physiological explanations: hysteria might be caused by alterations in cortical nutrition or secondary derangement of the lower nerve centres.[42] The prominence of the theory of psycho-physical parallelism, discussed in the previous chapter, meant that this cut-and-paste approach did not seem odd to Cole or his readers.

British doctors normalized Janet's diagnostic creation of psychasthenia in a similar fashion. Janet described psychasthenia as a psychological disorder in which depression, phobias, and obsessions coexisted with somatic symptoms.[43] In pre-war discussions of functional disease, British doctors often listed psychasthenia alongside hysteria and neurasthenia, and even occasionally presented it as a synonym of

[40] Ormerod, 'Two Theories of Hysteria', 286–7; T. Loveday, 'The Role of Repression in Forgetting (IV)', British Journal of Psychology, 7:2 (September 1914), 163.
[41] Raitt, 'Early British Psychoanalysis'. Paul Lerner suggests that responses to psychoanalysis may have followed a similar pattern in Germany, with 'many psychiatrists and neurologists … influenced by certain parts of psychoanalytic theory, while other doctors experimented with forms of psychoanalysis in the clinical environment without subscribing to the entirety of Freudian thought'. Lerner, Hysterical Men, pp. 165, 187–8.
[42] Cole, Mental Diseases [1913], pp. 216–9.
[43] P. Janet, Mental State of Hystericals: A Study of Mental Stigmata and Mental Accidents, trans. C. Corson (New York: G.P. Putnam's Sons, 1901), pp. 519–21; S. Shamdasani, 'Claire, Lise, Jean, Nadia, and Gisèle: Preliminary Notes Towards a Characterization of Pierre Janet's Psychasthenia', in Gijswit-Hofstra and Porter (eds.), Cultures of Neurasthenia, pp. 367–70.

neurasthenia.[44] Some doctors who tried to make sense of neurasthenia by carving up its symptoms for redistribution among other diagnostic categories saw psychasthenia as its psychological counterpart or believed the two syndromes coexisted in the 'shadowy borderlands' of functional disease and could not be entirely separated out.[45] However, Cole and others reconfigured psychasthenia to accommodate a physical basis, such as 'physiological error in the mechanism controlling the emotions', or 'a weakened state of health in a predisposed individual' which disrupted cortical functioning.[46] Janet conceived psychasthenia as a psychological disorder, but British uses of this term did not signal understanding or acceptance of his model of psychological functioning. This adherence to a somatic paradigm indicates the weakness of psychological modes of thought in pre-war British medical discourse, but also hints at processes of change. As diagnostic categories and psychological theories devised outside the British tradition were gradually incorporated within it, the tradition itself mutated. Despite their apparent misappropriation, the gradual incursions of psychological theories opened up new spaces within British psychological medicine.

British doctors did not read the theories of Janet or Freud quite as these authors intended. But the expositions of Cole and other doctors were not just misapprehensions or misappropriations which distorted the "true" nature of these theories. Rather, these apparently inconsistent readings are evidence of a now-alien interpretative strategy pursued by doctors who did not perceive psychological and physiological categories of explanation as irreconcilable. In this respect, they were open-minded about psychological theories, although their flexibility was ultimately limited by adherence to the somatic paradigm. This approach to psychological theories was possible because of the strong empirical tendency of British psychological medicine as well as the working modes of classification (such as 'functional disease') and explanation through which doctors simultaneously admitted and covered for their lack of knowledge. In the European theories they read, doctors sought practical solutions to problems of diagnosis and treatment, and were markedly less bothered about intellectual satisfaction or precision. The frequent substitution of 'subconscious' for 'unconscious' in discussions of Freud shows not only

---

[44] Ormerod, 'Two Theories of Hysteria', 279; E.L. Ash, 'The Combined Psycho-Electrical Treatment of Neurasthenia and Allied Neuroses', *Practitioner*, 91:1 (July 1913), 123.

[45] H. Macnaughton-Jones, 'The Relation of Puberty and the Menopause to Neurasthenia', *Lancet*, 29 March 1913, 879; Anon., 'Medical Societies: Nottingham Medico-Chirurgical Society', 1338.

[46] H. Thursfield, 'Review of Children's Diseases', *Practitioner*, 87:1 (July 1911), 118–19; Cole, *Mental Diseases* [1913], p. 225.

that the former concept was comprehended and accepted while the latter was not, but also that British commentators afforded the difference little weight in comparison with those aspects of Freud's theories they believed to be useful.[47] The consequence of such recastings was the piecemeal incursion of psychological theories into the somatic framework of understanding. The groundwork had been laid for the acceptance of psychological paradigms before "shell-shock" burst onto the psychiatric scene.

The Symptom, the Illness, and the Patient

These gradual shifts within the category of functional disease demonstrate that even before the war, a space for psychological theorization had opened up within the somatic paradigm of British psychological medicine. However, this period was marked by another trend which might seem to tug against increased openness to psychological thought: the entrenchment of biological modes of explanation. These approaches were not as contradictory as they first seem. An avowedly anti-theoretical stance enabled British doctors to sceptically engage with psychological theories, and to cut and paste elements of these theories into a somatic framework regardless of apparent logical inconsistencies, but also led them to focus on the patient rather than the disease.[48] This meant that doctors could acknowledge "psychic" components of illness, and even recommend treatments targeting these symptoms, but still insist the original fault lay in the body rather than the psyche. Moreover, although British doctors took pride in contrasting their own native tradition of empiricism with European colleagues' airy-fairy tendency to abstract thought, this hid their own enthralment to Darwinian evolutionism, among the greatest unprovable theories of all time.

This combination of factors led British doctors to shelve theoretical questions in favour of empirical accounts, but to base their discussions on premises derived from the evolutionary framework of understanding; to focus on manifestations of illness within particular patients rather than the nature of illnesses as abstract entities, but to understand illness as an indicator of individual and social failure; and to allow physical and "psychological" elements of thought to sit uneasily next to each other in their own accounts, with no acknowledgement of contradictions, while

---

[47] H.C. Thomson, 'Mental Therapeutics in Neurasthenia', *Practitioner*, 86:1 (January 1911), 77–9; Anon., 'Modern Views of Hysteria', 951.

[48] As Suzanne Raitt states, 'many doctors saw psychoanalysis more as a set of techniques than as a philosophy of mind, and ... for this reason it was easily incorporated into sessions with patients in which hypnotic or waking suggestion or "re-education" were also being freely used'. Raitt, 'Early British Psychoanalysis', 78.

pointing out all the apparent flaws in the logic and evidence of European theorists. This approach led doctors to view hysteria and neurasthenia as qualities of particular kinds of people rather than as distinct illnesses. It is no coincidence that etymologically, the hysterical and the hysteric precede hysteria. The English adjective "hysterical" dates from 1615; "hysteric" was used to describe a person prone to certain symptoms from 1657; but the first known use of the English noun "hysteria" was not until 1801.[49] It almost seems that hysteria was a disease incidental to hysterics rather than the necessary precondition of describing someone as hysterical. The association between neurasthenia and specific character traits was not quite as strong, but doctors did make similar judgements about the personalities of sufferers. One physician even suggested that doctors 'had frequently to deal with a neurasthenic temperament – not really a disease'.[50] Hysteria and neurasthenia were such large and ill-defined categories that, in the absence of an identifiable pathology, only the concept of the neurotic temperament or personality held each together as a discrete clinical entity.

The symptoms of hysteria and neurasthenia were described almost as mere extrusions of the individual personality. Hysterics were unstable, excitable, emotional, weak-willed, suggestible, and 'egoistic'.[51] Neurasthenics were hypochondriac, self-obsessed, 'exacting in their demands', and 'apt to be irritable, aggressive and quarrelsome'.[52] Indeed, doctors asserted, there were clear similarities between hysterics, neurasthenics, the insane, and malingerers.[53] In these unsympathetic portrayals, patients were seen as partially responsible for the production of illness, whether the "psychic" symptoms of hysteria or the nervous exhaustion of neurasthenia. In both cases, culpability was linked to faulty operation of the will. The neurasthenic patient's exhaustion left him 'unduly facile in response to all extraneous influences', and therefore unable to make reasoned judgements. As a result, he suffered from phobias, suggestibility, hypersensitivity, and emotional disturbances.[54]

[49] H. King, 'Once Upon a Text: Hysteria from Hippocrates', in S. Gilman et al., Hysteria Beyond Freud (Berkeley, Los Angeles, and London: University of California Press), pp. 73–4.
[50] Anon., 'Medical Societies: Medical Society of London', Lancet, 22 and 29 November 1913, 1469.
[51] Stoddart, Mind and Its Disorders [1908], pp. 370–3.
[52] Ibid., p. 363; G. Ward, 'A Few Consecutive Cases from General Practice', King's College Hospital Gazette, 4 (1925), 165.
[53] Ritchie, 'Neurasthenia', 117.
[54] Anon., 'Medical Societies: Medical Society of London', 1543; Anon., 'Review: La Neurasthénie Rurale by Dr Raymond Belbèze', Lancet, 30 September 1911, 351; A.J. Brock, '"Ergotherapy" in Neurasthenia', EMJ, 6 (January–June 1911), 430–4; A.F. Tredgold, 'Neurasthenia and Insanity', Practitioner, 86:1 (January 1911), 86; Potts, Nervous and Mental Diseases, p. 410.

Hysterics shared some of these "symptoms": two of the defining features of the hysteric personality were emotionality and suggestibility (understood as credulous susceptibility to suggestions regardless of reason).[55] In hysteria and neurasthenia, loss of the directing and controlling power of will resulted in excess of emotion and consequent diminution of reasoned thought, leaving the mind open to suggestion. The character traits of hysterics and neurasthenics therefore deviated from those of the ideal "civilized" European adult.

This view of regressive loss of will was far more prominent in descriptions of hysteria than in accounts of neurasthenia.[56] Although hysteria was sometimes portrayed as consisting of an excess of will (wilfulness), this was pathological and quite different from the reasoned self-control of the "civilized" adult. The will of the hysteric was depicted as utterly inflexible, immovable, and beyond the conscious control of the patient – and therefore not the self-directed will of the rational and free agent. This power of will existed outside the control of the subject, and so to all intents and purposes, the hysteric had no will to call her own. A standard announcement was, 'It is not that the patient will not, but that she cannot will'.[57] This absence of will excused the hysteric of the charge of malingering. She was described as 'an actress [who] does not know that she is acting'; if a supposedly paralysed limb stirred in sleep, the 'movements are volitional only in appearance ... the conscious ego does not participate therein'.[58] This dubious pardon denied the hysteric an existential reality beyond her disease and negated her identity by confounding it with that of her parasite. Indeed, Théodule Ribot insisted that the will had never 'constituted itself' in hysterics, whose 'constitutional impotency of the will' kept them in a permanent state of 'disequilibriation and ... moral ataxy'.[59]

Abnormal willpower and emotionalism defined the hysterical personality and were preconditions as well as consequences of hysteria. In his exposition of Janet's theory, Joseph Ormerod underlined the symbiosis of emotion and will in hysteria. Ormerod explained that restriction of the field of personal consciousness prevented certain memories from being integrated with the hysteric's perceptions of the present, and led to the development of a 'secondary consciousness'. The hysteric was both

[55] Stewart, *Diagnosis of Nervous Diseases*, p. 308; Stoddart, *Mind and Its Disorders* [1908], p. 368.
[56] Nagel, *Nervous and Mental Diseases*, p. 166; Cole, *Mental Diseases* [1913], p. 218; Cobb, 'Neurasthenia', 227; Stoddart, *Mind and Its Disorders* [1908], p. 378.
[57] Ormerod, 'Lumleian Lectures. II', 1236.
[58] Wilson, 'Some Modern French Conceptions of Hysteria', 314, 329.
[59] Ribot, 'Will, Disorders of', p. 1368.

stunted and freed by this relationship to the past, 'at once less checked and governed by past experiences than a normal person'. She was unable to take a 'comprehensive view of facts and motives', and therefore 'reasoned volition becomes replaced by impulsiveness, and she is said to suffer from weakness of will'. Consequently emotion not only *caused* the pathological condition of hysteria, but also manifested pathologically *within* the disease. The hysterical patient was 'not emotional, in the sense of readily responding with conscious emotion to the circumstances of the present'. Rather the 'emotions she exhibits are really old ones, relating to circumstances of the past, which have become automatic – old tune [sic], played in her subconscious mind, as if on a barrel organ'.[60] This description configured the emotion present in hysteria as doubly lower: the hysteric existed in a state of pure emotion (in that for medicine, her disease was her self) which was yet beyond emotion. Her symptoms were recrudescences of emotion, the frozen yet mutant remnants of a self both past and present, simultaneously dissociated from the self which had continued to develop and a barrier to normal, healthy growth. Just as the insane in asylums were throwbacks to a past stage of evolution, the hysteric personality was a living survival of a past stage in the patient's own mental evolution.

The existence of hysteria or neurasthenia was perceived to demonstrate mental and moral regression, and as will be seen, these judgements carried over into the diagnosis of "shell-shock". The lack of will of suggestible adults marked them out as fundamentally flawed. Commentators argued that suggestibility existed in 'inverse proportion to ... sanity and strength of will'.[61] Hugh Crichton-Miller (who hyphenated his surname from the 1920s), defined hysteria as 'the disease of inadequate inhibition, particularly characterized by pose and suggestibility' and listed a host of negative attributes which resulted from this lack of inhibition: sexual abnormalities, unreasonable emotional fits, poor concentration, and 'mental attainments chiefly along artistic lines' (!)[62] Arthur Brock (1879–1947), a general practitioner from Edinburgh, compared the neurasthenic to a 'backward infant', easily demoralized by failure, who responded to obstacles with attempts at evasion. In Brock's view, neurasthenics were weak-willed because they did not exercise effort and shrank from life's struggles rather than facing them head-on.[63] While children were naturally suggestible because they had not fully developed

---

[60] Ormerod, 'Two Theories of Hysteria', 272–3.
[61] Wilson, 'Some Modern French Conceptions of Hysteria', 323; H. Bernheim, 'Suggestion and Hypnotism', in Tuke (ed.), *Dictionary of Psychological Medicine*, vol. 2, pp. 1213–14.
[62] H. Crichton-Miller, 'Rest-Cures in Theory and Practice', *Practitioner*, 89 (July–December 1912), 836.

powers of reason or self-control, adults who displayed this quality of mind must be suffering from some pathological condition such as hysteria, neurasthenia, alcoholism, or general paralysis.[64] Within the dominant explanatory frameworks of British psychological medicine, it was not possible to be simultaneously weak-willed and "normal".

The perception of hysterics and neurasthenics as suggestible and mentally weak led to disagreements over the suitability of suggestion (including suggestion by hypnosis) as a cure for these disorders. In pre-war psychological medicine, suggestion was often understood quite broadly as the power to positively influence the patient rather than as a specific psychotherapeutic technique. It was defined as 'the setting up or prompting an idea which by constant reinforcement is turned into a dominant one leading to action in its own direction'.[65] Before 1914, doctors debated the proper uses of suggestion; these disputes were replayed when physicians began to experiment with suggestive techniques in the treatment of "shell-shock". Some physicians believed that the suggestibility of hysteric and neurasthenic patients made them ideal candidates for this form of treatment.[66] Others objected to the technique for exactly the same reason: using suggestion on already suggestible patients would only aggravate this undesirable condition. Instead, doctors should aim to strengthen the patient's self-control through positive measures and thereby equip him to cure himself.[67] British doctors rarely referred to this technique as "persuasion", but it closely followed the lines of treatment developed under this name by Swiss neurologists Paul Charles Dubois (1848–1918) and Joseph Jules Déjerine (1849–1917). The reformulations of British doctors emphasized the need to strengthen the will and to morally cleanse the patient. David Ferrier (1843–1928), a specialist in physiology and neuropathology, described the ideal treatment for neurasthenia as 'the cultivation of

[63] Brock, '"Ergotherapy" in Neurasthenia', 430–4; Brock, 'Habit as a Pathological Factor', 138.
[64] Wilson, 'Some Modern French Conceptions of Hysteria', 307–9, 316, 323–5.
[65] T. C. Shaw, 'Considerations on the Occult', *BMJ*, 18 June 1910, 1476. William McDougall provided another definition: 'Suggestion is a process of communication resulting in the acceptance with conviction of the communicated proposition in the absence of logically adequate grounds for its acceptance'. W. McDougall, *An Introduction to Social Psychology* (Bristol and Tokyo: Thoemmes Press and Maruzen, 1998) [1908], p. 97.
[66] G. Holmes, 'The Sexual Element in the Neurasthenia of Men', *Practitioner*, 86:1 (January 1911), 59; C.F. Fothergill, 'The Treatment of Neurasthenia', *Practitioner*, 92 (January–June 1914), 725; Thomson, 'Mental Therapeutics in Neurasthenia', 82; Russell, 'Treatment of Neurasthenia', 1454.
[67] Stewart, *Diagnosis of Nervous Diseases*, p. 309; Crichton-Miller, 'Rest-Cures in Theory and Practice', 843; Ross, 'Nature and Treatment of Neurasthenia', 306–7.

stoicism, self-control, and a reasoned disregard of the symptoms to which he has been attaching so much and such unnecessary importance'.[68] As with the rest cure, the ideal treatment for hysteria and neurasthenia should deal with the whole patient rather than the illness.

Race, Nation, and Politics: Hysteria, Neurasthenia, and the Neurotic Temperament

Views of hysteria and neurasthenia as character flaws resulting from failure of the will demonstrate the influence of evolutionary modes of understanding. Within the evolutionary framework, all nervous and mental disorders were conceived as forms of regression because they involved the loss of will, the most distinctively human faculty of mind. Medical constructions of such disorders were saturated with assumptions about the evolutionary value of certain behaviours, and therefore also with judgements about race, class, and gender. Heredity and race loomed large in doctors' lists of predisposing and exciting causes of hysteria and neurasthenia. Almost all agreed on 'neuropathic tendency', 'inheritance', or 'taint' as an underlying predisposing cause of hysteria and neurasthenia. This 'taint' was usually defined as the existence of some neurosis or neurotic disease in the family.[69] Through the aspect of heredity, which emphasized a dialogue between the body and the environment conceived in various ways (the environment of the individual body, of the family, of the race, and of the nation), medical constructs of hysteria and neurasthenia took on social and political dimensions.

The identification of heredity as the most important factor in the development of hysteria and neurasthenia meant that the *ultimate* cause of the disorder lay in the individual rather than in the social environment. The emphasis on heredity neutralized the significance of specific exciting causes. Doctors stated that a specific, external stimulus was always necessary for the *actual* development of hysteria or neurasthenia. However, once the disorder had developed, it was portrayed as a pre-existing potential of the individual which had merely been latent until the right circumstances for its expression arose. The apparent and immediate cause was always at most only 'a coefficient, and often merely serves as the spark which falls into the explosive matter'.[70] In practice, once the

[68] D. Ferrier, 'Neurasthenia and Drugs', *Practitioner*, 86:1 (January 1911), 14; Brock, '"Ergotherapy" in Neurasthenia', 434.

[69] Nagel, *Nervous and Mental Diseases*, pp. 163, 171; Potts, *Nervous and Mental Diseases*, pp. 414–5; Clarke, *Hysteria and Neurasthenia*, pp. 5–11, 176; Stoddart, *Mind and Its Disorders* [1908], pp. 362, 368.

[70] F.W. Mott, 'Preface', *Archives of Neurology*, 3 (1907), iii–iv.

disorder was diagnosed, doctors saw the specific stimulus as of secondary importance only. They did not see the social environment as completely insignificant, but conceived of its importance mainly in terms of possible modifications to prevent the manifestation of nervous disorder rather than as a way to permanently effect change in the nervous individual. The nervous child was 'born not made', even though some further spur was required to turn such a child into a fully fledged hysteric or neurasthenic.[71]

Biological determinism became more entrenched in the years immediately before the war. This is demonstrated by changing uses of analogies to plant life, a recurrent motif in discussions of nervous disorders. In 1892, one contributor to Daniel Hack Tuke's *Dictionary of Psychological Medicine* described neurasthenia as 'to a certain degree the starting-point of all the more severe nervous disorders, and the soil from which they grow'.[72] Another, the obstetrician and gynaecologist William Playfair (1835–1903), argued that the 'rank weeds of neurotic disease will only grow and flourish in suitable soil – that is, in a state of depressed vitality; improve the soil, and the unhealthy growth will disappear'.[73] This was an essentially positive outlook: the 'bad soil' of nervous exhaustion fostered neurotic disorders, but if the right measures were taken, more serious disorders could be prevented. Nervous exhaustion was an illness which affected the individual, not a pathology which defined her. Only a few years later, the metaphor was used quite differently to describe how 'the seeds' of neuroses were 'sown by stupid or ignorant parents or nurses through want of recognition of the signs of the nervous predisposition and temperament of the child'.[74] Here, the ultimate cause of the neurosis was the child's 'nervous predisposition and temperament'; the social environment was no more than a factor which allowed and encouraged the disorder to develop. Like original sin, this illness was embodied rather than contracted, and the aim was not to cure, but only to prevent the manifestation of its worst potentialities.

The key term in these descriptions is 'temperament'. In pre-war British medical discourse, temperament was often conceived as biological destiny rather than mere personality trait. Robert Jones (later Armstrong-Jones), superintendent of Claybury Asylum, stated that in the individual, temperament was determined by nation and race, and it therefore

---

[71] C. Riviere, 'Neurasthenia in Children', *Practitioner*, 86:1 (January 1911), 38.

[72] Arndt, 'Neurasthenia', 840, 842.

[73] W.S. Playfair, 'Neuroses, Functional, the Systematic Treatment of (So-called Weir Mitchell Treatment)', in Tuke (ed.), *Dictionary of Psychological Medicine*, vol. 2, p. 853.

[74] H. Macnaughton-Jones, 'The Sexual Element in the Neurasthenia of Women', *Practitioner*, 86:1 (January 1911), 69; Clarke, *Hysteria and Neurasthenia*, p. 7.

differed according to the level of evolutionary development.[75] His colleague, the neuro-pathologist Frederick Mott (1853–1926), put forward
a similar definition of the 'neuropathic temperament' as an inborn tendency determined by biological inheritance.[76] This concept of the neurotic temperament was deeply entrenched in medical accounts of hysteria
and neurasthenia and dovetailed with older conceptions of the hysteric or
neurasthenic character. The construction of the neurotic temperament as
a biologically determined quality meant that the actual appearance of
hysteria or neurasthenia was merely the final stage of a preordained
process, the disease itself simply a confirmation of a pathological identity
embedded so deep within that no autopsy or microscope would ever
uncover it. At the core of these amorphous diagnostic categories, what
was left when all the extraneous symptoms and abstruse jargon had been
removed, was the neurotic temperament. This was the internal environment on which the outside world acted either to stunt or develop, but
never to *cause*, the neurosis. The concept of the neurotic temperament
proved the difference between the neurosis as an essential manifestation
of self or as an attack from without, an invading agent which altered the
self. This difference is essential to understanding perceptions of the
threat hysteria and neurasthenia posed to "modern civilization", and
which "modern civilization" posed to the stability and right functioning
of the human body and mind. It is also essential to understanding what
was at stake in medical theories of "shell-shock" as a disorder predominantly afflicting those susceptible through existing biological or "psychological" weakness. This issue recurs in later chapters.

In the early years of the twentieth century, medical commentators
often argued that as 'the general level of culture and civilization in a race'
rose, so did the incidence of nervous disorders.[77] The sights, sounds, and
pace of modern life shook an exquisitely sensitive human nervous system
that had been fine-tuned over millennia of evolution. In Britain and
Europe, these fears were inextricably bound up with theories of biological
degeneration.[78] The rise of eugenics, particularly from the turn of

[75] [Armstrong-]Jones, 'Address on Temperaments', 1–2.
[76] F.W. Mott, *Nature and Nurture in Mental Development* (London: John Murray, 1914), pp. 68–71; Russell, 'Treatment of Neurasthenia', 1453–4.
[77] Anon., 'The Increase of Nervous Instability', *Lancet*, 2 December 1911, 1572.
[78] R.A. Fleming, 'Neurasthenia and Gastralgia', *Practitioner*, 86:1 (January 1911), 32–3; Tredgold, 'Neurasthenia and Insanity', 95; G.F. Drinka, *The Birth of Neurosis: Myth, Malady and the Victorians* (New York: Simon and Schuster, 1984), pp. 213–4; M. Micale, *Approaching Hysteria: Disease and Its Interpretations* (Princeton, NJ: Princeton University Press, 1995), pp. 205–20; R. Nye, 'Degeneration, Neurasthenia and the Culture of Sport in *Belle Époque* France', *Journal of Contemporary History*, 17 (1982), 51–68.

century, encouraged the view that nervous disorders such as hysteria and neurasthenia signalled the beginning of biological, and therefore social, political, and imperial decline.[79] Because hysteria and neurasthenia were thought to be biologically determined, they were increasingly seen as social dangers. If nervous disorders were both 'a special outcome of modern civilization' and 'the starting-point of an unstable nervous condition in a stock' bound to intensify under the continued influence of an unfavourable environment, then Britain was in trouble.[80] Fears of latent nervous and mental instability were apparent even in accounts which attempted to strike a more optimistic note. The eminent psychiatrist Sir George Savage (1841–1921) warned against believing too much in 'the tyranny of the organism', arguing that the right conditions were necessary for the development of insanity. To make this point, he compared heredity to 'the mycelium of the mushroom', which 'spreads far and wide and is not recognized till suitable conditions lead to what we call the mushroom which comes to the surface'. His audience probably took little comfort from his conclusion that similarly, 'the neurotic inheritance spreads far and wide and is deeply seated, but the occasion for its development may be wanting': after all, if this were true, what would happen in a national crisis?[81]

Hysteria and neurasthenia were framed as indicators of national and political health. A 1910 comment piece in the *Lancet* took issue with the French neurologist Déjerine's contention that the most important factor in the development of hysteria was emotional shock. The British author argued that as individuals and in the aggregate, the Latin races were less emotionally stable than the Teutonic, using this "fact" to explain the prevalence of both hysteria and social upheavals in France. It was well known that the Parisian mob became 'inflamed by any passing wind of emotion', while such events were uncommon in England. These dissimilarities could only be explained as the result of 'national and racial differences'. As a nation, the English were 'less emotional, less exuberant, less gesticulative': in short, less hysterical.[82] The physician and neurologist Samuel Kinnier Wilson (1874–1937) put forward a similar argument, pointing to the moment in the Sino-French War (1883–5) when 'the telegraphic announcement of an insignificant reverse at Langson [sic]

[79] G. Searle, *Eugenics and Politics in Britain, 1900–1914* (Leyden: Noordhoff, 1976); D. Pick, *Faces of Degeneration: A European Disorder, c. 1848–c. 1918* (Cambridge: Cambridge University Press, 1989), pp. 189–203.

[80] F.W. Mott, 'Is Insanity on the Increase?', *Sociological Review*, 6:1 (January 1913), 26–8.

[81] Savage, 'An Address on Mental Disorders', 1136.

[82] Anon., 'Emotion as a Factor in the Development of Neuropathic and Psychopathic Symptoms', *Lancet*, 20 August 1910, 572.

provoked a fury in Paris and France, and brought about the instantaneous overthrow of the Government', whereas 'a much more serious reverse undergone by our English expedition to Khartoum produced only a slight emotion, and no ministry was overturned'.[83] Here hysteria moved from individual to social and political pathology and was constructed as a fundamentally un-English disorder. As might be expected from such statements, hysteria was deemed to be more prevalent among Jews as well as the Latin races; the former were also seen as more liable to neurasthenia.[84] By association, English neurotics were not part of the nation, but aligned with the threatening forces clustered on its borders, awaiting their chance to attack or, worse, silently infiltrate the body politic.

It is therefore no coincidence that on the eve of the war, dialogues between medicine and politics featured hysteria and neurasthenia, both as actual diagnoses and as linguistic tropes. Historians usually locate three main sources of disruption to British political life in 1914: the threat posed to industrial productivity by trade union activity, the militant suffrage campaign, and the crisis around Home Rule for Ireland.[85] As regards the first of these, the relationship between medicine, the state, and the labour force was still being recalculated in the wake of the Workmen's Compensation Acts (1897, 1900, and 1906). One of the most vexed aspects of these debates, in which hysteria and neurasthenia were clearly implicated, was the issue of compensation for traumatic neurosis.[86] The militant suffragettes, meanwhile, were stigmatized as hysterical for their 'unwomanly' violence to private property and, by extension, the state.[87] Although the Celtic races were usually seen as

---

[83] Wilson, 'Some Modern French Conceptions of Hysteria', 322.

[84] Clarke, *Hysteria and Neurasthenia*, pp. 4–5; Stewart, *Diagnosis of Nervous Diseases*, p. 308; Oldfield, 'Some Pelvic Disorders', 335. Among the cases of functional neuroses treated at King's College Hospital in 1900, it was noted that among those for whom 'no definite cause' could be found, '1 was of French and another of Jewish extraction'. R.M. Leslie, 'Medical Report for the Year 1901', *KCHR*, 8 (1901), 97.

[85] D. Read, *The Age of Urban Democracy: England 1868–1914*, rev. edn (Essex: Longman, 1994), pp. 483–97; Hynes, *War Imagined*, pp. 6–7; Herringham, *Physician in France*, pp. 20–4.

[86] F.S. Palmer, 'Traumatic Neuroses and Psychoses', *Practitioner*, 86 (1911), 808–20; W. Thorburn, 'Presidential Address: The Traumatic Neuroses', Neurological Section, *Proceedings of the Royal Society of Medicine (PRSM)*, 7:2 (1913), 1–14; J.W.G. Grant, 'The Traumatic Neuroses – Some Points in Their Aetiology, Diagnosis, and Medico-Legal Aspects', *Practitioner*, 93 (1914), 26–43; K. Figlio, 'How Does Illness Mediate Social Relations? Workmen's Compensation and Medico-Legal Practices, 1890–1940', in P. Wright and A. Treacher (eds.), *The Problem of Medical Knowledge: Examining the Social Construction of Medicine* (Edinburgh: Edinburgh University Press, 1982), pp. 192–6.

[87] A. Wright, *The Unexpurgated Case against Woman Suffrage* (New York: Paul Hoeber, 1913), pp. 166–88; Shaw, 'Lecture on the Mental Processes in Sanity and Insanity', 214.

more liable to hysteria and neurasthenia, such labels were not applied to figures in the debates on the Irish Question.[88] However, when seeking to explain the mechanism of hysterical dissociation in early 1914, Ormerod plucked a prescient metaphor from political life: in the hysterical mind, he wrote, the 'central government is weak, and there results a turbulent home rule all round'.[89]

Conclusion

Diagnostic categories were not only pragmatic modes of organizing knowledge, but also alive with social, political, and cultural dimensions relevant outside the medical world. Because we know what happened next, it is tempting to "tidy up" past medical theories and fit them into our own explanatory categories. This blinds us to the fact that if we cannot make sense of earlier theories, it is because doctors understood these illnesses in ways alien to us. We do not need to "tidy up", but rather to recognize strangeness and understand the purposes which messiness served. Before 1914, British psychological medicine was in a state of flux. The psychological and somatic elements of functional disorders such as hysteria and neurasthenia were in continual interplay, extension, and retreat. There was little agreement on the ultimate causes of these disorders, but doctors acknowledged the presence of somatic and "psychic" elements within these diagnostic categories. Doctors remained formally committed to somatic explanations of nervous and mental disorders and were often sceptical about the value of European psychological theories. Their inability to find an organic basis for functional disorders led British doctors to focus on symptoms, patients, and the immediate problems of cure. The practical bent of the British medical tradition therefore left doctors open, often in contradictory and complex ways, to the influence of psychological theorization. Although European theories were often both unwittingly transformed and quite consciously chopped up into digestible chunks in their "translation" into the native idiom, engagement with these ideas also stretched and altered the somatic paradigm. Contradictions and tensions in the diagnosis of "shell-shock" were therefore partly a product of new questions opened up by the war, but also replicated and deepened the instability inherent in existing understandings of nervous and mental disorders.

---

[88] Clarke, *Hysteria and Neurasthenia*, pp. 4–5, 175.
[89] Ormerod, 'Lumleian Lectures. II', 1236.

Doctors who treated "shell-shock" fell back on old knowledges and fitted the awful novelties of war into existing frameworks of understanding as best they could. The uncertainties of pre-war understandings of nervous and mental disorders carried over into wartime, and the limitations of pre-war knowledge of hysteria and neurasthenia shaped early approaches to "shell-shock". Although the war wrought many changes, because doctors used older diagnostic classifications to make sense of "shell-shock", the ambiguities, contradictions, and blind spots within these categories carried over into their pronouncements on the sufferings of soldiers. Doctors disagreed on whether an event of such horrific magnitude as the war could be the sole cause of breakdown or whether it merely acted as the stimulus which precipitated breakdown and revealed latent weakness. The evolutionary framework of pre-war psychological medicine shaped concepts of hysteria and neurasthenia as it did other diagnoses, and its influence extended into wartime medical discourse. Questions concerning the nature of human identity and civilization were worked out through disorders such as hysteria and neurasthenia before 1914 and continued to be debated through the prism of "shell-shock" during the war. Because hysteria and neurasthenia were viewed as the product of biological "taint", both were related to prevalent sociopolitical concerns and were thus highly charged categories on the eve of the war. The pathology of the neuroses was always social. Before 1914, medical discourse implied that neurotic Britons were not just ill or bad, but unpatriotic. They were enemy aliens at the most basic biological level, latent lesions on the body of the nation which might erupt and threaten the health of the whole at the first serious crisis. This crisis came with the First World War, when doctors were forced to negotiate and reassess a prior set of values and meanings attached to illnesses such as hysteria and neurasthenia in order to make sense of the war neuroses.

3 Body and Mind in "Shell-Shock"
War and Change within Psychological Medicine

As the war went on, doctors reflected on the status of knowledge about "shell-shock", and constructed narratives about the progress of medical understanding of the disorder. These narratives were articulated in the neutral language of science, and presented as fact rather than interpretation. In July 1918, the anthropologist-neurologist-psychologist W.H.R. Rivers put forward his view:

> In the early days of the war the medical profession, in accordance with the materialistic outlook it had inherited from the latter part of the nineteenth century, was inclined to emphasise the physical aspect of the antecedents of a war neurosis. As the war has progressed the physical conception has given way before one which regards the shell explosion or other catastrophe of warfare as, in the vast majority of cases, merely the spark which has released long pent up forces of a psychical kind.[1]

In this simple and authoritative statement, Rivers presented "what happened" as established fact, as uncontroversial as the acknowledgement that Britain declared war on Germany on 4 August 1914. This kind of deceptively "objective" statement hides the subject position of the author and implicitly refuses the possibility of disagreement. Rivers' own stance on the war neuroses, the elaboration of a modified psychoanalytic theory and therapy, was both highly individual and related to the "analytic" school associated with Maghull Military Hospital.[2] The account which opens this chapter is taken from his preface to the Canadian psychologist John T. MacCurdy's *War Neuroses* (1918), the most directly Freudian explanation of "shell-shock" published in wartime. Rivers' interpretation of wartime developments does not represent majority medical opinion.

In fact, there was no medical consensus on the physical or psychological origins of "shell-shock": not at the outset of the war, not in 1918,

[1] W.H.R. Rivers, 'Preface', in J.T. MacCurdy, *War Neuroses* (Cambridge: Cambridge University Press, 1918), p. vi.
[2] The "analytic" school is discussed in depth in Chapter 5.

and not for some decades afterwards. Narratives of linear transition from physical to psychological understandings of the war neuroses are not supported by the evidence of wartime medical discourse on "shell-shock", despite the central place of this claim in most histories of the disorder, and in arguments that the war caused a fundamental reorientation of medical approaches to mental illness.[3] This chapter explores physical theories of causation in medical explanations of "shell-shock" and assesses the extent of transition to psychological modes of understanding during the war. Undoubtedly, the experience of "shell-shock" complicated medical views of psychological processes, mind–body relations, and the interaction of heredity and environment in nervous and mental disorders. However, physical theories of causation did not dominate early medical approaches to "shell-shock". Initial interpretations emphasized the diversity of potential physical and psychological causes of the disorder, as well as the interaction of body and mind in the production, maintenance and treatment of symptoms. When we remember that many "shell-shock" doctors were not specialists in mind, nerves, and brain, this lack of clearly formulated preliminary causal explanations is unsurprising. Although the war did cause an important shift in medical opinion, this was not the transition from physical to psychological modes of understanding. Rather, it was the emergence of distinctly articulated forms of physical and psychological explanations out of the useful chaos of the diagnostic strategies of pre-war psychological medicine.

The crucial effect of the war was to make manifest the latent potential for fully psychological modes of understanding within categories such as functional disorder. One order of conceptualization did not *replace* another. The coherent articulation of physical and psychological modes of understanding developed out of older, more equivocal approaches and bore the hallmarks of this tradition, not least in the continued importance of heredity (as individual or racial inheritance) across the spectrum of medical opinion. Newer explanations coexisted with older forms of understanding. As demonstrated by the most popular methods of treatment for "shell-shock", there was no binary division between physical and psychological modes of explanation in wartime psychological medicine. Therapeutic conservatism remained common, and even treatments which directly targeted the mind usually demonstrated naïve conceptions of psychology. The absence of physical explanations of "shell-shock" did not mean the presence of sophisticated forms of psychological thought.

---

[3] See my earlier discussion on historiographical constructions of the war as a catalyst for the adoption of psychodynamic approaches in Loughran, 'Shell-Shock and Psychological Medicine'.

Indeed, the publication of more complex psychological theories by a handful of doctors sparked a minor backlash against psychodynamic approaches. This demonstrates the practical benefits, even as it reveals the limitations, of the ambiguous accommodations common within pre-war psychological medicine. Furthermore, the differentiation of physical and psychological modes of explanation heralded another important shift, which at least partially countered tendencies towards greater understanding of psychological pain: the displacement of responsibility for "shell-shock" from the war onto the individual soldier. When doctors emphasized the importance of hereditary weakness *or* earlier psychological maladaptation in the production of "shell-shock", they implicitly denied that breakdown was most often a legitimate and understandable response to the war itself.

Early Medical Responses to the Nervous and Mental Disorders of War, 1914–1916

In November 1914 the earliest reports of cases of 'nervous and mental shock' among soldiers appeared in the British medical press. These reports did not mention the physical effects of bursting shells but explained soldiers' symptoms as the result of 'exposure and the severe strain and tension of the fighting line' or 'the depressing effect of the horrible sights and sounds of modern battlefields'. The authors also described some cases as 'traumatic hysteria'.[4] Over the next few months, doctors noted similarities between the symptoms of war shock and those found in victims of industrial and railway accidents.[5] The nervous and mental disorders of war were immediately assimilated into the diagnostic categories of pre-war psychological medicine. At the same time, doctors struggled to understand how the war environment contributed to the production of symptoms in soldiers. In the first eighteen months of the war, the interplay of pre-war modes of explanation with attempts to comprehend the effects of battle on soldiers shaped medical responses to "shell-shock". This approach militated against the ascription of purely physical aetiologies to the disorder. The pre-war diagnostic categories

---

[4] Anon., 'Mental and Nervous Shock among the Wounded', *BMJ*, 7 November 1914, 802; Anon., 'French Wounded from Some Early Actions', *BMJ*, 14 November 1914, 854.

[5] T.R. Elliott, 'Transient Paraplegia from Shell Explosions', *BMJ*, 12 December 1914, 1005; Anon., 'The War and Nervous Breakdown', *Lancet*, 23 January 1915, 189; E.F. Buzzard in 'Discussion: The Psychology of Traumatic Amblyopia Following Explosion of Shells', Neurological Section, *PRSM*, 8:2 (1914–1915), 66; Anon., 'Shell Explosions and the Special Senses', *Lancet*, 27 March 1915, 663; W. Harris, *Nerve Injuries and Shock* (London: Oxford University Press, 1915), pp. 51, 123.

employed to understand similar symptoms were too ambiguous to allow uniform implementation of physical explanations, while the essential novelty of industrial warfare compelled doctors to explore factors beyond the effects of shell explosions.

Aetiological ambiguity is conspicuous in early medical reports on the nervous and mental disorders of war. Authors deliberately avoided mono-causal theories. Instead, they resorted to elaborate descriptive categories: 'men who came back from the front with nerves shattered'; 'the dumb and the deaf, the paralysed, and the insane from shell explosions and shock'; and 'military cases of hysteria, hystero-traumatism, traumatic neurosis, and nervous troubles due to suggestion'.[6] A bill proposed in the House of Commons in April 1915 to facilitate the early treatment of mental dis-orders replicated this deliberate inclusiveness, referring to those 'suffering from mental disorder of recent origin arising from wounds, shock, disease, stress, exhaustion, or any other cause'.[7] The desire for precision without commitment to definite causes tied some authors in knots. One account discussed 'cases labelled more or less definitely as "nervous breakdown," "collapse," "shell shock," "shell concussion," "traumatic hysteria," "trau-matic neurasthenia," where the symptoms are insomnia, battle dreams, disturbances of the special senses, "functional" palsies and anaesthesias, emotional overreaction, defects of mental synthesis, mental instability or disequilibrium, even paramnesia and hallucinations'.[8] Another medical commentator gave up in despair, concluding that no existing label adequately described diverse cases of 'nervous shock under a single heading'.[9] It is easy to see the appeal of "shell-shock" as a term which attributed miscellaneous symptoms to war conditions but refused further efforts at diagnostic precision.[10]

Many medical commentators were reluctant to ascribe first causes to "shell-shock" because they lacked knowledge, or found it difficult to think beyond the ambivalence of familiar modes of explanation. But it is also crucial to appreciate that in the early months of the war, the appearance of symptoms *in soldiers* was more important than other

---

[6] Anon., 'Medical Notes in Parliament: The Naval and Military War Pensions Bill', *BMJ*, 17 July 1915, 107; Osler, 'Address on Science and War', 798; Anon., 'The Neurology of War', *BMJ*, 14 August 1915, 264.

[7] Anon., 'Medical Notes in Parliament: Early Treatment of Mental Disorder', *BMJ*, 1 May 1915, 777.

[8] Anon., 'Lord Knutsford's Special Hospitals for Officers', *Lancet*, 27 November 1915, 1201.

[9] Anon., 'The Commotional Syndrome in War', *BMJ*, 31 July 1915, 186.

[10] Myers, 'Contribution to the Study of Shell Shock', 320; G.R. Jeffrey, 'Some Points of Interest in Connection with the Psychoneuroses of War', *JMS*, 66: 273 (April 1920), 132.

aspects of their manifestation. It is partly because men serving their country suffered these symptoms that doctors resisted reducing war syndromes to their exact pre-war counterparts but instead portrayed such conditions as the outcome of immersion in war, which incorporated the totality of embodied experience.[11] Any number of factors might lead soldiers to break down: anxiety, fatigue, lack of food, 'the horrors of the battlefield', concussion, strain and tension, or 'the sight of blood, of suffering, and of death'.[12] Doctors saw war as the supreme causative agent of "shell-shock", and therefore explored the emotional, "psychic" and physical pressures of warfare. Although they realized that therapeutic efficacy would depend on more precise knowledge, at this early stage of hostilities doctors also emphasized the shared origin of these conditions above their different manifestations. What really mattered was not whether symptoms resulted from 'psychical or physical traumata', but that they were 'the product of modern warfare under modern conditions'.[13]

Of course, rigid distinctions between physical and psychological disorders had little place in the workable ambiguities of pre-war psychological medicine. The theory of psycho-physical parallelism allowed for psychological or somatic explanations, as well as considerable latitude in assigning the ultimate causes of mental disorder. This flexible approach was reflected in the diagnostic categories and language used to describe soldiers' nervous and mental illnesses in the early months of the war, which had shifting connotations in pre-war medical discourse and were all open to interpretation. In describing symptoms as "traumatic", doctors referred soldiers' conditions to a diagnostic category with acknowledged physical and "psychic" elements, but no accepted theory of causation.[14] They also spoke of "nerves", another concept occupying the shadowy hinterland between brain and mind, psyche and soma.[15] The same ambiguity is evident in extensive references to "shock", another concept which skirted the ground between the "psychic" and

[11] See, for example, A. Feiling, 'Loss of Personality from "Shell Shock"', *Lancet*, 10 July 1915, 63; Anon., 'Mental and Nervous Shock among the Wounded', 802.

[12] Anon., 'War and Nervous Breakdown', 189; Anon., 'Insanity and the War', *Lancet*, 4 September 1915, 553; H.S. Pemberton, 'The Psychology of Traumatic Amblyopia Following the Explosion of Shells', *Lancet*, 8 May 1915, 967; W.A. Turner, 'Remarks on Cases of Nervous and Mental Shock Observed at the Base Hospitals in France', *BMJ*, 15 May 1915, 835.

[13] Anon., 'Lord Knutsford's Special Hospitals for Officers', *Lancet*, 27 November 1915, 1201.

[14] See Chapter 4 for an extended discussion of the traumatic neuroses.

[15] G.S. Rousseau, *Nervous Acts: Essays on Literature, Culture and Sensibility* (Basingstoke: Palgrave Macmillan, 2004), pp. 65–6.

the physiological, manifested in many different forms ('surgical shock, psychical shock, apoplectic shock, commotio cerebri, diaschisis'), and had uncertain origins.[16]

Above all, in the early months of the war, the default diagnosis for these conditions was functional disorder. Indeed, at this stage in the war, on the rare occasions when doctors did propose physical theories of causation they assumed widespread acceptance of the functional nature of most cases. Before 1916, physiologist Thomas Elliott (1877–1961) and ophthalmologist John Evans (1871–1941) put forward the two most detailed expositions of physical theories. Both physicians adopted the same rhetorical strategy, arguing that the majority of cases were undoubtedly functional, but it was nevertheless possible that some resulted from actual organic lesions. They explicitly aimed to highlight alternative physical explanations for the nervous and mental disorders of war and to provide aids for differential diagnosis.[17] At this point, it seems that doctors considered the potential organic origin of symptoms only after functional disorder had been ruled out, or after therapeutic methods based on this diagnosis had failed.[18] Throughout the war, the belief persisted that some doctors too readily assumed the functional nature of these conditions, although others pointed out the dangers of misdiagnosing "psychic" conditions as organic injuries.[19] Most doctors also accepted the coexistence of functional and organic injuries, including wounds.[20]

---

[16] J.G. Wilson, 'The Effects of High Explosives on the Ear', *BMJ*, 17 March 1917, 353; H.W. Page, 'Shock from Fright', in Tuke (ed.), *Dictionary of Psychological Medicine*, vol. 2, p. 1158.

[17] Elliott, 'Transient Paraplegia'; J.J. Evans, 'Organic Lesions from Shell Concussion', *BMJ*, 11 December 1915, 848.

[18] A. Hertz [Hurst], 'Paresis and Involuntary Movements Following Concussion Caused by a High Explosive Shell', Neurological Section, *PRSM*, 8:2 (1914–15), 84.

[19] On the potential misdiagnosis of organic cases, see Anon., 'Medical Societies: Brighton and Sussex Medico-Chirurgical Society', *Lancet*, 20 May 1916, 1042; Anon., 'Reviews: "War Shock"', *BMJ*, 5 April 1919, 414. On the potential misdiagnosis of functional cases, see M. Culpin, 'Practical Hints on Functional Disorders', *BMJ*, 21 October 1916, 548–9; E.G. Fearnsides, 'Essentials of Treatment of Soldiers and Discharged Soldiers Suffering from Functional Nervous Disorders', Neurological Section, *PRSM*, 11 (1917–18), 43.

[20] It is a myth that wounded men did not develop "shell-shock". See G. Holmes and W.T. Lister, 'Disturbances of Vision from Cerebral Lesions, with Special Reference to the Cortical Representation of the Macula', *Brain*, 39:1–2 (June 1916), 34; E. Bramwell, 'Recent Advances in Medical Science: Neurology', *EMJ*, 15 (July–December 1915), 436; A.F. Hewat, 'Clinical Cases from Medical Division, Royal Victoria Hospital, Netley', *EMJ*, 18 (January–June 1917), 211–12; J.S.B. Stopford, 'So-Called Functional Symptoms in Organic Nerve Injuries', *Lancet*, 8 June 1918, 795–6; R. Eager, 'Head Injuries in Relation to the Psychoses and Psycho-Neuroses', *JMS*, 66:273 (April 1920), 123–4, 130.

As in pre-war psychological medicine, diagnosis of functional disorder did not necessarily mean that doctors viewed conditions as psychological. A report on 'the pathology of shell concussion' from August 1915 argued that rapid and dramatic changes in atmospheric conditions could cause instantaneous death and pondered whether 'acute neurasthenia' resulted from similar but less extensive damage to the nervous system sustained in shell explosions.[21] In theories of "shell-shock", doctors continued to exploit the conceptual fissures inherited from pre-war modes of explanation, as when "psychological" explanations were coupled with nominal allegiance to the existence of an underlying physical pathology. For example, John Herbert Parsons, ophthalmic consultant to the home troops, described cases of traumatic amblyopia (blurry vision) as 'wounds of consciousness' because he could find 'no demonstrable organic lesion' but cautiously added that 'this does not imply that there is no neural lesion to account for the psychological disorder, but merely that it has hitherto escaped observation'.[22] This was not mere rhetoric designed to appease thoroughgoing materialists. The entire mode of medical thought tended to break down distinctions between physical and psychological damage and to stress interchange between body and mind in functional disorders. Some doctors held that functional disturbance might eventually become 'structural and permanent'; others maintained that when physical damage healed, purely functional symptoms might remain; still others argued that hysterical symptoms, such as transient paraplegia, might be grafted on to organic disorders.[23] Most doctors believed it was impossible to draw hard-and-fast lines between "psychic" and somatic damage in "shell-shock".

When doctors debated the possible physical causes of wartime functional disorders, their discussions extended beyond the effects of shell explosions. At meetings of the laryngological section of the Royal Society of Medicine held in 1915 and 1916, doctors considered military cases of functional aphonia (inability to produce voice): some diagnosed 'pure' functional disorder, some argued that functional elements coexisted with anatomical irregularities, and others suggested incipient or developed

---

[21] Anon., 'The Pathology of Shell Concussion', *BMJ*, 14 August 1915, 265; A. Miles and J.S. Fowler, 'Editorial Notes: Annus 1915', *EMJ*, 16 (January–June 1916), 3.

[22] J.H. Parsons, 'The Psychology of Traumatic Amblyopia Following Explosion of Shells', Neurological Section, *PRSM*, 8:2 (1914–15), 56–7.

[23] Anon., 'The Disabled Soldier in France', *BMJ*, 7 October 1916, 499; W.H. Jessop in 'Special Discussion on Shell Shock Without Visible Signs of Injury', Sections of Psychiatry and Neurology (Combined Meeting), *PRSM*, 9:3 (1915–16), xxxvi; Turner, 'Remarks on Cases of Nervous and Mental Shock', 835; Anon., 'Shell Explosions and the Special Senses', 663.

tubercular disease as the cause.[24] Of course, physicians did linger on the possible effects of continual exposure to shell explosions, the most novel and dramatic feature of modern warfare – but they saw these effects as extending beyond damage to the nervous system. Even at a very early stage in the war, doctors conjectured that often, shell explosions did no more than tip exhausted and emotional men over the edge into definite breakdown.[25] Some speculated that prolonged shelling caused sensory overload which inhibited the function of the special senses, leading to loss of sight, hearing, or smell.[26] One report compared functional deafness in soldiers to auditory problems in 'boilermakers, riveters, blacksmiths, and people working on railways'.[27] The battlefield could be configured as a gross extension of the pathological modern industrial environment.

In the first years of the war, physical theories of causation did not dominate medical discourse on "shell-shock". Instead, physical theories of causation sat alongside other forms of explanation which emphasized the interaction and coexistence of physical and "psychic" elements.[28] Even doctors who believed in the physical origins of some cases of "shell-shock" noted that sometimes symptoms were caused by terrifying 'psychical experiences' and anxiety over the performance of duty.[29] Neurologists did not rush to insist on physical aetiologies; the neurological journal *Brain* published no articles on "shell-shock" until 1919. On the other hand, some doctors put forward relatively complex psychological theories in the initial stages of the war. In March 1915, the

[24] See, for example, C. Potter, 'Case of Gunshot Wound of the Neck with Laryngeal Symptoms for Diagnosis and Opinions as to Treatment', Laryngological Section, *PRSM*, 8:2 (1914–15), 116; 'Discussion on Functional Cases', Laryngological Section, *PRSM*, 8:2 (1914–15), 117–20; W. Milligan, 'A Note on Treatment of "Functional Aphonia" in Soldiers from the Front', Laryngological Section, *PRSM*, 9:2 (1915–16), 83–5; C. Potter, 'Case of Aphonia in a Soldier', Laryngological Section, *PRSM*, 9:2 (1915–16), 90–2; L.H. Pegler, 'Case of (?) Nervous or Functional Aphonia', Laryngological Section, *PRSM*, 9:2 (1915–16), 118–20.

[25] Turner, 'Remarks on Cases of Nervous and Mental Shock'; Anon., 'Special Hospitals for Officers: Lord Knutsford's Appeal', *Lancet*, 20 November 1915, 1155; H. Campbell, 'War Neuroses', *Practitioner*, 96:5 (May 1916), 501.

[26] W. Milligan and F.H. Westmacott, 'Warfare Injuries and Neuroses: Introductory Paper', Laryngological Section, *PRSM*, 8:2 (1914–15), 114; Parsons, 'Psychology of Traumatic Amblyopia', 62–3; Harris, *Nerve Injuries and Shock*, pp. 109, 121.

[27] Anon., 'Shell Explosions and the Special Senses', 663.

[28] Anon., 'Special Hospitals for Officers', 1157; J. Collie, 'Neurasthenia: What It Costs the State', *Journal of the RAMC*, 26:4 (April 1916), 526; T.E. Harwood, 'A Preliminary Note on the Nature and Treatment of Concussion', *BMJ*, 15 April 1916, 551; T.E. Harwood, 'Three Cases Illustrating the Functional Consequences of Head-Injuries', *Lancet*, 2 September 1916, 431; Harris, *Nerve Injuries and Shock*, pp. 5, 31, 50, 93 and 98.

[29] Turner, 'Remarks on Cases of Nervous and Mental Shock', 833 and 835.

neurological section of the Royal Society of Medicine discussed traumatic amblyopia. No participants referred to concussion or commotion (the theory that dynamic force exerted by explosions caused decompression within the organism).[30] One claimed the disturbance was 'purely mental and belonged to the region of ideas'; another referred to a case in which this 'mental condition' had been caused by the man's anxiety over the welfare of his wife and children; the final respondent, Hugh Crichton-Miller (1877–1959) talked about 'defence' and 'anxiety' mechanisms produced by intolerable mental conflict.[31] A few months later the gastro-enterologist Adolphe Abrahams explained a patient's hysterical paraplegia as an 'anxiety-neurosis' originating in the soldier's fear that he would be permanently crippled and become a burden to his family.[32] Although this kind of familiarity with sophisticated psychological language was unusual in this period, realization of the emotional strain of warfare was not. The more elaborate psychological theories formulated in the later years of the war evolved out of these moments of simple recognition.

1916: Differentiation, Opposition, and Displacement

In 1916, debates on the war neuroses moved up a gear, with nearly treble the number of articles published on "shell-shock" in the medical press as in the previous year. When the sections of neurology and psychiatry of the Royal Society of Medicine held a special combined meeting on 'shell-shock without visible signs of injury' in January 1916, there was a new seriousness to the discussions and clear commitment to grappling with "shell-shock" as a scientific problem. Doctors now had considerable experience in diagnosing and treating "shell-shock", and consequently could develop more sustained arguments and conclusions. Moreover, it was now evident that Britain was in the war for the long haul. As the numbers of "shell-shocked" men increased and the rate of volunteers for the army slowed, the "shell-shock" epidemic could not be viewed apart from the looming manpower crisis. Renewed medical engagement with the nervous and mental disorders of war reflected urgent fears about the mental health of the army and the potential consequences of psychiatric failure for the fighting strength of the nation.

---

[30] On the longer history of the concept of commotion, see W. Schivelbusch, *The Railway Journey: The Industrialization of Time and Space in the 19th Century* (Leamington Spa, Hamburg and New York: Berg, 1986), p. 137.

[31] E.F. Buzzard, L. Paton, and H. Crichton-Miller in 'Discussion: The Psychology of Traumatic Amblyopia Following Explosion of Shells'.

[32] A. Abrahams, 'A Case of Hysterical Paraplegia', *Lancet*, 24 July 1915, 179.

This more serious approach manifested in increased criticism of "shell-shock" as a viable diagnostic label. Although the initial appeal of "shell-shock" lay in its aetiological ambiguity, it rapidly became apparent that this vagueness could also limit its usefulness as a diagnostic category. Doctors needed to return patients to military service or productive civilian work as quickly as possible and to obtain replicable results. The deferred aetiological judgements and hit-and-miss therapeutic measures of pre-war psychological medicine did not serve these purposes. Less than a year after the first appearance of "shell-shock" in print, neurologist Henry Head impatiently complained that 'heterogeneous . . . nervous affects from concussion to sheer funk, which have merely this much in common that nervous control has at last given way', should not be bracketed together. Dealing with all these conditions under one label, Head claimed, was 'to sweep up the various fruits which fall from the trees in a strong wind and then to discuss them without first stating that some fell from an apple and some from a pear tree'.[33] This rejection of "shell-shock", a term which accorded primacy to the origins of suffering in war rather than more specific causes or particular symptoms, was necessary to doctors' more vigorous attempts to discriminate between different mental and nervous disorders of war.[34]

These efforts resulted in increased differentiation between physical and psychological theories of causation. The exploratory ethos of the first half of the war, when doctors attempted to blend physical and "psychic" causes and symptoms, did not entirely vanish: it survived in individual accounts, and in the trend for physiological theories of emotion.[35] However, from 1916 inclusiveness ceased to be the dominant approach to "shell-shock". In the second half of the war, some doctors began to elaborate complex theories of physical causation for the first time, while others formulated intricate and explicitly psychological theories.[36] These developments were two sides of the same coin: the

---

[33] Anon., 'A Discussion on Shell Shock', *Lancet*, 5 February 1916, 306; F.W. Mott, 'Opening Paper and Concluding Response: Special Discussion on Shell Shock without Visible Signs of Injury', Sections of Psychiatry and Neurology, *PRSM*, 9:3 (1915–16), xli.

[34] Campbell, 'War Neuroses'; W.A. Turner, 'Arrangements for the Care of Cases of Nervous and Mental Shock Coming from Overseas', *Lancet*, 27 May 1916, 1073; W. Garton, 'Shell Shock and Its Treatment by Cerebro-Spinal Galvanism', *BMJ*, 28 October 1916, 584–6; E.F. Buzzard, 'Warfare on the Brain', *Lancet*, 30 December 1916, 1096.

[35] Physiological theories of "shell-shock" are discussed in Chapter 6.

[36] On psychological theories, see M.D. Eder, 'An Address on the Psycho-Pathology of the War Neuroses', *Lancet*, 12 August 1916, 264–8; C.S. Myers, 'Contributions to the Study of Shell Shock (II): Being an Account of Certain Cases Treated by Hypnosis', *Lancet*, 8 January 1916, 65–9; R.G. Rows, 'Mental Conditions Following Strain and Nerve Shock', *BMJ*, 25 March 1916, 441–3; G.E. Smith, 'Shock and the Soldier. I',

methodical exposition of physical theories provoked similarly detailed articulation of psychological theories in response, and vice versa. Alongside this differentiation, another movement occurred in both forms of theorization: displacement of responsibility for mental breakdown from the war itself onto the individual soldier, the material it worked upon. The war could be exculpated in two ways. Some psychological theorists located the origins of breakdown in the patient's unique mental make-up and life history, rather than in the distressing experiences of war alone. War *could* cause even the strongest individual to break down, but often simply set the spark to flammable material in the patient's own psyche.[37] Other doctors emphasized that breakdown usually occurred in men with inherently weak and unstable nervous systems.[38] These forms of explanation often merged: most physicians maintained that heredity and life experience were both important factors in the production of neurosis, but in their own theories focused on one over the other.[39] Theories of "shell-shock" that were radically different in almost all other respects shared this tendency to absolve the war of ultimate responsibility for breakdown.[40]

This was not an intentional move, but emerged from attempts to resolve the question of why some men broke down while others did not. The war alone ceased to be sufficient explanation for "shell-shock"

Lancet, 15 April 1916, 813–17; G.E. Smith, 'Shock and the Soldier. II', *Lancet*, 22 April 1916, 853–7.

[37] C.S. Myers, 'Contributions to the Study of Shell Shock (III): Being an Account of Certain Disorders of Cutaneous Sensibility', *Lancet*, 18 March 1916, 610–11; C.S. Myers, 'Contributions to the Study of Shell Shock (IV): Being an Account of Certain Disorders of Speech, with Special Reference to Their Causation and Their Relation to Malingering', *Lancet*, 9 September 1916, 466; W. Brown in 'Special Discussion on Shell Shock', xxvii–xxx.

[38] Campbell, 'War Neuroses', 501–3; J.M. Clarke, 'Some Neuroses of the War', *Bristol Medico-Chirurgical Journal*, 34:130 (July 1916), 59; G.H. Savage, 'Mental Disabilities for War Service', *JMS*, 62:259 (October 1916), 653; 'Discussion: Mental Disabilities for War Service', *JMS*, 62:259 (October 1916); Anon., 'Reports of Societies: Mental Disabilities for War Service', *BMJ*, 5 August 1916; see the contributions of Stansfield and Fearnsides to 'Special Discussion on Shell Shock', xxx, xxxix.

[39] For example, Smith and Pear denied that they were 'out-and-out environmentalists': G.E. Smith and T.H. Pear, 'Letters to the Editor: Shell Shock and Its Lessons', *Nature*, 100 (September 1917–February 1918), 65; G.E. Smith, 'Correspondence: "The Psychoneuroses of War"', *BMJ*, 22 September 1917, 402. See also W.H.R. Rivers, 'War-Neurosis and Military Training', *Mental Hygiene*, 2:4 (October 1918), 18, fn 1, 513–33.

[40] Simon Wessely argues that the most novel aspect of the construct of post-traumatic stress disorder when introduced into the psychiatric canon in 1980 was the view that the 'insanity of war' alone, rather than genetic predisposition or upbringing, could cause protracted and severe psychiatric breakdown. S. Wessely, 'Twentieth-Century Theories on Combat Motivation and Breakdown', *Journal of Contemporary History*, 41:2 (2006), 281–2.

and instead became seen as a contributory factor in breakdown: more severe than most, perhaps, with more direct influence on some cases than others, but nevertheless an agent which worked on the latent suscepti-bilities of the individual rather than a horrific event which alone accounted for these men's disorders. In 1916 conscription was intro-duced: this was the year of the Somme, the year in which the crisis visibly deepened and the unity of the war effort became ever more important. In this context, doctors across the spectrum of medical opinion reframed "shell-shock" as a pathological individual reaction rather than an unavoidable response to the environment of war.

This shift in medical discourse is all the more striking because in the early months of the war, doctors rarely even hinted that soldiers might break down due to existing nervous instability.[41] The temporary retreat from heredity as a viable explanation for (war-related) nervous and mental disorders was the most surprising aspect of medical discussions in 1914 and 1915, especially as the experience of war did not dent hereditarian beliefs elsewhere in Europe.[42] However, in Britain doctors initially judged the conditions of industrial warfare sufficient explanation for most breakdowns, partly because they optimistically believed that selection procedures prevented unstable individuals from joining up. Medical men emphasized that the 'terrible stresses' of trench warfare made "shell-shock" an entirely different order of experience to civilian nervous disorders. Broken soldiers should 'be regarded and spoken of as mentally war wounded'.[43] This position arose out of the strong voluntary tradition in Britain.[44] In the earliest days of the war, soldier heroes were almost always represented as willing volunteers. Having proved their moral worth through the act of joining up, such men were less vulnerable to medical suspicions of hereditary taint. It is notable that the resurgence of hereditary explanations occurred after the Military Service Act 1916, although the legacy of voluntarism continued to shape public portrayals of masculine courage and doctors rarely mentioned conscription in their wartime publications.

This retreat from hereditarian explanations for breakdown constituted a complete revolution from the dominant position of pre-war psycho-logical medicine, but was short-lived. In the later years of the war,

---

[41] Exceptions are Myers, 'Contribution to the Study of Shell Shock', 317; Anon., 'War and Nervous Breakdown', 189; Anon., 'Special Hospitals for Officers', 1155–6.

[42] Thomas, *Treating the Trauma of the Great War*, pp. 10, 18; Lerner, *Hysterical Men*, pp. 215–21.

[43] Anon., 'The Mental Treatment Bill', *BMJ*, 1 May 1915, 772; Anon., 'Insanity and the War', 553.

[44] Voluntarism is discussed further in Chapter 5.

medical authors frequently commented on the prevalence of 'neuro-pathic or psychopathic disposition' or 'hereditary taint' among soldiers suffering from mental or nervous disorders.[45] As with physical and psychological theories of causation, elaborate investigations into the role of heredity in "shell-shock" were a product of the second half of the war and afterwards.[46] Some doctors compiled statistics demonstrating the prevalence of personal and family histories of nervous and mental instability among "shell-shocked" soldiers; when results showed little direct correlation between heredity and war-related breakdown, they argued that the methods of investigation must have been unreliable, and the actual incidence of predisposition was undoubtedly higher.[47] Alex Watson suggests that the realization that psychiatric disorders affected only a small minority of the men exposed to similar stressing factors spurred doctors to investigate hereditary predisposition.[48] This explains the impulse to research heredity but not the results of these investigations. If some doctors believed the war had shown that any man could break down, for others the "shell-shock" epidemic had revealed 'the large number of neuropathic persons there are who "carry on" in civilian occupations, battling with their feelings of self-insufficiency as best they may, and the still more numerous others in whom these

---

[45] See, for example, E.D. Adrian and L.R. Yealland, 'The Treatment of Some Common War Neuroses', *Lancet*, 9 June 1917, 868; Anon., 'Reports of Societies: Shell Shock', *BMJ*, 21 July 1917, 81; R.D. Hotchkis, 'Renfrew District Asylum as a War Hospital for Mental Invalids: Some Contrasts in Administration. With an Analysis of Cases Admitted during the First Year', *JMS*, 63:261 (April 1917), 246; F.W. Burton-Fanning, 'Neurasthenia in Soldiers of the Home Forces', *Lancet*, 16 June 1917, 907; W.A. Turner, 'The Bradshaw Lecture on Neuroses and Psychoses of War', *Lancet*, 9 November 1918, 613; L.A. Weatherly, 'The War and Neurasthenia, Psychasthenia and Mild Mental Disorders. I', *The Medical World (TMW)*, 11 (July–December 1918), 217; C. McDowall, 'The Genesis of Delusions: Clinical Notes', *JMS*, 65:270 (July 1919), 187–8; R. Eager, 'A Record of Admissions to the Mental Section of the Lord Derby War Hospital, Warrington, from June 17th, 1916, to June 16th, 1917', *JMS*, 64:266 (July 1918), 277, 280, 284, 290; F. Golla, 'The Organic Basis of the Hysterical Syndrome', Section of Psychiatry, *PRSM*, 16 (1923), 2. See also the post-war claim of a consulting physician for nervous and mental diseases to the Eastern Command that 'a large proportion' of "shell-shocked" men had pre-existing nervous troubles resulting from excessive masturbation: T.E. Knowles, 'An Address on Some of the Causes of Our C3 Population', *BMJ*, 17 December 1921, 1023.
[46] J.M. Wolfsohn, 'The Predisposing Factors of War Psycho-Neuroses', *Lancet*, 2 February 1918, 177–80; H.L. Gordon, 'Eye-Colour and the Abnormal Palate in Neuroses and Psychoses', *Lancet*, 5 July 1919, 9–10.
[47] R. Eager, 'War Psychoses Occurring in Cases with a Definite History of Shell Shock', *BMJ*, 13 April 1918, 422–5; O.P.N. Pearn, 'Psychoses in the Expeditionary Forces', *JMS*, 65:269 (April 1919), 101–2.
[48] A. Watson, *Enduring the Great War: Combat, Morale and Collapse in the German and British Armies, 1914–1918* (Cambridge and New York: Cambridge University Press, 2008), pp. 35–9.

conditions are latent'.[49] The tendency to fall back on hereditarian explanations reflects doctors' pre-existing prejudices and underscores how remarkable it was that doctors neglected heredity in the early years of the war.

The later emphasis on heredity was not universal. Neurologist Howard Tooth (1856–1925) pointed out that given the horrendous strain of warfare, it spoke 'well for the mental stability of the British soldier that there are not five times as many neurasthenics as there are'.[50] Other doctors believed that hereditary predisposition increased the likelihood of breakdown, and might even be an operative factor in most cases, but nevertheless maintained that the experience of trench warfare might 'shatter' even 'the strongest nervous system'.[51] Millais Culpin (1874–1952) believed that 'given enough of the strain of modern warfare, any man whatsoever will eventually break down', but also claimed to have discovered increased incidence of predisposition (not necessarily hereditary) among patients as the war went on. He concluded that 'the number of patients whose symptoms are due entirely to war experiences acting upon a mentally sound organism is likely to be small'.[52] On the other hand, for Frederick Dillon (1887?–1965) the war showed that mental disorder did not necessarily result from 'inborn predisposition'. Instead, 'We are all of us potentially or latently susceptible to neurotic manifestations'.[53]

The doctrine of hereditary predisposition was undermined to some extent by the experience of war, but there were limits to this process. The conclusions of the Report of the Committee of Enquiry into "Shell-Shock" (1922), based on the expert testimony of both military and medical witnesses, provide a useful guide to dominant opinion at the end of the war. The Report stated that 'pre-disposition plays an immense part in the incidence of shell shock' but also listed several other factors which increased the likelihood of breakdown, including environment, training, and education in childhood.[54] This widened the definition of

[49] C.H. Bond, 'The Position of Psychological Medicine in Medical and Allied Services', JMS, 67:279 (October 1921), 431.
[50] H.H. Tooth, 'Neurasthenia and Psychasthenia', Journal of the RAMC, 28:3 (March 1917), 339.
[51] J.S. Bury, 'Remarks on the Pathology of the War Neuroses', Lancet, 27 July 1918, 98; A.F. Grimbly, 'Neuroses and Psycho-Neuroses of the Sea', Practitioner, 102:5 (May 1919), 244; summary of findings, RWOCESS, p. 144; Macpherson et al., History of the Great War, p. 14.
[52] M. Culpin, Psychoneuroses of Peace and War (Cambridge: Cambridge University Press, 1920), p. 122.
[53] F. Dillon, 'The Methods of Psychotherapy', JMS, 71:292 (January 1925), 58.
[54] Summary of findings, RWOCESS, p. 148.

'predisposition' in accordance with the latest psychological thinking but
did not discount the importance of heredity in breakdown. The eugeni-
cist Alfred Tredgold (1870–1952) claimed that although 'mental stress'
played some part in "shell-shock", 'in most of the sufferers a definite
predisposition to this breakdown was present', as some 'were never near
to the firing line, nor had they seen or heard an exploding shell'.[55] As late
as 1940, Charles Myers echoed these conclusions, explaining that often
"shell-shock" was dependent 'on a previous psycho-neurotic history and
inherited predisposition, on inadequate examination and selection ...
and on the lack of proper discipline and *esprit de corps*'.[56] To the end of
the war and beyond, medical belief in hereditary weakness as a predisposing factor in the production of "shell-shock" remained widespread.

Concussion and Commotion: Frederick Mott and Physical Theories of Causation

One doctor whose view on the importance of heredity in nervous and
mental disorders was not changed at all by the war was the neurologist
and pathologist Frederick Mott. Mott is best known as the most influential British proponent of physical theories of causation for "shell-
shock".[57] Although he did not publish directly on "shell-shock" until
1916, by the end of the war Mott had produced more articles on the topic
than any other physician. He conducted lengthy investigations into the
potential commotional origins of "shell-shock" and insisted until his
death that some cases had a purely physical basis. Mott's interventions
decisively shaped medical debates on "shell-shock". Although physical
theories of causation were tentatively touted from the early months of the
war, from 1916 many more doctors confidently asserted the organic basis
of at least some cases of "shell-shock", almost always citing Mott's
research in support of this position.[58] At around the same time, other

---

[55] Anon., 'Mental Disorder in Relation to Eugenics', *BMJ*, 26 February 1927, 386. See
also W. Salisbury Sharpe's comments in Anon., 'Traumatic Neurasthenia and the
"Litigation Neurosis"', *BMJ*, 17 December 1927, 1145: 'The worse case of so-called
shell shock he had seen was that of a man who had been for nearly ten years wholly
incapacitated by a purely functional paralysis, and yet who had been at no time nearer
the war than Plymouth'.

[56] Myers, *Shell Shock in France*, p. ix; see also A.F. Hurst, *Medical Diseases of War*, 4th edn
(London: Edward Arnold, 1944), pp. 1, 3. This emphasis on heredity contrasted with
Hurst's claim in the immediate post-war period that the majority of war hysterics had 'no
personal or family history of neuroses'; 'The War Neuroses and the Neuroses of Civil
Life', *Guy's Hospital Reports*, 70 (1922), 142.

[57] Leese, *Shell Shock*, pp. 52, 70; Jones and Wessely, *Shell Shock to PTSD*, p. 23.

[58] For arguments by other authors published in 1916 in support of the theory of
commotion, see Campbell, 'War Neuroses'; Turner, 'Arrangements for the Care of

physicians started to firmly refute physical theories of "shell-shock".[59] Mott's elaboration of physical theories provided a clear statement for other doctors to support or argue against, and so boosted the differentiation of physical and psychological modes of explanation from 1916 onwards. However, even Mott never argued that all cases of "shell-shock" resulted from organic damage to the nervous system. Indeed, his earliest discussion of the nervous and mental disorders of war concentrated on "psychic" conditions.[60] This should warn us not to assume the existence of neat divisions between physical and psychological theories.

Mott put forward his most sustained exposition of physical theories of causation in the Lettsomian lectures delivered in February and March 1916. He set out three classes of injury to the central nervous system caused by high explosives: immediate fatality, including death without visible injury; non-fatal wounds and injuries of the body which did not exhibit functional disturbances; and injury to the central nervous system without visible effects, including 'functional neuroses and psychoses'. Mott acknowledged that some war-related functional disorders were not caused by the effects of shell explosions but justified the inclusion of functional disorders in this discussion because any "psychic" disturbance must have a physical counterpart, even it was undiscoverable.[61] By mid-1917, Mott believed he had clearly identified a class of 'true' or 'real' "shell-shock" caused by concussion, commotion, or gas inhalation, which should be separated from purely functional cases.[62] However, he also insisted that there was no fixed division between these two classes, and that 'emotional' and 'commotional' factors could play a part in the same case; for example, he diagnosed one soldier as a case of 'shell shock and psychic trauma from witnessing death of comrades; psychic trauma maintained by terrifying experiences and dreams;

Cases of Nervous and Mental Shock', 1073; Anon., 'The War: Nervous and Mental Shock', *BMJ*, 10 June 1916, 830–2; Clarke, 'Some Neuroses of the War', 49–50; Garton, 'Shell Shock and Its Treatment by Cerebro-Spinal Galvanism'.

[59] See Myers, 'Contributions to the Study of Shell Shock (IV)', 464; H. Wiltshire, 'A Contribution to the Etiology of Shell Shock', *Lancet*, 17 June 1916, 1207–12; Buzzard, 'Warfare on the Brain', 1097–8.

[60] F.W. Mott, 'The Psychic Mechanism of the Voice in Relation to the Emotions', *BMJ*, 11 December 1915, 846.

[61] F.W. Mott, 'The Lettsomian Lectures on the Effects of High Explosives Upon the Central Nervous System. I', *Lancet*, 12 February 1916, 331.

[62] F.W. Mott, 'The Chadwick Lecture on Mental Hygiene and Shell Shock during and after the War', *BMJ*, 14 July 1917, 41; F.W. Mott, 'The Microscopic Examination of the Brains of Two Men Dead of Commotio Cerebri (Shell Shock) without Visible Injury', *Journal of the RAMC*, 29:6 (December 1917), 671.

nervous predisposition'.[63] Mott, the staunchest supporter of physical theories of causation, believed mind and body were both implicated in the production of many cases of war-related nervous and mental disorder.

A similar line of argument was pursued in other detailed researches on "shell-shock". In 1919, Alfred Carver (d. 1950), an RAMC captain who served at Maghull Military Hospital, published the results of experiments into commotional shock. Carver observed the effects of high explosives on fish, rats and mice, and humans. He aimed to correct 'the present tendency to regard the neuroses of war as of exclusively emotional origin', and to gain 'a more general recognition for the underlying physical basis demonstrable in a considerable proportion of them'.[64] Carver concluded that 'physical or "commotional" factors' were present in many cases, but emphasized that 'under the conditions of modern warfare the soldier is continually subjected both to physical and emotional causes of shock, and that the two factors operate in conjunction'. Crucially, although physical or emotional causes might initially dominate in any given case, 'the individual, once sensitized by either, remains for a long time, perhaps always, hypersensitive to both forms of stimulation, and a vicious circle is thus established'.[65] Carver was not a crank: he presented papers to the neurological section of the Royal Society of Medicine, and published in *Brain*, the *British Journal of Psychology*, and the *Lancet*. Nor did he stubbornly cling to physical theories: in the post-war period his research extended in more clearly psychological directions.[66] Rather, he explored different approaches to "shell-shock", and placed physical theories on a wider spectrum of potential explanations. Carver's experimental methods were unusual, but his arguments were consonant with broader trends in wartime medical debates.

Accounts which insisted on the interdependence of physical and "psychic" factors fitted with pre-war approaches to nervous and mental disorders. Continuity in modes of explanation is also evident in Mott's work. Mott's research into "shell-shock" extended his existing interest in

---

[63] Quotation Mott, 'Opening Paper', xxi–xxii and xiii; see also F.W. Mott, *War Neuroses and Shell Shock* (London: Hodder and Stoughton, 1919), pp. 2, 22, 30, 35; F.W. Mott, 'The Lettsomian Lectures on the Effects of High Explosives Upon the Central Nervous System. II', *Lancet*, 26 February 1916, 441; F.W. Mott, 'Punctiform Haemorrhages of the Brain in Gas Poisoning', *BMJ*, 19 May 1917, 637–41.

[64] A. Carver and A. Dinsley, 'Some Biological Effects due to High Explosives', Section of Neurology, *PRSM*, 12 (Parts 1 and 2) (1918–1919), 51.

[65] Ibid., 36; A. Carver, 'Some Observations Bearing Upon the Commotional Factor in the Aetiology of Shell Shock', *Lancet*, 2 August 1919, 195–6.

[66] A. Carver, 'The Search for a Kingdom', Medical Section, *British Journal of Psychology*, 2:4 (1922), 273–91; A. Carver, 'Primary Identification and Mysticism', *British Journal of Medical Psychology*, 4:2 (1924), 102–14.

the causes of insanity, which incorporated active campaigning for research into the early treatment of mental disorders.[67] These efforts were driven by his conviction that the apparent increase in insanity was one of the most pressing social issues of the day and formed part of his wider concern with the social aspects of health and illness.[68] Mott's research on alcohol and syphilis emphasized the interaction of physical, environmental, temperamental, and "psychic" factors in the production of addiction, illness, and disease.[69] His publications on "shell-shock" furthered these explorations and fit seamlessly with his longer-established concerns and research methods. Likewise, the manner of Mott's engagement with psychological theorists illustrates the persistence of older approaches. Mott was not a sophisticated psychological thinker. In his efforts to understand the human mind and behaviour he drew on diverse sources, from classical texts to Jung and Freud, without acknowledging the contradictions between apparently opposed theories of mind.[70] This eclecticism was typical of pre-war British medicine and only began to seem outdated after the war.

Mott's war experience did cause him to modify his views about the prevalence of commotional "shell-shock". At the outset of the war, he believed that a substantial number of cases had suffered organic damage to the central nervous system, although he did not state a precise figure at this time.[71] In 1918 he estimated the ratio of emotional to commotional cases as 10:1, and in 1922 he revised this upwards to 5:1, following the conclusions of the Report of the Committee of Enquiry into "Shell-Shock".[72] This reassessment of the level of commotional "shell-shock"

[67] Mott, 'Preface', iii–vii; Anon., 'The Maudsley Hospital', *BMJ*, 13 January 1917, 51; F.W. Mott, 'The Second Maudsley Lecture', *JMS*, 67:278 (July 1921), 319–25; Anon., 'Obituary: Sir Frederick Mott', *Lancet*, 19 June 1926, 1228–30.

[68] See the bibliography of Mott's work in J.R. Lord (ed.), *Contributions to Psychiatry, Neurology and Sociology Dedicated to the Late Sir Frederick Mott, K.B.E.* (London: H.K Lewis, 1929), pp. 391–401. For comments on insanity as a social problem, see F.W. Mott, 'Sanity and Insanity', *Journal of the Royal Sanitary Institute*, 33 (1912–13), 228; F.W. Mott, 'A Study of the Neuropathic Inheritance', *American Journal of Insanity*, 69 (1912–13), 907–38.

[69] F.W. Mott, 'On Alcohol and Insanity', *BMJ*, 28 September 1907, 797; F.W. Mott, *Syphilis of the Nervous System* (London: Henry Frowde and Hodder and Stoughton, 1910), p. 11 and pp. 193–8.

[70] F.W. Mott, 'The Study of Character by the Dramatists and Novelists', *JMS*, 61:254 (July 1915), 339–44; E. Jones, *Free Associations: Memories of a Psycho-Analyst* (London: Hogarth Press, 1959), p. 123.

[71] Mott, *War Neuroses and Shell Shock*, p. 35.

[72] Mott in 'Discussion: War Psychoses and Psychoneuroses', *JMS*, 64:265 (April 1918), 237; F.W. Mott, 'The Neuroses and Psychoses in Relation to Conscription and Eugenics', *Eugenics Review*, 14:1 (April 1922), 13; *RWOCESS*, p. 112. See pp. 100–19 for a summary of evidence on concussion and commotion shock.

followed the general trend of medical opinion.[73] After 1917, most articles on "shell-shock" focused on emotional and psychological theories, even if they did not deny the existence of commotional shock. Although the concept of invisible injury to the central nervous system continued to merit some attention in articles,[74] books,[75] correspondence,[76] and reports of public lectures and meetings of medical societies,[77] discussions usually concluded that 'true' "shell-shock" constituted only a small proportion of cases. This remained the position of most post-war medical literature. The official medical history of the war published in 1923 stated that approximately 2.5 per cent of cases 'showed evidence of a possible lesion of the nervous system'.[78] Even in the 1940s, some former "shell-shock" doctors still insisted that 'men of stout heart' had broken down through 'the blast of a shell which damaged their brains', and that 'when a man is hit he deserves more consideration than when he is frightened'.[79] Arguably, such theories have never completely disappeared: there are definite similarities between the diagnostic categories of commotional shock and

---

[73] Anon., 'The Treatment of War Psycho-Neuroses', *BMJ*, 7 December 1918, 634.

[74] Tooth, 'Neurasthenia and Psychasthenia', 339–40; Wilson, 'The Effects of High Explosives on the Ear'; J.G. Wilson, 'Further Report on the Effects of High Explosives on the Ear', *BMJ*, 5 May 1917, 578–9; R. Armstrong-Jones, 'The Psychology of Fear and the Effects of Panic Fear in War Time', *JMS*, 63:262 (July 1917), 369, 372–3; A.F. Hurst, 'Observations on the Etiology and Treatment of War Neuroses', *BMJ*, 29 September 1917, 413; Eager, 'Record of Admissions', 287 8; J. Collie, 'The Management of Neurasthenia and Allied Disorders Contracted in the Army', *Journal of State Medicine*, 26:1 (January 1918), 2–3; E.W. White, 'Observations on Shell Shock and Neurasthenia in the Hospitals in the Western Command', *BMJ*, 13 April 1918, 422; Bury, 'Remarks on the Pathology of War Neuroses', 97; Turner, 'Bradshaw Lecture', 614–15; W. Johnson, 'Hysterical Tremor', *BMJ*, 7 December 1918, 627–8; Grimbly, 'Neuroses and Psycho-Neuroses of the Sea', 248; W. Hale-White, 'An Address on Some Applications of Experience Gained by the War to the Problems of Civil Medical Practice', *BMJ*, 23 August 1919, 229; H. Davy, 'An Address on Some War Diseases', *BMJ*, 27 December 1919, 837.

[75] A.F. Hurst, *Medical Diseases of the War* (London: Edward Arnold, 1917), pp. 3–6; A.F. Hurst, *Medical Diseases of the War*, 2nd edn (London: Edward Arnold, 1918), pp. 44–59; H.C. Marr, *Psychoses of the War, Including Neurasthenia and Shell Shock* (London: Henry Frowde and Hodder & Stoughton, 1919), pp. 49, 110–19.

[76] J.L. Thomas, 'Correspondence: Death from High Explosives without Wounds', *BMJ*, 5 May 1917, 599; L. Hill, 'Correspondence: Death from High Explosives without Wounds', *BMJ*, 19 May 1917, 665.

[77] Anon., 'Shell Shock, Gas Poisoning, and War Neuroses', *BMJ*, 19 May 1917, 656; Anon., 'The Management of Neurasthenia and Allied Disorders in the Army', *TMW*, 8 (January–June 1917), 642–3; Anon., 'Reports of Societies: Shell Shock', 81; Anon., 'British Medical Association Special Clinical Meeting, Section of Medicine: War Neuroses', *Lancet*, 26 April 1919, 709–11.

[78] Macpherson *et al.*, *History of the Great War*, pp. 18-9.

[79] Lord Moran, *The Anatomy of Courage* (London: Sphere Books, 1968) [1945], 18-19, 35-7; Hurst, *Medical Diseases of War* [1944], pp. 121–30.

mild traumatic brain injury (MTBI), claimed to be the signature injury of recent conflicts in Iraq and Afghanistan.[80]

Of course, it does matter that interest in physical theories peaked at the mid-point of the war and that the promotion of these theories continued after the war's end: this demonstrates there was no linear or absolute transition from physical to psychological modes of understanding. Likewise, Mott's physical theories of causation are important because they spurred the articulation of explicitly psychological theories and so helped to draw out the latent "psychological" potential in pre-war modes of explanation. But we should not use physical theories of causation as the litmus test of change within psychological medicine. Apart from a brief flare of excitement in 1916–17, these theories formed a minor part of medical discourse on "shell-shock" from the outset of the war until decades after its end. Physical theories were put forward in response to a novel feature of industrialized warfare, the use of massive quantities of high explosives. It is not really surprising that there was a short-lived vogue for these forms of explanation, or that most doctors preferred to develop other theoretical frameworks which emphasized "psychic", psychological, or emotional factors, or that some doctors refused to discount physical theories of causation some decades after the war. It makes more sense to ask how doctors employed, adapted, or rejected older forms of explanation for nervous and mental disorders. Here we must return to the role of heredity in theories of "shell-shock".

Mott's views on the prevalence of commotional shock changed over the course of the war. His belief in heredity as the most important predisposing factor in mental disorders did not.[81] In his 1916 lectures, Mott argued that the material and emotional conditions of trench warfare could 'exhaust and eventually even shatter the strongest nervous system'.[82] This acknowledgement seemed to mark a retreat from his pre-war insistence on heredity as the single most reliable determinant of mental disorder.[83] However, Mott continually undermined this apparently radical conclusion by insisting that 'neuropathic' individuals were more likely than the 'neuro-potentially sound' to break down in response to shell fire or other aspects of trench warfare.[84] In 1918 he instigated an investigation into the family and personal history of patients at the

---

[80] E. Jones, N.T. Fear, and S. Wessely, 'Shell Shock and Mild Traumatic Brain Injury: A Historical Review', *American Journal of Psychiatry*, 164 (2007), 1641–5.

[81] F.W. Mott, 'War Psychoses and Psychoneuroses', *JMS*, 64:265 (April 1918), 234.

[82] Mott, 'Lettsomian Lectures. I', 331.

[83] F.W. Mott, 'Heredity and Insanity', *Eugenics Review*, 2:4 (January 1911), 258; F.W. Mott, *Nature and Nurture in Mental Development*, pp. 64–5.

[84] Mott, 'Opening Paper', iii–v; 'Lettsomian Lectures. II', 448; 'Chadwick Lecture', 40.

Maudsley Hospital, which purported to discover 'a family history of neurotic or psychopathic stigmata' in 74 per cent of 'psycho-neurotic cases'.[85] For Mott, this statistic held the status of gospel truth.[86] Overall, hereditary predisposition played a more important part in Mott's theories of "shell-shock" than organic damage to the nervous system.[87] He believed that it contributed to breakdown in both emotional and commotional cases of "shell-shock": 'neuropathic' individuals would collapse under physical or emotional strain more quickly and severely than healthy men. Doctors sceptical of physical theories of causation put forward similar arguments.[88] Again, the absence of a physical explanation does not guarantee the presence of psychological approaches.

Although Mott reassessed his views on the pervasiveness of commotional shock, he never evolved a more sophisticated psychological position. His pre-war research on alcoholism and syphilis acknowledged the part of "psychic" factors in the production of disease as did his first publications on "shell-shock", but his attempts at psychological understanding were always naïve. Right up until his death, heredity remained the central pillar of his arguments about the causation of mental disorder.[89] It is even possible that the experience of treating "shell-shock" strengthened Mott's belief in the importance of heredity. In wartime, Mott displayed brisk sympathy for soldier patients, but his post-war work dissected the inadequacies of the conscript army. When the patriotic fervour surrounding "shell-shock" had faded, Mott publicly stated that the war had 'shown that a very considerable percentage of the male population are potential neuropaths, and it only required the necessary stress of fear and exhausting nervous strain to reveal the same'.[90] He lamented the sad consequences of treating these 'neuropaths': the

---

[85] Wolfsohn, 'Predisposing Factors of War Psycho-Neuroses', 180.

[86] F.W. Mott, 'Two Addresses on War Psycho-Neurosis. (I) Neurasthenia: The Disorders and Disabilities of Fear', *Lancet*, 26 January 1918, 127; F.W. Mott, 'Alcohol and Its Relations to Problems in Mental Disorders', in E.H. Starling, *The Action of Alcohol on Man* (London: Longmans, Green, 1923), p. 207.

[87] At least one obituarist identified Mott's finding that the war neuroses usually occurred in those of a 'constitutionally neuropathic disposition' as the most important aspect of his wartime research, and did not even mention his support for commotional theories. Anon., 'Obituary: Sir Frederick Mott', 1229.

[88] Wiltshire, 'Contribution to the Etiology of Shell Shock', 1209–10 explicitly argues against theories of concussion and commotion, but identifies 'neuropathic predisposition' or 'taint' as one of the most important factors in the production of war neurosis.

[89] F.W. Mott, 'Heredity in Relation to Mental Disease and Mental Deficiency', *BMJ*, 19 June 1926, 1023–6.

[90] F.W. Mott, 'The Psychopathology of Puberty and Adolescence', *JMS*, 67:278 (July 1921), 301; Anon., 'British Medical Association Special Clinical Meeting', 709; F.W. Mott, 'Body and Mind: The Origin of Dualism', *Lancet*, 7 January 1922, 4.

government now struggled with a crippling pensions bill, and inferior men had not been 'killed off to anything like the degree that the A1 physically and mentally sound men were'. War no longer stimulated 'the purifying effect that it had in ancient times when in the struggle for existence the mentally and physically strong alone could survive'.[91] Audiences listened to this crude and repugnant social Darwinism without protest. In Mott's case, the war did not foster greater psychological understanding. It hardened existing prejudices, and convinced him that civilization was in the throes of decline.

Suggestion, Hypnosis, and Therapeutic Conservatism

The uneven and complex effects of the war on British psychological medicine are perhaps most evident in the therapies deployed, created, revived, and adapted to manage and cure "shell-shock". From one perspective, medical treatment of "shell-shock" looks deeply conservative. Peter Leese has shown that the most common home front treatments for "shell-shock" consisted of conventional measures such as rest, massage, diet, and drugs.[92] Versions of Weir Mitchell's rest cure were still popular, especially for cases of neurasthenia and nervous exhaustion. Doctors removed the gross symptoms of hysteria using suggestion and hypnosis, but remained committed to rest and diet as measures to foster long-term improvement. Treatments based on mental and physical relaxation aimed to repair "nerves" by helping bodies to recover from exhaustion and providing a soothing atmosphere for minds troubled by war.[93] As in pre-war psychological medicine, diagnosis of the "psychic" origins of a disorder coexisted with conservative therapies which targeted the body. Mainstream therapeutic practice shows up the limitations of psychological knowledge.

The picture is quite different if we examine public discussion of therapies, which represented a different form of knowledge about "shell-shock" and often served different purposes. Conservative treatments did not attract much attention in the medical press. Archival records tell us about

---

[91] Mott, 'Psychopathology of Puberty and Adolescence', 302; Mott, 'The Neuroses and Psychoses in Relation to Conscription and Eugenics', 16.

[92] Leese, "Why Are They Not Cured?" On medicinal treatments, see L.A. Weatherly, 'The War and Neurasthenia, Psychasthenia and Mild Mental Disorders. II', *TMW*, 11 (July–December 1918), 265–6; P.C.C. Fenwick, 'Entero-Spasm Following Shell Shock', *Practitioner*, 98:4 (April 1917), 391.

[93] Anon., 'British Medical Association Special Clinical Meeting', 711; Hewat, 'Clinical Cases from Medical Division, Royal Victoria Hospital, Netley', 211–3; Hurst, 'War Neuroses and the Neuroses of Civil Life'; W. Harris, 'The Value of Sleep', *Practitioner*, 122:1 (January 1929), 19; Dillon, 'Neuroses among Combatant Troops', 66; Humphries and Kurchinski, 'Rest, Relax and Get Well'.

practice on the ground, but do not capture important differences between pre-war and wartime medical discourse on treatments for nervous and mental disorders, or how this discourse may have helped to change therapeutic practice. At the public level, the focus was on therapeutic experimentation, albeit usually within established bounds. The impetus for this experimentation was the need to return "shell-shocked" soldiers to productive roles within or outside the military. The results of these experiments were disseminated through the medical press, causing some doctors to adapt their approaches, and exposing many more to new ideas. This kind of influence cannot be precisely calculated.

For the most part, experimental treatments followed lines familiar within pre-war psychological medicine, and therefore remained within certain boundaries. The absence of physical theories and rejection of conservative therapies rarely led to adoption of sophisticated psychological theories and treatments. Most doctors readily accepted that "shell-shock" often constituted a "psychic" or emotional response to war experience. However, this acceptance was compatible with simplistic models of "psychic" functioning. In this view, war was terrifying; it scared and horrified men; fear and horror were expressed as hysterical or "nervous" symptoms, especially among those predisposed to neurotic illness; the doctor should remove symptoms, reassure the man that he was not "really" ill, and return him to productive service. As with physical, "psychic", and psychological theories, the important division is not between treatments focused on the body and those aimed at the mind. The relevant distinction is between treatments employing simplistic models of mental functioning and crude methods such as suggestion to remove hysterical manifestations, and those employing complex and fully articulated models of psychological functioning to tackle problems at the level of psychological process rather than that of the symptom. Most often, those wartime treatments which were not exclusively concerned with building up nervous strength aimed only to remove symptoms, most often through suggestion.

Applications of suggestion usually adhered to principles established within pre-war psychological medicine. This approach was used from the early months of the war, although over time suggestion attracted greater publicity and was employed more widely. Physicians often mixed methods of suggestion depending on symptom type or perceptions of likely responsiveness to particular procedures.[94] In the most basic form of this treatment, doctors made direct suggestions to the patient, often

---

[94] J.L.M. Symns, 'Hysteria as Seen at a Base Hospital', *Practitioner*, 101:2 (August 1918), 90–6.

supported by the creation of an 'atmosphere of cure' (by banning crutches and other visible signs of disability or showing patients other men previously cured by the same methods).[95] Another technique involved forcing the lost function into action, thereby demonstrating to the patient that there was nothing physically wrong with him. To this end, doctors stimulated the muscles of paralysed men using electricity, and put mute patients under anaesthesia in the hope that they would drift into speech.[96] In contrast to direct methods, some forms of suggestion were fundamentally dishonest, and tricked the patient into believing that a particular medical procedure had cured his somatic illness. William Reynell (1885–1948), neurological specialist to a Ministry of Pensions clinic, told patients suffering from hysterical vomiting that the insertion of a stomach tube before meals prevented stomach contractions after eating.[97] Although all suggestive techniques aimed only to remove symptoms, different methods incorporated quite different views of the doctor–patient relationship and the ethical responsibility of the physician to his patient.

The most notable champion of suggestion for "shell-shock" was Arthur Hurst (1879–1944), who served as consultant to the British forces in Salonika, neurologist to the Royal Victoria Hospital, Netley, and then as commanding officer of the Seale Hayne Military Hospital at Newton Abbot. Hurst initially employed eclectic methods including hypnotic suggestion and deception (he pretended to perform operations on soldiers suffering from hysterical deafness in order to convince them that he had dealt with a physical problem and thereby restored their hearing).[98]

[95] A.F. Grimbly, 'The Cure of Spinal Concussion in Warfare by Suggestion', *Practitioner*, 100:3 (March 1918), 292; Johnson, 'Hysterical Tremor'; F.W. Mott, 'The Lettsomian Lectures on the Effects of High Explosives Upon the Central Nervous System. III', *Lancet*, 11 March 1916, 553; F.W. Mott, 'Mental Hygiene in Relation to Insanity and Its Treatment', *Lancet*, 14 October 1922, 795; Anon., 'High Explosives and the Central Nervous System', *Nature*, 97 (March 1916), 114.

[96] Hewat, 'Clinical Cases from Medical Division, Royal Victoria Hospital, Netley', 211–12; Fraser, 'War Injuries of the Ear', 118-19; Stopford, 'So-Called Functional Symptoms in Organic Nerve Injuries', 796; Herringham, *A Physician in France*, p. 136. A form of "treatment" based on similar principles was jolting the patient out of his symptom through 'some novel and unexpected emotional or physical shock', although it seems that this was more often observed as an accidental effect of surprise than pursued as deliberate medical policy. See for example Leonard Guthrie in 'Special Discussion on Shell Shock', xli.

[97] W.R. Reynell, 'Hysterical Vomiting in Soldiers', *Lancet*, 4 January 1919, 18–20.

[98] Hurst, 'Observations on the Etiology and Treatment of War Neuroses'; A.F. Hurst and E.A. Peters, 'A Report on the Pathology, Diagnosis, and Treatment of Absolute Hysterical Deafness in Soldiers', *Lancet*, 6 October 1917, 517–9; A.F. Hurst and J.L.M. Symns, 'The Rapid Cure of Hysterical Symptoms in Soldiers', *Lancet*, 3 August 1918, 139–41; A.F. Hurst, 'The Bent Back of Soldiers', *BMJ*, 7 December 1918, 621–3. Unsurprisingly, other doctors decried fake operations as dishonest and dangerous. See C.S. Myers, 'Correspondence: The Justifiability of Therapeutic Lying', *Lancet*, 27 December 1919, 1213–14.

By the end of the war, Hurst and his co-workers had concluded that most patients could be cured through persuasion and re-education alone.[99] But before this, Hurst gained a short-lived reputation for "miracle" cures, partly based on the propaganda film *War Neuroses* (1917) which used re-enactments and judicious editing to showcase his successes.[100] Hurst and his medical officers were disappointed if they had not removed hysterical symptoms 'within twenty-four hours of admission', and boasted that one aphonic patient had been dispatched in 'thirty seconds'.[101] Although few could match this speed, supporters of suggestion often emphasized its swiftness.[102] Opponents argued that removal of symptoms did not deal with their underlying causes, whether nervous exhaustion or severe emotional disturbance, and therefore suggestion did not achieve lasting cures.[103] Charles Myers likened the use of suggestion to the practice of 'a surgeon who might attempt to get rid of an abscess by opening it where it pointed, neglecting to follow up the pus to the original source from which it had tracked'.[104]

Similar objections were raised against hypnosis, but here the opposition was much more virulent.[105] Hypnosis struck at the ideals of

[99] In Hurst's version of persuasion and re-education, the doctor appealed to the patient's reason to establish recovery and then taught him to perform the lost function again. Symns, 'Hysteria as Seen at a Base Hospital', 96; Hurst, *Medical Diseases of the War* [1918], p. 33; Shephard, *War of Nerves*, pp. 78–80.

[100] A.F. Hurst, 'Cinematograph Demonstration of War Neuroses', Section of Neurology, *PRSM*, 11:2 (1917–18), 39–42; E. Jones, 'War Neuroses and Arthur Hurst: A Pioneering Medical Film about the Treatment of Psychiatric Battle Casualties', *Journal of the History of Medicine and Allied Sciences*, 67:3 (2012), 345–73; J.B. Köhne, 'Visualising "War Hysterics": Strategies of Feminization and Re-Masculinization in Scientific Cinematography, 1916–1918', in C. Hämmerle, O. Überegger and B. Bader Zaar (eds), *Gender and the First World War* (Basingstoke and New York: Palgrave Macmillan, 2014).

[101] Anon., 'Reports of Societies: War Neuroses', *BMJ*, 23 March 1918, 345; Anon., 'Reviews: The Treatment of Hysteria', *BMJ*, 9 November 1918, 516; C.H.L. Rixon, 'The Hysterical Perpetuation of Symptoms', *Lancet*, 15 March 1919, 417–9.

[102] P.R. Cooper, 'Correspondence: Treatment of "Shell Shock"', and W. Milligan, 'Correspondence: Treatment of "Shell Shock"', *BMJ*, 12 August 1916, 242–3; H. Smurthwaite, 'War Neuroses', Laryngological Section, *PRSM*, 11 (Parts 1 and 2) (June 1918), 182–5; G.L. Scott, 'Hysterical "Paralysis" of Long Standing', *Practitioner*, 101:2 (August 1918), 97.

[103] Davy, 'Address on Some War Diseases', 837; see also letters under the heading 'Correspondence: Treatment of War Neuroses', *Lancet*, 17 August 1918, 219; 7 September 1918, 341–2; and 14 September 1918, 370–1; T.A. Ross, 'The Prevention of Relapse of Hysterical Manifestations', *Lancet*, 19 October 1918, 516–7; W. Brown, 'Hypnosis, Suggestion, and Dissociation', *BMJ*, 14 June 1919, 734–6; E. Prideaux, 'Stammering in the War Psycho-Neuroses', *Lancet*, 8 February 1919, 217–18.

[104] C.S. Myers, *Present-Day Applications of Psychology with Special Reference to Industry, Education and Nervous Breakdown* (London: Methuen, 1918), pp. 40–1.

[105] For accounts of hypnotic treatment, see A.W. Ormond, 'The Treatment of "Concussion Blindness"', *Journal of the RAMC*, 26:1 (January 1916), 44; J.B.

rationality, autonomy, and self-control – indeed, at the very heart of manly character. Alongside Freudian psychoanalysis, hypnosis was the most controversial form of treatment for "shell-shock".[106] The disreputable heritage of hypnosis – the charlatanism of Mesmer, the predatory powers of Svengali and, most recently, the menace of Freudianism – was never far from the minds of medical critics.[107] Use of hypnosis in cases of "shell-shock" often prompted outrage, although some doctors defended its employment in the exceptional circumstances of wartime.[108] Antagonists argued that hypnosis deepened tendencies towards suggestibility and dissociation, and warned against suppressing the subject's capacity for willed action.[109] Hypnosis involved no effort from the patient, and so tended 'towards deterioration and weakness' rather than 'development and strengthening of the character'.[110] This analysis of medical power could be extended to all forms of suggestion. As Paul Lerner notes, all such techniques 'sought to restore the patient's control over his own body, but paradoxically, in doing so ... demanded that the doctor wield full control and authority over the patient's mind and body'.[111]

Wartime doctors were aware of these power dynamics. Even proponents of suggestion agreed that the method worked through 'the dominance of a strong mind over a weak one', and boiled down to 'essentially a contest between the physician's personality and that of the hysterical patient'.[112] Most freely acknowledged that suggestion was an unsophisticated method. At best, deliberate use of suggestion was depicted as heightening the element of suggestive hope present in all forms of

Tombleson, 'An Account of Twenty Cases Treated by Hypnotic Suggestion', *Journal of the RAMC*, 29:3 (September 1917), 340–6; Myers, 'Contributions to the Study of Shell Shock (II)'.

[106] In Germany, the hypnotic 'miracle cures' of hysterical soldiers achieved by the neurologist Max Nonne provoked similar fears and objections. See P. Lerner, 'Hysterical Cures: Hypnosis, Gender and Performance in World War I and Weimar Germany', *History Workshop Journal*, 45 (1998), 79–101.

[107] See R. Harris, *Murders and Madness: Medicine, Law, and Society in the Fin de Siècle* (Oxford: Clarendon, 1989); D. Pick, *Svengali's Web: The Alien Enchanter in Modern Culture* (New Haven, CT, and London: Yale University Press, 2000); D. Forrest, *Hypnotism: A History* (London: Penguin, 1999).

[108] See correspondence under the heading 'Hypnosis in Hysteria', *Lancet*, 21 September 1918, 404–5; 28 September 1918, 433; and 5 October 1918, 471; under the heading 'Hypnotism', *Times*, 22, 23 and 25 April 1919; and under the heading 'Hypnotism, Suggestion, and Dissociation', *BMJ*, 12 May 1919, 561; 19 May 1919, 592–3; 17 May 1919, 624–5; and 31 May 1919, 693.

[109] Shaw, 'Considerations on the Occult', 1474.

[110] Anon., 'Reviews: Sane Psycho-Therapy', *BMJ*, 23 October 1915, 605.

[111] Lerner, *Hysterical Men*, p. 122.

[112] Anon., 'Medical Societies: Royal Society of Medicine', *Lancet*, 23 March 1918, 438; Stewart, 'Treatment of War Neuroses', 20.

medical treatment.[113] At worst, it was portrayed as a "primitive" art form.[114] Rivers concluded a lecture series on 'Medicine, Magic and Religion' by stating that from 'the psychological point of view the difference between the rude arts I have described in these lectures and much of our own medicine is not one of kind, but only of degree'.[115] Although suggestion worked on the mind, it did not constitute a properly psychological form of treatment. However, practical familiarity with suggestion encouraged some doctors to ask further questions about the operation of the mind, and so fostered greater engagement with the psychological. In itself, suggestion was not radical, but its practice set some doctors on the road to radical conclusions. Suggestion demonstrated the manipulability of the mind, and encouraged doctors to try to replicate or extend its results using methods not open to the same objections. It therefore inspired exploration of psychological processes. As doctors conceded that suggestion did not tackle the ultimate cause of neurosis and therefore could not prevent relapse, they sought forms of explanation and modes of treatment which might achieve what suggestion could not.

Psychodynamic and Psychoanalytic Approaches

Doctors unsatisfied with physical remedies or suggestive techniques often explored psychodynamic approaches, most notably psychoanalysis. Many historians now argue that the experience of "shell-shock" did not, as was once thought, overturn the dominant explanatory frameworks of British psychological medicine by encouraging mass conversions to Freudianism.[116] Certainly, psychoanalysis "proper" did not enter the medical mainstream in wartime, and even the most committed British doctors significantly modified Freudian theories in their own approaches to "shell-shock". The reviewer who described Charles Myers as advancing 'a point of view that approximates towards that of psychoanalysis' nicely captured the tentative nature of British explorations of

---

[113] Anon., 'The Psychical Factor in Therapeutics', *BMJ*, 22 December 1917, 836–7.

[114] R.R. Marett, 'The Primitive Medicine-Man', Section of the History of Medicine, *PRSM*, 11 (Parts 1 and 2) (1917–18), 49; Anon., 'Some Methods of Treatment Exercised by the Ancient Australian Medicine Men', *King's College Hospital Gazette*, 3 (October 1924), 508–11.

[115] W.H.R. Rivers, 'The Fitzpatrick Lectures on Medicine, Magic, and Religion. II', *Lancet*, 15 January 1916, 122.

[116] J. Bourke, *Dismembering the Male: Men's Bodies, Britain and the Great War* (London: Reaktion Books, 1999), p. 121; D.J. Poynter, '"Regeneration" Revisited: W.H.R. Rivers and Shell Shock during the Great War', in M. Hughes and M. Seligmann (eds.), *Leadership in Conflict 1914–1918* (Barnsley, South Yorkshire: Leo Cooper, 2000), p. 237; Jones and Wessely, 'Impact of Total War', 136–7.

Freudianism.[117] Wartime revisions of psychoanalytic theory and practice demonstrate the continuing influence of pre-war modes of thought and the limitations of medical engagement with Freud. However, the war did cause an upsurge of critical interest in psychodynamic approaches to mind which built on the conceptual assimilations of the pre-war period and steadily ripened in the decades after the armistice. This process of change was multidirectional, complex, and accommodated many apparent contradictions.

A case in point is British modifications to Freudian theory, especially the radical rejection of an exclusively sexual aetiology for war-related neurosis.[118] Even Ernest Jones (1879–1958), Freud's most active British disciple, claimed at times that the instinct of self-preservation was more important than the sexual instinct in the development of "shell-shock".[119] Although British objections to Freud did not focus exclusively on the sexual elements of his theory, these definitely provoked more extreme hostility than other aspects of psychoanalysis. When the physician David Forsyth (1877–1941) postulated a psychoanalytic interpretation of "shell-shock", diagnosing one patient as 'a case of unconscious homosexuality with well-marked anal eroticism' and another as 'anxiety hysteria, together with a strong Oedipus complex', he prompted a four-month-long debate in the correspondence columns of the *Lancet*.[120] The most antagonistic comments centred on the corruption of innocent patients by psychoanalytic 'filth'.[121] The vituperative response to Forsyth's article was at odds with the accommodation of psychodynamic theories in pre-war medical

[117] Anon., 'Reviews: Charles Myers, Present-Day Applications of Psychology with Special Reference to Industry, Education and Nervous Breakdown', *British Journal of Psychology*, 9:2 (October 1918), 259.

[118] W.H.R. Rivers, 'A Case of Claustrophobia', *Lancet*, 18 August 1917, 239; F. Dillon, 'The Analysis of a Composite Neurosis', *Lancet*, 11 January 1919, 57–60; T.A. Ross, 'Certain Inter-Relations between Peace and War Neuroses', Section of Neurology, *PRSM*, 12 (Parts 1 and 2) (1918–19), 20.

[119] E. Jones, 'War Shock and Freud's Theory of the Neuroses', Section of Psychiatry, *PRSM*, 11:3 (April 1918), 31–3. He later criticized Rivers' 'simplistic' insistence on the primacy of the instinct of self-preservation in the causation of war neurosis. See E. Jones, 'The Psychopathology of Anxiety', *British Journal of Medical Psychology*, 9:1 (1929), 24, fn. 1.

[120] D. Forsyth, 'Functional Nerve Disease and the Shock of Battle: A Study of the So-Called Traumatic Neuroses Arising in Connexion with the War', *Lancet*, 25 December 1915, 1402.

[121] C.A. Mercier, 'Correspondence: Functional Nervous Disease', *Lancet*, 15 January 1916. See other correspondence under this heading, *Lancet*, 22 January 1916, 210–11; 29 January 1916, 265; 5 February 1916, 318; 12 February 1916, 373; 19 February 1916, 430; 11 March 1919, 588–9; 29 April 1916, 933–4; and 6 May 1919, 971. For a similarly antagonistic response to psychoanalytic approaches, see 'Correspondence: Psycho-Analysis', *BMJ*, 6 January 1917, 32–3; 13 January 1917, 64–5; and 20 January 1917, 102–4.

discourse. Venomous refutations of Forsyth's analysis further demonstrate the process of differentiation between approaches to "shell-shock": full articulation of a psychoanalytical interpretation of war neurosis prompted the elaboration of opposing views. However, this furore was also prompted by the application of a fairly straightforward Freudian interpretation *to* *soldiers*. The rejection of sexual aetiologies, especially in W.H.R. Rivers' thoughtful and extended discussions, was applauded by those unsympathetic towards Freud, and probably convinced some members of the medical community to engage more closely with other aspects of psychoanalytic theory.[122] But in point of fact, most psychoanalytically oriented doctors did not reject the sexual aetiology of neurosis lock, stock, and barrel. Rather, they argued that the sexual origins of neurosis might be important in civilian cases, even if Freud had concentrated too exclusively on this aspect, but that the shock and strain of warfare was sufficient to explain breakdown in otherwise "normal" men.[123]

This emphasis on war as a stressor of abnormal severity helps to explain an apparently paradoxical fact about the potential role of "shell-shock" as a catalyst for change within British psychological medicine: although as a consequence of the war many doctors read Freud more closely and started to formulate psychodynamic theories of mind, this did not lead to the adoption of complex psychotherapeutic methods. Of course, war conditions were not conducive to full-blown psychoanalysis. Doctors had little time and even fewer resources, and needed to treat or discharge men as quickly as possible. But more important was the belief that breakdown in soldiers had been triggered, if not caused, by recent war experience, and so treatment did not need to unearth 'hidden psychical trauma and its buried complexes'.[124] Even David Eder, one of the founder members of the London Psycho-Analytical Society, accepted this view and treated only five patients from a series of one hundred cases by psychoanalysis.[125] Mass breakdown in apparently

---

[122] Burton-Fanning, 'Neurasthenia in Soldiers', 911; Hurst, *Medical Diseases of the War* [1918], pp. 73–5.

[123] M.D. Eder, *War-Shock: The Psycho-Neuroses in War Psychology and Treatment* (London: William Heinemann, 1917), p. 12; W.H.R. Rivers, *Instinct and the Unconscious: A Contribution to a Biological Theory of the Psycho-Neuroses* (Cambridge: Cambridge University Press, 1920), pp. 136–8; Mott, 'Two Addresses on War Psycho-Neurosis. (I)', 128.

[124] Harris, *Nerve Injuries and Shock*, p. 106; Stewart, 'Treatment of War Neuroses', 16, 24; Collie, 'Management of Neurasthenia', 10; E.F. Ballard, 'The Psychoneurotic Temperament and Its Reactions to Military Service', *JMS*, 64:267 (October 1918), 374–5; Eager, 'Record of Admissions', 294–5; R. Eager, 'The Early Treatment of Mental Disorders', *Lancet*, 27 September 1919, 559.

[125] Eder, 'Address on the Psycho-Pathology of the War Neuroses', 268.

healthy young men encouraged doctors to explore unfamiliar approaches to mind, but the existence of war as the factor decisively tipping men into psychiatric illness discouraged the full application of psychoanalytic therapies. Ultimately, most doctors believed that war itself precipitated the development of "shell-shock" – sooner in the physically or mentally unstable, later in the physically and mentally sound, but eventually it would weaken all men. The therapeutic rationale of psychoanalysis was undermined by this combination of wartime constraints on practice and the belief that latent weakness had risen to the surface only through the extreme stress of war. The war simultaneously provoked, limited, and contained the potentially radical effects on psychological medicine of intellectual engagement with psychoanalytic theory.

The incomplete application of analytic therapies to "shell-shock" also extended the characteristic conceptual and practical strategies of pre-war psychological medicine. As shown in Chapter 2, popular therapies for functional disorders reflected views of mind and body as indissolubly linked and sought to strengthen body, mind, and character. This approach to treatment assumed no strict correlation between the dominant causative factor in illness – partly because this was ultimately unknown – and specific therapeutic measures. The pragmatism of pre-war British psychological medicine left doctors open to engagement with psychological theorization, but limited their embrace of it. The same process is seen in wartime flirtations with psychoanalysis.[126] Walter Duncanson Chambers (1886?–1958), an asylum psychiatrist who served with the RAMC in France, diagnosed an 'oedipus-complex' in one young officer; his treatment extended no further than sending the man back to his unit 'to look for his manhood once more'.[127] Paul Bousfield, physician to the Lancaster Clinic of Psychotherapy, introduced examples of 'an abnormal erotic condition', 'infantile fixations', and 'a strong "father complex"' into his discussion of treatment of the war neuroses through lowering blood pressure (he did not claim this was the only possible method of treatment).[128] The "translations", accommodations, and partial assimilations of pre-war approaches to psychological theories carried over into wartime.

This is illustrated by responses to W.H.R. Rivers' theory of the role of repression in war neurosis. Rivers argued that the most severe symptoms

---

[126] Fearnsides, 'Essentials of Treatment', 47.

[127] W.D. Chambers, 'Mental Wards with the British Expeditionary Force: A Review of Ten Months' Experience', *JMS*, 65:270 (July 1919), 171.

[128] P. Bousfield, 'The Relation of Blood-Pressure to the Psycho-Neuroses', *Practitioner*, 101:5 (November 1918), 270.

of war neurosis were caused by attempts to banish distressing memories from consciousness, and that the recovery and reintegration of these memories into a coherent personal narrative of war experience could significantly relieve symptoms.[129] In 1919, Millais Culpin, a surgical specialist who retrained in psychology as a result of his war experience, concluded that the therapeutic value of the revival of repressed memories was 'the most important lesson taught us by the war'. But Culpin also complained that this topic was not even mentioned by other participants at a recent meeting on the war neuroses.[130] As this suggests, some physicians either did not understand Rivers' argument or denied its validity. When Rivers first delivered his paper on the repression of war experience to the psychiatric section of the Royal Society of Medicine, one respondent suggested that talking about war experiences perpetuated symptoms, and recommended trout-fishing as a way to dispel memories of warfare.[131] Acknowledgement of the emotional origins of war neurosis easily coexisted with recommendations for doctors 'to induce "self-for-getfulness"' and teach patients *not* to think about their war experi-ences.[132] However, doctors who did agree with Rivers also "translated" into more familiar terms his argument that expression of emotion relieved symptoms. Laughton Scott (1887?–1953), another physician to the Lancaster Clinic of Psychotherapy, spoke quite simply of the benefits of 'confession'.[133] This selective appropriation of elements of Rivers' theory, as well as the specific language of assimilation, echoes pre-war approaches to Freudian psychoanalysis.

---

[129] W.H.R. Rivers, 'An Address on the Repression of War Experience', *Lancet*, 2 February 1918, 173–7.

[130] M. Culpin, 'Correspondence: The Discussion on War Neuroses', *BMJ*, 19 April 1919, 501. Culpin admitted that when he had been unable to find a cause for patients' mental conflicts, he too had fallen back on the advice to repress their troubles; Culpin, *Psychoneuroses of Peace and War*, p. 121. For further controversy over the value of the theory of repression, see A. Carver, 'Forgetting: Psychological Repression', *BMJ*, 10 January 1920, 46–7, and subsequent correspondence under the heading 'Forgetting: Psychological Repression', *BMJ*, 17 January–21 February 1920.

[131] C.M. Tuke in 'Discussion: The Repression of War Experience', Section of Psychiatry, *PRSM*, 11:3 (1917–18), 20.

[132] J.E. Middlemiss, 'Correspondence: The Treatment of War Psycho-Neuroses', *BMJ*, 21 December 1918, 700; Anon., 'Treatment of War Psycho-Neuroses'; F.C. Forster, 'The Management of Neurasthenia, Psychasthenia, Shell-Shock, and Allied Conditions', *Practitioner*, 100:1 (January 1918), 86–8; R.T. Williamson, 'Remarks on the Treatment of Neurasthenia and Psychasthenia Following Shell Shock', *BMJ*, 1 December 1917, 715; White, 'Observations on Shell Shock and Neurasthenia', 422; Hale-White, 'Address on Some Applications of Experience', 229.

[133] G.L. Scott, 'The Anxiety State – An Aspect of Treatment', *Practitioner*, 102:4 (April 1919), 222, 224.

Assimilation and "translation" characterized wartime encounters with psychoanalysis. Although the word 'psychoanalysis' appeared in the medical press frequently from 1918, this usually indicated little more than lip service to the talking cure. Quite often, when doctors referred to 'psychoanalysis' in their own practice, they meant only that the physician should have a long conversation with the patient about his war experiences, and continued to stress their distance from Freud's theories and techniques.[134] This stratagem was noted by other doctors, who saw it as evidence that despite all the chatter about novel "psychic" theories, new names only cloaked older approaches and explanations.[135] Accommodation without fundamental revision – described previously as welding rather than assimilation – is also evident. The second edition of R.H. Cole's textbook of nervous and mental disorders, published in 1919, was scattered with new references to Freud. But these involved no more than a sentence or two inserted into the existing text. Cole took account of the surge of interest in Freudian and other psychological theories, but did not alter his general framework of explanation as a result of exposure to these ideas.[136]

Because so few "shell-shock" doctors fully endorsed psychoanalysis, the qualified and tentative characterization "analytic" best describes those who engaged with psychoanalytic ideas. "Analytic" is not a synonym for "psychoanalytic". Military doctors did not employ psychoanalysis "proper" as a treatment for "shell-shock". "Analytic" is used here as an umbrella label for doctors who displayed keen interest in the psychodynamic theories of Continental physicians, and sought to understand how their therapeutic techniques might be modified to provide effective care in wartime conditions. These "analytic" doctors also drew on modes of conceptual assimilation familiar from pre-war psychological medicine, and employed an eclectic mix of therapeutic methods which did not neatly match up to particular theories of mind.

[134] D.E. Core, 'Some Mechanisms at Work in the Evolution of Hysteria', *Lancet*, 9 March 1918, 369; Fearnsides, 'Essentials of Treatment', 47–8; R.H. Trotter, 'Neurasthenic and Hysterical Cases in General Military Hospitals', *Lancet*, 23 November 1918, 704; Stewart, 'Treatment of War Neuroses', 16, 24; Collie, 'Management of Neurasthenia', 10; Ballard, 'Psychoneurotic Temperament', 374–5; Eager, 'A Record of Admissions', 294–5; Eager, 'Early Treatment of Mental Disorders', 559.

[135] R. Armstrong-Jones in 'Discussion: Observations on the Rolandic Area in a Series of Cases of Insanity', *JMS*, 64:267 (October 1918), 363; see Anon., 'Review: *The New Psychiatry* by W.H.B. Stoddart', *EMJ*, 16 (January–June 1916), 152.

[136] Cole, *Mental Diseases: A Text-Book of Psychiatry for Medical Students and Practitioners* [1913], pp. 28, 216, 221; 2nd edn [1919], pp. 31, 220, 225.

"Analytic" doctors worked with a sophisticated model of psychological functioning which incorporated understanding of unconscious processes and the complex interaction of previous events in the patient's life history with the effects of more recent war experience in the formation of neurosis. They employed psychological analysis, including techniques derived from psychoanalysis, for diagnostic purposes. Most tried to elicit patients' lost memories and to prevent the repression of emotion associated with distressing incidents, but also treated patients with non-analytic therapies such as suggestion, persuasion, and re-education.[137] Apart from Rivers, few "analytic" doctors provided elaborate theorizations of mental processes. They drew lightly on the technical vocabulary of psychology, instead using plain language such as 'interview' and 'heart-to-heart discussion' to describe therapeutic encounters. It was common to underplay the specialist skills necessary for analysis, and to claim that drawing out a patient's war experience demanded no 'expert knowledge, but simply common sense, discreet sympathy, and tact'.[138] Finally, these doctors made sense of psychological theories and therapies through analogies to other scientific and medical activities such as chemical analysis, anatomical dissection, diagnosis of physical ailments, and surgical operations.[139] Such comparisons tamed and normalized psychodynamic theories.

These modes of presentation might be viewed as mere rhetorical strategies designed to soften the public reception of controversial material. The psychologist T.H. Pear (1886–1972), co-author of *Shell-Shock and Its Lessons* (1917), one of the major wartime publications in the "analytic" mould, claimed as much in his unpublished reminiscences.[140] Wartime outbreaks of hostility towards psychoanalysis led some sympathizers to dissociate themselves from Freudianism. For example, Millais Culpin displayed thoughtful fascination with Freudian dream interpretation in his publications, but felt compelled to disavow descriptions of his methods as 'psycho-analytical'.[141] However, the separation between

---

[137] See, for example, Eder, *War-Shock*, pp. 132–4; C. McDowall, 'Mutism in the Soldier and Its Treatment', *JMS*, 64:264 (January 1918), 63–4. On therapeutic eclecticism, see Jones, 'Shell Shock at Maghull and the Maudsley', 388.

[138] Smith, 'Shock and the Soldier. I', 814; Ross, 'Prevention of Relapse', 517; C. McDowall, 'Functional Gastric Disturbance in the Soldier', *JMS*, 63:260 (January 1917), 88; 'Discussion: Functional Gastric Disturbance in the Soldier', 147.

[139] Smith, 'Shock and the Soldier. I', 816; G.E. Smith and T.H. Pear, *Shell Shock and Its Lessons*, 2nd edn (Manchester: Manchester University Press, 1918), pp. 54–7; Eder, *War-Shock*, pp. 4, 115, 130, 139.

[140] Jones, 'Shell Shock at Maghull and the Maudsley', 384.

[141] M. Culpin, 'Dreams and Their Value in Treatment', *Practitioner*, 102:3 (March 1919), 162; Culpin, 'Correspondence: The Discussion on War Neuroses', 501. Grafton Elliot

diagnostic theory and therapeutic practice in the work of "analytic" doctors cannot be simply written off as a tactical posture. There is evidence of genuine scepticism towards certain elements of psychoanalysis, as when Grafton Elliot Smith (1871–1937) uncompromisingly described Freudian dream interpretation as a mass of 'repulsive excrescences'.[142] But most importantly, there is no fundamental contradiction between the view that "analytic" doctors pursued certain rhetorical strategies in their presentation of psychodynamic theories, and the view that these modes of presentation demonstrate continuities with the conceptual approaches of pre-war psychological medicine. The witting and unwitting choice of particular rhetorical strategies reveals the existence in British medical culture of shared ways of thinking and approaching problems. For example, "analytic" doctors were not the only physicians to compare psychotherapy to surgical operations: the same comparison was made by psychoanalysts defending their claim to scientific expertise, and by medical men warning their colleagues about the dangers of amateur investigations into the unconscious.[143] In war as in peace, British doctors integrated psychological modes of explanation with existing approaches to mind and its disorders.

Conclusion

In 1919, Robert Armstrong-Jones attempted to elucidate some of the newer theories of mind for a general medical audience. He explained that 'the simile has been advanced that the Mind is a constant running stream of consciousness, like a mighty river'. To help his readers understand what this comparison meant, Armstrong-Jones proposed an act of imagination:

If we could picture for one moment the river Thames as frozen solid from its source to its outlet, and we were to divide it across, say, at Blackfriars Bridge, then if we could turn up each divided end and look at it, we should get a view of our own consciousness at a particular time and place; but if we were to contemplate the whole course of the river, then we should have the whole human mind during any one life-time.[144]

Smith and Thomas Pear also denied they were psychoanalysts: G.E. Smith, 'Correspondence: Functional Nervous Disease', Lancet, 6 May 1916, 971; Smith and Pear, 'Letters to the Editor', 64.

[142] G.E. Smith, 'Preface', in W.H.R. Rivers, Conflict and Dream (London: Kegan Paul, Trench, Trubner 1923), p. vii.

[143] E. Jones, 'Correspondence: Functional Nervous Disease', Lancet, 11 March 1916, 589; Robertson, 'Teaching of Mental Diseases in Edinburgh', 234.

[144] R. Armstrong-Jones, 'Mental and Nervous States in Connection with the War and Their Mechanism', Practitioner, 103:5 (November 1919), 325–6.

If the stream of consciousness is the paradigmatic metaphor of psycho-dynamic psychology, then freezing the stream and chopping it up into separate components represents equally well the characteristic response of mainstream British psychological medicine to the challenges posed by new forms of psychological thought and practice.[145] For the most part, British doctors struggled to assimilate psychodynamic approaches to mind, and employed the same conceptual strategies for handling psychological theories already in use before 1914.

At the same time, the effects of the "shell-shock" epidemic on British psychological medicine were more complex than sometimes assumed. At the beginning of the war, doctors did not adopt exclusively and uncompromisingly organicist positions on the likely origins of "shell-shock". Elaborate physical theories of causation emerged alongside "psychological" explanations of the war neuroses. Although psychological modes of understanding became more prominent in the later years of the war, they did not displace physical theories of causation. Older forms of explanation emphasizing the interplay of "psychic" and somatic elements in nervous and mental disorders remained commonplace throughout the war. Theorists who concentrated on physical factors in the development of "shell-shock" did not exclude emotional and psychological elements from their accounts, and those who focused on "psychological" explanations did not deny the potential role of physical factors in at least some cases.[146] Moreover, after a temporary suspension of (public) belief in heredity as a significant aetiological factor in war-related breakdown, many doctors reverted to their pre-war positions on the importance of inherited predisposition. The differentiation of physical and psychological modes of understanding proved crucial in the long-term development of British psychological medicine, but there was not steady progress towards psychological thought. The processes of change were uneven, multidirectional, and never complete.[147]

---

[145] Armstrong-Jones approached the study of the stream of consciousness in the manner of an anatomist or pathologist. John Herbert Parsons explained why this method was not appropriate to psychology: 'In dealing in this manner with a living moving stream, such as the stream of human consciousness, the anatomical method fails through freezing everything into a static condition. The anatomist's dry bones can be made to live only by the physiologist's study of the parts in motion – the play of the muscles, the circulation of the blood, the telegraphic impulses along the nerves, and so on. So the psychologist, though he is forced to study mental processes by a method of analysis, must correct the distortions which he thus artificially produces by constant reference to the everlasting and continuous flow of consciousness'. Parsons, *Mind and the Nation*, pp. 60–1.

[146] Jones, 'Shell Shock at Maghull and the Maudsley', 381–2.

[147] See Mathew Thomson's excellent short discussion of some of these issues: *Psychological Subjects*, pp. 182–6.

What really matters is not whether a psychological revolution occurred within the span of four years, but what those four years meant for British psychological medicine over the longer period. The war exposed doctors who had not previously specialized in nervous and mental disorders to the frailties of the human mind and demanded that they do everything possible to patch up broken men. As a result, doctors engaged with new theories of mind and rejected prejudices against older forms of treatment such as suggestion. The effects of "shell-shock" on British psychological medicine cannot be reduced to what happened in the moment of war. This is partly because the war simultaneously provoked and constrained radical reassessments. It forced doctors to reconsider the causes of breakdown, but provided a ready-made and exceptional explanation for "shell-shock". It demanded they find methods of treatment, but allowed them no time to explore more elaborate psychotherapeutic measures. It made them realize that any man could break down, but provided no answers as to why not every man did. The effects of war on psychological thought cannot be neatly wrapped up, quantified, and confined to a discrete period of time. War familiarized doctors with new ways of thinking about psychological problems, but these innovatory approaches coexisted with older therapeutic measures and modes of understanding. The experience of 1914–18 stretched rather than broke the explanatory frameworks of pre-war psychological medicine. But stretched far enough, any shape will eventually become unrecognizable.

4   Reading Silences
Gender and Class in Medical Discourse on "Shell-Shock"

Introduction

In keeping with their preferred self-image as men of science, early twentieth-century doctors were not much given to public declamations of poetry. An exception was made at the inaugural meeting of the 1910–11 session of the King's College Hospital Medical Society, which concluded with a reading of 'a new and stirring poem by Rudyard Kipling entitled "If–"'.[1] The poem paid tribute to the 'heroic' colonial statesman Leander Starr Jameson (1853–1917), now usually remembered for his role in a failed raid against the Boer government in 1895. The victorious tone of the poem belies its origins in military defeat, and 'If –' is often seen as emblematic of a certain brand of blithely unreflective and blindly confident imperial masculinity.[2] The poem is a verse shopping list of components to build the ideal man, one who can:

> ... force your heart and nerve and sinew
> To serve your turn long after they are gone,
> And so hold on when there is nothing in you
> Except the Will which says to them: 'Hold on!'

Above all, Kipling's masculine ideal was characterized by self-control and willpower.[3] This representation chimed with the values of certain audiences in Britain, where it became a set piece for rote learning in public schools, and worldwide: it was soon translated into twenty-seven languages.[4] The model of manly behaviour set out in the poem also clearly appealed to members of the King's College Hospital Medical

---

[1] KCHMSA: KHU/C1/M8, Opening Meeting, KCH Medical Society (14 October 1910).
[2] On the masculine stereotype, see G. Mosse, *The Image of Man: The Creation of Modern Masculinity* (New York and Oxford: Oxford University Press, 1996).
[3] P. Kaarsholm, 'Kipling and Masculinity', in R. Samuel (ed.), *Patriotism: The Making and Unmaking of British National Identity. Volume 3: National Fictions* (London: Routledge, 1989), pp. 215–26.
[4] R. Kipling, *Something of Myself: For My Friends Known and Unknown* (London: Penguin, 1988) [1937], p. 146.

Society. The enthusiastic reaction to 'If–' in this setting gives some clue as to the aspirant visions of masculinity that inspired doctors to join up and shaped their clinical encounters with "shell-shocked" men.

'If–' hymned the values of a middle-class model of masculinity.[5] Some historians have argued that this model, centred on the attributes of physical vigour, independence, self-restraint, honour, and commitment to work and home, was seriously damaged by the experience of war.[6] "Shell-shock" transformed the upright bearers of stiff upper lips to quivering, jerky, stuttering messes of men. It is a striking visual symbol of the fractured carapace of bourgeois Edwardian masculinity.[7] As an emblem of the devastation of war, "shell-shock" slots neatly into debates on war and social change. From the 1960s onwards, historians began to emphasize the disruptive effects of war on established class and gender relations.[8] However, it is now more common for scholars to underline the temporary, contingent, and limited nature of wartime shifts in class and gender relations.[9] Where does "shell-shock" fit into these debates?

This chapter probes how doctors exploited the ambivalences of pre-war diagnostic categories to construct highly gendered and classed concepts of "shell-shock", but simultaneously denied the operation of gender or class in the disorder. This denial looks very radical when placed against pre-war medical discourse saturated with assumptions

---

[5] On bourgeois masculinity, see J. Tosh, 'Masculinities in an Industrializing Society: Britain, 1800–1914', *Journal of British Studies*, 44 (2005), 332–5.

[6] Light, *Forever England*, pp. 66–75; J. Rutherford, *Forever England: Reflections on Race, Masculinity and Empire* (London: Lawrence and Wishart, 1997), pp. 72–3; Barham, *Forgotten Lunatics of the Great War*, pp. 161–4.

[7] G. Koureas, *Memory, Masculinity and National Identity in British Visual Culture, 1914–1930: A Study of 'Unconquerable Manhood'* (Aldershot: Ashgate, 2007), pp. 118–19.

[8] On class, see Marwick, *Deluge*, pp. 300–5; Winter, *Great War and the British People*, pp. 279–81; G. Robb, *British Culture and the First World War* (Basingstoke and New York: Palgrave, 2002), pp. 67–95. For debates on war, gender, and social change, see G. Braybon, 'Winners or Losers: Women's Symbolic Role in the War Story', in G. Braybon (ed.), *Evidence, History, and the Great War: Historians and the Impact of 1914–18* (Oxford: Berghahn Books, 2003), pp. 86–112; L. Doan, 'A Challenge to Change? New Perspectives on Women and the Great War', *Women's History Review*, 15:2 (April 2006), 337–43.

[9] See G. Sheffield, *Leadership in the Trenches: Officer-Man Relations, Morale and Discipline in the British Army in the Era of the First World War* (Basingstoke and New York: Macmillan Press, 2000), pp. 61–164; J. Bourne, 'The British Working Man in Arms', in H. Cecil and P.H. Liddle (eds.), *Facing Armageddon: The First World War Experienced* (London: Leo Cooper, 1996), pp. 336–52; Gregory, *Last Great War*; Bourke, *Dismembering the Male*; S. Grayzel, *Women's Identities at War: Gender, Motherhood, and Politics in Britain and France during the First World War* (Chapel Hill, NC and London: University of North Carolina Press, 1999); M. Roper, 'Nostalgia as an Emotional Experience in the Great War', *Historical Journal*, 54:2 (2011), 421–51.

about the role of class and gender in mental health. This position was entirely contingent on wartime circumstances and therefore temporary. It represented fragile efforts towards democratization based on belief in the equality of sacrifice, but did not represent doctors' deepest beliefs about the relative susceptibilities of "shell-shocked" men. Wartime experiences did not fundamentally overturn medical prejudices about class, gender, and mental illness. However, as demonstrated by these temporary efforts towards democratization, the war did provoke a *potentially* radical questioning of established attitudes. To that extent, "shell-shock" opened up space for alternative medical conceptualizations of the individual, social, and moral worth of those who broke down, in much the same way that the category of functional disorder had opened up space for psychological theorizing within the dominant somatic paradigm of pre-war psychological medicine.

This argument, that medical discourse on "shell-shock" implicitly confirmed the wider wartime rhetoric of democratization, conflicts with the virtuoso expositions of Eric Leed and Elaine Showalter, which portrayed medical responses to "shell-shock" as structured around class and gender differences. In this view, doctors divided "shell-shock" into the component diagnoses of hysteria and neurasthenia, respectively applied to ranking men and officers, and punished hysterical men through painful "disciplinary" therapies while sympathetically treating officers with "talking cures".[10] However, the separate elements of this interpretation do not hold up.[11] In wartime medical discourse, several diagnostic categories other than hysteria and neurasthenia fed into conceptualizations of "shell-shock". It was not standard practice to differentially diagnose officers and men, and when this did happen, diagnostic labels did not split neatly into hysteria and neurasthenia. Moreover, the distinction between "disciplinary" and "analytic" therapies is a retrospective historiographical construct (these terms were not used in the same sense by contemporaries), and only a minority of physicians practised either form of treatment.[12]

Attempts to create alternative accounts of the operation of class and gender in diagnostic constructions of "shell-shock" founder on a puzzling absence in wartime medical literature. *Most "shell-shock" doctors did not comment on class or gender at all.* This absence has not been

[10] Leed, *No Man's Land*, pp. 169–80; Showalter, *Female Malady*, pp. 167–94.
[11] Loughran, 'Shell-Shock in First World War Britain', 40–7, 99–123.
[12] Leese, '"Why Are They Not Cured?"'; L. Stryker, 'Mental Cases: British Shellshock and the Politics of Interpretation', in G. Braybon (ed.), *Evidence, History and the Great War: Historians and the Impact of 1914–18* (New York and Oxford: Berghahn Books, 2003), pp. 154–71; Humphries and Kurchinski, 'Rest, Relax and Get Well'.

identified in previous scholarship. Leed and Showalter focused on the few exceptions, the anomalous doctors who made class and gender central to their accounts or used overtly classed or gendered language. It has usually been taken for granted that these rare examples were representative of broader medical opinion, and this assumption has cloaked the far more startling absence of such commentary. The silence of medical discourse on class and gender in "shell-shock" has not been noticed and so has not been explained. It is possible that analysis of different forms of evidence, such as unpublished case notes, could reveal more explicit discussion of these aspects of identity: but even so, the question of why doctors wrote class and gender out of their public accounts of "shell-shock" would still remain.

This chapter identifies and interrogates silences on gender and class within wartime medical literature on "shell-shock" and tries to explain what work such silences performed. I refer to this absence in the medical literature as "silence" – a conscious, or at least partially conscious, writing out of class and gender – for two reasons. First, officers and men were treated separately in both the state wartime treatment network and in private institutions.[13] At a fundamental level, assumptions about class difference structured medical encounters with "shell-shocked" men. These assumptions did not manifest in simplistic divisions in treatment modalities: conservative treatments were most common for officers and men alike, while one of the most innovative sites of "analytic" treatment, Maghull Military Hospital, treated ranking men. Nevertheless, given that the treatment network was structured around military rank, it is odd that wartime doctors did not comment on class difference more often. Second, before 1914, doctors routinely discussed gender and class in relation to hysteria, neurasthenia, traumatic neurosis, and other disorders; and from the 1920s onwards, some gradually incorporated commentaries on gender and class into their accounts of "shell-shock". The relative absence of such discussion in wartime medical literature is apparent when we consider practices in the immediate past and the post-war future, and it then demands explanation. In other words, we are not dealing with the same lack of *explicit* attention to particular concepts routinely encountered by historians mining sources for information beyond the conscious intentions of their authors. This absence within wartime medical discourse seems closer to decision than accident. Neither description quite captures the set of unarticulated beliefs which caused this absence, but any term we use should contain

---

[13] Reid, *Broken Men*, pp. 30–4.

the possibility at least of deliberate writing out or withholding of opinion. "Silence" is not a perfect description, but it is the best available.

To a certain extent, reading any historical source is an exercise in listening to silences. Ordinary difficulties are magnified when silences are our main concern, when what we really want to know is what was *not* said or *not* recorded. Any interpretation of the unsaid is necessarily tentative, and persuasive only insofar as it fits with the best available evidence. This chapter compares wartime silences on gender and class in medical discourse on "shell-shock" with pre-war discussion of similar diagnostic categories and discusses the limited references to class and gender in post-war literature on war neurosis. I argue that medical silence on these matters testifies to doctors' strength of belief in the equality of sacrifice of serving soldiers. In turn, this illustrates medical commitment to both the war itself and the values and behaviour enshrined in the masculine ideal.[14] Ultimately, in containing the potentially radical challenge "shell-shock" posed to the existing social and cultural order, these silences maintained and reinforced conservative views of gender and class identities.

This interpretation, like all interpretations of silence, is speculative. But silence is never meaningless. What is taken for granted is rarely explicitly articulated, and sometimes the most powerful influences are assumed rather than elaborated. Even when not spoken about, gender is everywhere, and in advanced industrial societies, the same holds true for class. In both public representation and lived experience, class and gender are inextricably entwined. Aspects of identity coexist in individual subjectivity and in the structures of social relations. At different times, particular facets of the self hold more prominence in individual consciousness; awareness of certain aspects of identity is sharper in certain social contexts; and, depending on the concerns of the author, different historical sources say more or less about class, gender, race, or sexuality. But people are whole entities. Aspects of identity continue to exist when not the focus of immediate attention, and they shape what is said, thought, and felt no less powerfully when operating in silence.

The published medical literature on "shell-shock" is silent on some matters which nevertheless shaped all that was written and structured the doctor–patient relationships behind the text. Acknowledgement of these formative silences must precede further acts of interpretation.

---

[14] On sacrificial ideals of masculinity, see J. Horne, 'Masculinity in Politics and War in the Age of Nation-States and World Wars, 1850–1950', in S. Dudlink, K. Hagemann, and J. Tosh (eds.), *Masculinities in Politics and War: Gendering Modern History* (Manchester and New York: Manchester University Press, 2004), p. 32.

In itself, the relative absence of direct reference to class reveals the privileged position of those who constructed medical discourse.[15] This silence hides the position of power that military doctors held over patients: the enormous imbalance between the number of surviving sources produced by doctors and those penned by patients testifies most eloquently to the inequalities in this relationship. As a professional group drawn mainly from the middle classes, wartime doctors occupied an unusual position in the social and military hierarchies. Although often from humbler social backgrounds than their officer patients, doctors as temporary officers in the RAMC held military authority over these social "superiors". In relation to ranker patients, the professional expertise and social status doctors enjoyed in peacetime coalesced with the naked exercise of power enjoined by military command. Structural inequalities pervaded the medical system and were barely noticed by most doctors because they simply reflected the structural inequalities of everyday life. Silence hides power.

Gender and Class in Pre-War Medical Discourse on the Functional Disorders

Medical pronouncements on "shell-shock" were partially shaped by doctors' pre-war experiences of dealing with similar illnesses, including their existing ideas about the role of gender and class in functional disorders. One tactic for reading silences is the exploration of conceptual alignments in discussions of gender and class in pre-war and wartime medical discourse. The unexpected absence or presence of particular silences in wartime texts can illuminate the nature and extent of change in medical views of gender, class, and mental disorder. However, comparison of pre-war and wartime views is not straightforward. As with other aspects of functional disorders in the immediate pre-war period, there was considerable flux in perceptions of how gender and class shaped predisposition. Above all, instability in the class and gender identities of functional disorders arose out of the construction of complex models of male hysteria and shifts within the concept of traumatic neurosis.

Historically, hysteria has been viewed as the archetypal female malady, a disorder encapsulating traditions of female suffering, protest, and stigmatization.[16] There is more disagreement over the gendering of the nineteenth-century construct of neurasthenia. In North America, the

---

[15] See Barham, *Forgotten Lunatics of the Great War*, pp. 76–7.
[16] N. Tomes, 'Feminist Histories of Psychiatry', in M. Micale and R. Porter (eds.), *Discovering the History of Psychiatry* (Oxford and New York: Oxford University Press, 1994), pp. 348–83; Micale, *Approaching Hysteria*, pp. 161–8.

birthplace of the diagnosis, it was associated with the ills of overwork
and civilization and applied mainly to men. A diagnosis of neurasthenia
may have even conferred prestige on sufferers.[17] In Britain, it seems
that doctors most often perceived neurasthenia as more or less equally
distributed among the sexes, perhaps with a slight preponderance of
male sufferers.[18] Across nineteenth-century Europe and North America, these functional disorders were usually portrayed as bourgeois
malaises, most prevalent among the middle and upper classes.[19] But
in pre-war Britain, the class and gender identities of different functional
disorders were not assured or self-evident. By 1900, medical commentators agreed that working-class patients frequently displayed hysterical
and neurasthenic symptoms.[20] Yet the very need to emphasize that
these illnesses were found 'in all ranks and at all ages' suggests that
older beliefs about the class basis of functional disorders retained some
purchase.[21] Such statements, which simultaneously acknowledged and
controverted strongly held beliefs, point to instability in these diagnostic categories.

The most dramatic change in the medical profile of any functional
disorder in this period was the establishment, in the face of centuries of
medical tradition, of a complexly gendered model of male hysteria. By
the time of his death in 1893, Jean-Martin Charcot, *grand maître* of
hysteria, had achieved great success in his campaign for the medical
acceptance of male hysteria.[22] In Britain, Charcot's research was usually

---

[17] B. Sicherman, 'The Uses of a Diagnosis: Doctors, Patients, and Neurasthenia', *Journal of
the History of Medicine and Allied Sciences*, 32 (1977), 33–54; S. Wessely, 'Neurasthenia and
Fatigue Syndromes: Clinical Section', in G.E. Berrios and R. Porter (eds.), *A History of
Clinical Psychiatry: The Origin and History of Psychiatric Disorders* (London: Athlone, 1995),
pp. 509–32. This interpretation is disputed by T. Lutz, 'Neurasthenia and Fatigue
Syndromes: Social Section', in Berrios and Porter (eds.), *History of Clinical Psychiatry*,
pp. 536–7.

[18] Macnaughton-Jones, 'Relation of Puberty and the Menopause to Neurasthenia';
E. Clarke, 'Neurasthenia and Eyestrain', *Practitioner* 86:1 (January 1911), 25; Oldfield,
'Some Pelvic Disorders', 337; Ross, 'Nature and Treatment of Neurasthenia'. See also
C. Sengoopta, '"A Mob of Incoherent Symptoms"? Neurasthenia in British Medical
Discourse, 1860–1920', in Gijswijt-Hofstra and Porter (eds.), *Cultures of Neurasthenia*,
p. 99; M. Thomson, 'Neurasthenia in Britain: An Overview', in Gijswijt-Hofstra and
Porter (eds.), *Cultures of Neurasthenia*, p. 81.

[19] M. Gijswijt-Hofstra, 'Introduction: Cultures of Neurasthenia from Beard to the First
World War', in Gijswijt-Hofstra and Porter (eds.), *Cultures of Neurasthenia*, p. 23;
Micale, 'Hysteria and Its Historiography', 85–93.

[20] Micale, 'Hysteria and Its Historiography', 85–93; Sengoopta, '"Mob of Incoherent
Symptoms"?', 98–9; Neve, 'Public Views of Neurasthenia', 143–5.

[21] Fleming, 'Neurasthenia and Gastralgia', 31; Ritchie, 'Neurasthenia', 115.

[22] M. Micale, 'Charcot and the Idea of Hysteria in the Male: Gender, Mental Science, and
Medical Diagnosis in Late Nineteenth-Century France', *Medical History*, 34 (1990),
365–71.

the first point of reference in medical discussions of male hysteria.[23] The creation of a separate model of male hysteria did not dissolve its traditional gender identity, but there are some indications that male hysteria was normalized in this period. Medical accounts of male hysteria did not always comment on the peculiarity of the condition; they sometimes suggested that the condition was probably more common, even in strong and healthy men, than often supposed; and frequently they did not attribute effeminate qualities to the patient.[24] By 1911, physicians might even use the male pronoun throughout a general discussion on hysteria, although this remained the exception to the rule.[25] While change was slow, by 1914 male hysteria was neither ignored nor systematically stigmatized.

Of course, this is not the whole story. Certain features of the discussion of male hysteria in British medical discourse from around the turn of the century suggest that doctors continued to find the existence of the disorder problematic. In his research on male hysteria in nineteenth-century Europe, Mark Micale suggests that male physicians were unwilling to countenance hysterical weakness and emotionality in their own sex because it threatened their self-image as rational men of science. Consequently, their accounts of male hysteria were characterized by 'anxiety, ambivalence, and selective amnesia'.[26] Micale identifies 'techniques of avoidance' which enabled physicians to acknowledge the existence of male hysteria while minimizing its importance. Strategies of definition involved manipulating the clinical content of the hysteria diagnosis. These included acknowledging the existence of male hysteria but dismissing its incidence as statistically negligible; diagnosing certain symptoms as hysterical in women but finding another explanation for their appearance in men; ascribing speculative organic aetiologies to male, but not female, cases; employing hybrid diagnostic categories such as 'hystero-epilepsy' for men; describing symptoms as 'hysterical' without applying the label to the male patient himself; putting 'hysteria' in quotation marks when discussing male patients; and camouflaging the diagnosis with less derogatory, more technical language. Strategies of deployment controlled when, how often, and to whom the diagnosis

---

[23] E. Jacob, 'Remarks on Functional Aphemia', *BMJ*, 13 September 1890, 622–3; H.C. Bastian, 'On Different Kinds of Aphasia, with Special Reference to Their Classification and Ultimate Pathology', *BMJ*, 5 November 1887, 985–90; J. Wyllie, *The Disorders of Speech* (Edinburgh: Oliver and Boyd, 1894), pp. 42–4; Wilson, 'Some Modern French Conceptions of Hysteria', 294.

[24] Stewart, *Diagnosis of Nervous Diseases*, pp. 238–9.

[25] Wilson, 'Some Modern French Conceptions of Hysteria'. Usually, doctors referred to hysterics as 'she' and to sufferers from other nervous disorders as 'he'.

[26] M. Micale, *Hysterical Men: The Hidden History of Male Nervous Illness* (Cambridge, MA and London: Harvard University Press, 2008), p. 7.

was applied. These included restricting the diagnosis to supposedly effeminate or homosexual men; applying the diagnosis only to men from certain cities, cultures, or nations; and illustrating the diagnosis with cases drawn from socially, ethnically, or racially stigmatized populations.[27] In short, when male hysteria was not denied, it was qualified to the point of non-existence; and when acknowledged, the male hysteric was portrayed as effeminate and barely a man at all.

This reading of medical discourse focuses on elisions, ellipses, and exclusions rather than on positive statements. The same strategies of definition and deployment are found in pre-war British medical discourse on male hysteria. When doctors discussed male hysteria, they usually added that the disorder was much more prevalent among women.[28] If they noted that the incidence of male hysteria had risen in recent years, doctors insisted the increase was more apparent than real: impoverished men who contracted hysteria appeared in hospital records, but 'idle and well-to-do' women, constituting the majority of sufferers, did not.[29] Sometimes physicians implicitly coded male hysterics as feminine and scornfully dismissed them as 'highly sensitive and nervous gentlemen'.[30] Some doctors employed differential diagnosis, describing symptoms as hysterical in women, but applying alternative labels such as 'epileptiform convulsions' to men.[31] Often, doctors insisted that hysteria manifested differently in men and women. Hysteria was easily provoked in women, but followed severe shock or upset in men.[32] In men, slight symptoms proved the existence of hysteria, whereas women suffered from extreme manifestations of the disorder such as fits.[33] Or perhaps the reverse was true: women suffered from mild forms of hysteria, often not even meriting medical attention, but male hysteria was 'more serious

---

[27] Micale, *Hysterical Men*, pp. 193–208. On the use of these strategies in the British context, see M. Micale, 'Hysteria Male/Hysteria Female: Reflections on Comparative Gender Construction in Nineteenth-Century France and Britain', in M. Benjamin (ed.), *Science and Sensibility: Gender and Scientific Enquiry, 1780–1945* (Oxford: Basil Blackwell, 1991), pp. 215–26.

[28] Potts, *Nervous and Mental Diseases*, p. 414; Clarke, *Hysteria and Neurasthenia*, pp. 127–32; Nagel, *Nervous and Mental Diseases*, p. 163.

[29] H. Ellis, *Man and Woman: A Study of Human Secondary Sexual Characters*, 5th edn (New York and Melbourne: Walter Scott Publishing, 1914), p. 384.

[30] GHMSA: G/S7/38, [author unknown], 'On Hysteria and Its Simulations to Other Diseases', (16 December 1870), 18.

[31] Ash, 'Combined Psycho-Electrical Treatment', 131.

[32] F.P. Weber, 'The Association of Hysteria with Malingering: The Phylogenetic Aspect of Hysteria as Pathological Exaggeration (or Disorder) of Tertiary (Nervous) Sex Characters', *Lancet*, 2 December 1911, 1543; see also U. Link-Heer, '"Male Hysteria": A Discourse Analysis', *Cultural Critique*, 15 (1990), 214.

[33] Glynn, 'Abstract of the Bradshaw Lecture'.

and obstinate'.[34] Apparently contradictory claims affirmed the same conclusion: hysteria was part of the female condition, but a definite pathology in men. In these ways, medical men simultaneously acknowledged the existence and denied the importance of male hysteria. Their qualifications to the diagnosis reinforced rather than undermined traditional gender identities.

Gender, Class, and Traumatic Neurosis

The unwitting use of techniques of avoidance suggests that despite far greater attention to the condition in the early twentieth century, male hysteria had not been fully integrated into medical accounts of functional disorders. But in one context – and the most relevant for understanding wartime approaches to "shell-shock" – male hysteria was completely accepted. Across Europe, including Britain, medical responses to war neurosis drew on existing constructs of traumatic neurosis. Charcot's work on male hysteria had included extensive observations on traumatic accidents. Although hysteria remained a stigmatizing and highly gendered diagnostic category, in France there was 'a striking absence of commentary among doctors on the fact that the 1914–18 epidemic struck primarily a male population'.[35] In Germany, the concept of male hysteria emerged hand in hand with debates on traumatic neurosis. In the 1880s, industrial and railway accidents multiplied as a result of rapid industrialization. This coincided with Bismarck's social insurance legislation and more general concerns with collective health. The neurologist Hermann Oppenheim (1858–1919) argued that traumatic neurosis originated in material damage to the nervous system, while critics countered it was nothing more than hysteria. The question had important political implications: if symptoms were caused by the pathological mental processes of the individual, then the state or employers were not liable to pay compensation to accident victims. In Germany, the association of hysteria with work displaced its traditional gender identity and made it a preferable diagnosis for employers and the state. Initial responses to war neurosis in Germany were shaped by existing debates on traumatic

[34] Ellis, *Man and Woman*, p. 384.
[35] M. Roudebush, 'A Battle of Nerves: Hysteria and Its Treatments in France during World War I', in M. Micale and P. Lerner (eds.), *Traumatic Pasts: History, Psychiatry, and Trauma in the Modern Age, 1870–1930* (Cambridge: Cambridge University Press, 2001), pp. 254–5, 263; M. Micale, 'Jean-Martin Charcot and *les névroses traumatiques*: From Medicine to Culture in French Trauma Theory of the Late Nineteenth Century', in Micale and Lerner (eds.), *Traumatic Pasts*, pp. 119–22, 130–1; Thomas, *Treating the Trauma of the Great War*, pp. 48–51.

neurosis.[36] In both France and Germany, then, male hysteria was associated with the modern industrial environment and the masculine world of work.

In Britain too, the concept of traumatic neurosis was an important precursor of "shell-shock" and played a crucial part in displacing the conventional class and gender associations of hysteria. The earliest reports in the British medical press on the nervous and mental disorders of war drew attention to the aetiological role of 'shock' and described symptoms as analogous to those found in civilians after railway or industrial accidents.[37] Traumatic neurosis was the first point of reference for doctors trying to make sense of "shell-shock". Medical debates on traumatic neurosis demonstrate that even before 1914, a link had been forged between hysteria, public (male) environments, and the relations of the individual to the state. Ambivalences within this diagnostic construct carried over into "shell-shock". Just as accidents could happen to anyone, so in theory traumatic neurosis could manifest in anyone, regardless of class or sex. In practice, as the victims of workplace accidents, working-class men were over-represented in medical discourse on traumatic neurosis. Tensions between potential and actual applications of the diagnosis were replicated in debates on "shell-shock". This limited the radical implications of the admission that any man could break down under sufficient strain.

The main difference between traumatic neurosis and other functional disorders was aetiological. The symptoms of traumatic neurosis arose after a definite episode causing nervous or mental shock.[38] In Britain, the concept of traumatic neurosis was first developed in the mid-Victorian period through the diagnostic category of "railway spine". Initially, doctors believed that this condition, associated with railway accidents, resulted from organic injury to the spinal cord, but later decided that it was a nervous disorder produced by extreme shock and fear at the

[36] P. Lerner, 'From Traumatic Neurosis to Male Hysteria: The Decline and Fall of Hermann Oppenheim, 1889–1919', in Micale and Lerner (eds.), *Traumatic Pasts*; Lerner, *Hysterical Men*, pp. 15–85, 124–62; D. Kaufmann, 'Science as Cultural Practice: Psychiatry in the First World War and Weimar Germany', *Journal of Contemporary History*, 34 (1999), 129–34; H-P. Schmiedebach, 'Post-Traumatic Neurosis in Nineteenth-Century Germany: A Disease in Political, Juridical and Professional Context', *History of Psychiatry*, 10 (1999), 27–57; B. Holdorff and T. Dening, 'The Fight for "Traumatic Neurosis", 1889–1916: Hermann Oppenheim and His Opponents in Berlin', *History of Psychiatry*, 22:4 (2011), 465–76.
[37] See Anon., 'Mental and Nervous Shock among the Wounded'; Anon., 'French Wounded from Some Early Actions'; Anon, 'War and Nervous Breakdown'; Myers, 'Contribution to the Study of Shell Shock'; Anon., 'Shell Explosions and the Special Senses'.
[38] H.C. Thomson, 'Traumatic Neurasthenia', *JMS*, 59:247 (October 1913), 583.

moment of the accident. By the early 1900s, most British commentators agreed that traumatic neurosis *might* be caused by organic injury, but the emotional and psychological reactions of the sufferer contributed considerably to development of the disorder. Most often, doctors argued that auto-suggestion perpetuated and fixed experiences of shock or injury in the victim's mind.[39] However, physicians never perceived traumatic neurosis as a purely individual pathology. Because it originated in debates over railway accidents, the diagnosis was associated with anxieties about the cost and consequences of industrialization and "modernization".[40] These apprehensions carried over into later concepts of traumatic neurosis, whether the site of the accident was the industrial workplace or the industrial battlefield.

In the early 1900s, medical accounts of traumatic neurosis referred more often to workplace than to railway accidents. As a result, the patients whom doctors discussed were usually male and working-class. This shift played an important part in establishing the concept of male hysteria. In 1914 the surgeon John Geary Grant (1864-5?–1947) remarked that hysteria was 'formerly considered to belong almost exclusively to the gentler sex, but now it is quite frequently found as an "hysterical accident" in the male'. Grant's own case histories documented traumatic hysteria in 'sturdy workmen' including colliers, dock labourers, and plumbers.[41] Although doctors did not always explicitly make connections between male hysteria and accidents, hysterical men discussed in published medical literature nearly always had histories of traumatic injury. Female hysterics did not.[42] In the wake of the Employers' Liability Act (1890) and the Workmen's Compensation Acts (1897, 1900, and 1906), doctors argued that the desire for compensation

---

[39] Cole, *Mental Diseases* [1913], p. 234; Palmer, 'Traumatic Neuroses and Psychoses', 811–13; Thorburn, 'Presidential Address', 4, 7–8; Ritchie, 'Neurasthenia', 116; Grant, 'Traumatic Neuroses', 40.

[40] R. Harrington, 'The Railway Accident: Trains, Trauma, and Technological Crises in Nineteenth-Century Britain', in Micale and Lerner (eds.), *Traumatic Pasts*, pp. 43–51; Pick, *War Machine*, pp. 106–10, 113–35; Schivelbusch, *Railway Journey*, pp. 129–49.

[41] Grant, 'Traumatic Neuroses', 30, 38; Thomson, 'Traumatic Neurasthenia', 591. Medical discussions of traumatic neurasthenia often referred to miners. See Jacob, 'Remarks on Functional Aphemia', 623; H.W. Gardner, 'A Case of Periodic Paralysis', *Brain*, 35:3 (February 1913), 243; Anon., 'Medical Societies: Edinburgh Medico-Chirurgical Society', *Lancet*, 1 January 1910, 27–8. After the war, Myers noted the large number of cases of shell-shock among soldiers who were miners in peacetime and linked this to the prevalence of neurasthenia in mining communities. Myers, *Present-Day Applications of Psychology*, pp. 44–5.

[42] Leslie, 'Medical Report for the Year 1901', 97; E.F. Ballard, 'A Case of Aggravated Hysteroid Movements', *JMS*, 56:233 (April 1910), 317–20; J.E. Middlemiss, 'Notes on a Case of Hysteria', *JMS*, 56:234 (July 1910), 502–3; Ormerod, 'Two Theories of Hysteria', 274, 277.

fostered traumatic neurosis and subconsciously encouraged the maintenance of symptoms.[43] Some doctors focused on the alarming rise in
numbers of men suffering from traumatic neurosis following these acts,
but others commented that the number of women making claims for
traumatic neurosis had also increased.[44] In these discussions, doctors
associated the gendered aspects of traumatic neurosis with more widespread anxieties about the unsettled condition of relations between
employer and employed, men and women, and individual and state.[45]

In pre-war medical discourse, the diagnosis of traumatic neurosis therefore encompassed a version of hysteria particularly associated with public
(male) environments and experiences. However, as with other forms of
functional disorder, doctors believed that traumatic neurosis usually
developed in those of unsound mind or body, and portrayed patients as
emotional and suggestible. By the 1900s, most doctors believed that
emotional shock was the most important factor in the genesis of traumatic
neurosis. Crucially, they emphasized the importance of fear in provoking
neurosis, particularly the 'sights and sounds and elements of horror' found
in large-scale accidents.[46] Doctors argued that lurid newspaper coverage
of accidents created public fear and so prepared 'a fertile soil for nervous
disturbance in those who might themselves be injured at a later date'.[47]
Such comments imply that victims of traumatic neurosis were emotional
and suggestible even *before* their accidents. This undermined representations of the accident as the sole or main cause of symptoms and relocated
the pathology to the body and mind of the patient.[48]

Along similar lines, some doctors believed that most sufferers had an
inherited or acquired 'neuropathic tendency' which left them vulnerable
to traumatic neurosis.[49] As we have seen in previous chapters, before the
war, beliefs about hereditary weakness influenced theorizations of

---

[43] E. Bramwell, 'Recent Advances in Medical Science. Neurology', *EMJ*, 14 (January–June 1915), 477–8.

[44] A. James, 'Trauma as a Factor in Disease. II', *EMJ*, 8 (January–June 1912), 313; Thorburn, 'Presidential Address', 11, 13–14.

[45] See A.J. Hall, 'How Far Is Trauma a Possible Factor in the Production of Disease', *Practitioner*, 88:6 (June 1912), 832; Thorburn, 'Presidential Address', 12–13; Palmer, 'Traumatic Neuroses and Psychoses', 818.

[46] Grant, 'Traumatic Neuroses', 27; Anon., 'The British Medical Association Seventy-Ninth Annual Meeting in Birmingham: Section of Neurology and Psychological Medicine', *Lancet*, 12 August 1911, 450–1; Hall, 'How Far Is Trauma a Possible Factor in the Production of Disease', 839–40; Thomson, 'Traumatic Neurasthenia', 583–4.

[47] Thorburn, 'Presidential Address', 1, 9–10.

[48] Palmer, 'Traumatic Neuroses and Psychoses', 813; Grant, 'Traumatic Neuroses', 40.

[49] Thorburn, 'Presidential Address', 11; Hall, 'How Far Is Trauma a Possible Factor in the Production of Disease', 844; Anon., 'Medical Societies: Liverpool Medical Institution', 1001; Grant, 'Traumatic Neuroses', 37; Russell, 'Treatment of Neurasthenia', 1453.

hysteria and neurasthenia and, after a temporary lull, these preoccupations resurfaced in wartime theories of "shell-shock". Concern with heredity likewise threads through pre-war medical discourse on traumatic neurosis. Of particular relevance to wartime debates were attempts to understand the relative importance of latent weakness versus precipitating event in the formation of traumatic neurosis. Where the severity of symptoms seemed out of proportion to the seriousness of the accident, doctors were especially likely to fall back on the catch-all explanation of predisposition. In these cases, physicians insisted that the accident was only an 'agent provocateur', and problems really arose from the 'latent morbidity' of the patient's brain.[50] In practical terms, they argued that if hysterical symptoms could be attributed to pre-existing constitutional weakness, patients should not be allowed to claim damages or compensation. Discussions of emotion, suggestibility, and predisposition in traumatic neurosis foreshadowed later medical deliberations on "shell-shock". Exactly the same issues were debated again and again as doctors attempted to uncover the exact causes of the war neuroses and as politicians attempted to settle the vexed question of whether pensions should be awarded for wartime traumatic injury.

Wartime doctors drew on their pre-existing knowledge about traumatic neurosis to make sense of "shell-shock", and the industrial environment could easily be extended to include the modern battlefield. However, one of the most important factors shaping responses to the nervous and mental disorders of war was not positive knowledge but rather a peculiar ambivalence within the construction and application of the diagnosis of traumatic neurosis. Doctors unwittingly exploited and extended this ambiguity in their encounters with "shell-shock". It arose from the unacknowledged tension between conceptualizations of traumatic neurosis as itself an accident, a misfortune as arbitrary as the derailment of a train or the collapse of a mineshaft, and the actual class and gender profile of typical sufferers. In theory, anyone could develop a traumatic neurosis, but in practice, working-class men were the usual victims of routine industrial accidents. As existing medical paradigms favoured biological explanations for neurotic illnesses and held that working-class patients were inherently biologically inferior to those higher up the social scale, it did not take a considerable leap to confound greater exposure of a particular social group to workplace accidents with its (alleged) biological weakness. Moreover, in diagnosing functional

[50] Grant, 'Traumatic Neuroses', 40–3; H. Littlejohn and J.H.H. Pirie, 'Medical Jurisprudence: Mental Disturbances Following Traumatism', EMJ, 7 (July–December 1911), 88.

disorders, doctors had substantial scope for retrospective aetiological construction. If no alternative explanation could be found, if an accident did not seem sufficiently horrific to justify traumatic symptoms, if patients had an individual or family history of nervous weakness, then doctors could invoke "predisposition" as the cause of illness. The distinctive class and gender profile of victims of traumatic neurosis coexisted with the theoretical awareness that accidents could happen to anyone, just as the primacy of shock in the aetiology of traumatic neurosis coexisted with medical dependence on the concept of "predisposition". In practice, this left considerable room for doctors' personal and social prejudices to influence diagnostic decisions.

Class and Rank in "Shell-Shock"

The extension and exploitation of this ambivalence within the concept of traumatic neurosis helps to explain certain elements within wartime accounts of the role of class and/or rank in "shell-shock". Very few medical authors directly addressed the relation between rank, symptoms, and treatment in "shell-shock". The major exceptions to this rule were the Canadian psychologist John T. MacCurdy (1886–1947) and W.H.R. Rivers. Both expounded theories of war neurosis in which social differences between officers and ranking men were central.[51] Both doctors argued that hysteria was a crude response to mental conflict, overwhelmingly found in ranking men, in which a physical symptom satisfied the soldier's desire for escape from the trenches. Anxiety neurosis, the disorder of officers, was a more complicated reaction in which conflict was caused and maintained by a heightened sense of duty. This distinction was attributed partly to differences in military function and training, but more importantly to the greater intelligence, education, idealism, and social responsibility of officers.[52] There is clear class prejudice at work in the view that ranking men had simpler mental responses to combat experience, and that differences in the mental responses of officers and men were not attributable to military function alone. MacCurdy and Rivers published these theories late in the war, in 1918. Although doctors sometimes briefly commented on the role of class or rank in "shell-shock", no other wartime publications put forward systematic and

---

[51] On MacCurdy's relationship with Rivers, see J. Forrester, '1919: Psychology and Psychoanalysis, Cambridge and London – Myers, Jones and MacCurdy', *Psychoanalysis and History*, 10:1 (2008), 75–7.

[52] J.T. MacCurdy, *War Neuroses* (Cambridge: Cambridge University Press, 1918), pp. 17, 21, 23, 86, 88, 122–4; Rivers, 'War-Neurosis and Military Training', 514–19, 524–7.

comprehensive theories of rank or social difference.[53] The MacCurdy–
Rivers thesis on the influence of rank/class on symptom formation
attracted marginal support in the 1920s but became more established
in the 1930s and 1940s. How did this happen?

It is important to be clear on what the medical literature can and
cannot tell us. To begin with, it is impossible to make definitive
statements about the general class profile of those who suffered from
"shell-shock", far less the particular manifestations of the disorder such
as hysteria or neurasthenia. As noted elsewhere, doctors did not always
speak the same diagnostic language: there was no single accepted definition of "shell-shock" or of the causes, symptoms, or ideal treatment of
neurasthenia, anxiety neurosis, anxiety hysteria, conversion hysteria,
psychasthenia, traumatic neurosis, war neurosis, war shock, or the many
other terms which doctors employed in relation to soldier patients.
Furthermore, most of the time, doctors did not comment on the social
status of their patients at all. The published medical literature did not
routinely include this information. It was standard to note the rank of a
patient when discussing individual cases, but doctors also made general
statements about "shell-shock" without referring to particular cases or
mentioning rank at all. Moreover, the high rates of promotion in the
army as the war went on make it impossible to correlate class to rank with
any certainty. By 1918, 39 per cent of officers were from lower-middle
and working-class backgrounds.[54] Likewise, social class cannot be easily
correlated with behavioural norms: it seems likely that those selected for
promotion conformed, in at least some respects, to the bourgeois models
of masculinity valued within the military.

Although medical statistics collected during and after the war indicate
higher rates of breakdown among officers than ranking men, at best these
figures tell us about diagnostic practices rather than the actual incidence
of psychological collapse.[55] There are many potential reasons for differential rates of diagnosis. Greater social contact between officers and
RMOs provided more informal opportunities for diagnosis, while some
symptoms were perceived as more serious in officers because of their

[53] On the lack of wider support for the Rivers–MacCurdy thesis in the wartime medical
literature, see Loughran, 'Shell-Shock in First World War Britain', 40–7; Loughran,
'Hysteria and Neurasthenia', 35–7.

[54] Watson, *Enduring the Great War*, p. 121; G. Sheffield, 'Office-Man Relations, Discipline
and Morale in the British Army of the Great War', in H. Cecil and P.H. Liddle (eds.),
Facing Armageddon: The First World War Experienced (London: Leo Cooper, 1996),
p. 417; Leese, *Shell Shock*, pp. 85, 110–16.

[55] Macpherson *et al.* (eds.), *History of the Great War*, pp. 2, 17 (the evidence here is mixed);
Mitchell and Smith, *History of the Great War*, pp. 115–16.

greater responsibility for the safety of the unit.[56] We cannot know with any certainty how these factors operated because doctors did not record this information or even necessarily appreciate its significance. Nevertheless, the differential rate of diagnosis is important because it shows that rank was not irrelevant to the military doctor–patient relationship. This makes the relative absence of wartime comment on the role of class/rank in "shell-shock" even more puzzling and supports the interpretation that medical silence on the subject was at least semi-intentional.

So, it seems that class and rank did influence the doctor–patient relationship, but that most doctors chose not to comment on these aspects of their patients' identities or did not make them central to theories of "shell-shock". If this is the case, why were Rivers and Mac-Curdy exceptions to this rule? One compelling explanation is simply that both produced more extensive and elaborate theories than most other doctors, and therefore explicitly discussed class/rank in a manner that was less likely in brief or descriptive statements. Moreover, unlike most wartime "shell-shock" doctors, Rivers and MacCurdy were heavily influenced by psychoanalytic approaches. Because psychoanalysis was deeply contested and demanded extensive theoretical articulation, authors influenced by Freud expounded theories of "shell-shock" in more depth than doctors who saw themselves as working within accepted traditions.

This alone does not account for Rivers' and MacCurdy's views on class/rank, and especially not for the decision to make these factors fundamental to their theories of breakdown. As psychoanalysis has developed in subsequent decades, one of the perceived problems in its theoretical basis and practical application is that it does not allow sufficient space for the social, and so this often drops out of the discussion.[57] In wartime British medical discourse, however, psychoanalytically inclined authors produced the most sustained analyses of the social basis of war neurosis. There are several possible explanations for this. In its early years, the mainstream psychoanalytic movement paid more attention to the social environment than in subsequent decades. In the 1920s, dozens of free outpatient clinics were set up in Germany and Austria by psychoanalysts who saw their practice as a form of social activism which challenged social and political conventions.[58] While no such clinics

---

[56] Anon., 'The Mind of the Soldier', *BMJ*, 11 August 1917, 188–9; Young, *Harmony of Illusions*, p. 62; C. May, 'Lord Moran's Memoir: Shell-Shock and the Pathology of Fear', *Journal of the Royal Society of Medicine*, 91 (1998), 99; Thomson, 'Status, Manpower and Mental Fitness', p. 154.

[57] I am grateful to Michael Roper for this observation.

[58] E.A. Danto, *Freud's Free Clinics: Psychoanalysis and Social Justice, 1918–1938* (New York and Chichester, West Sussex: Columbia University Press, 2005).

were set up in Britain, and the Rivers–MacCurdy thesis was hardly inspired by a crusading spirit of social justice, the attention of both doctors to the social background of patients is not so out of step with trends in the international psychoanalytic movement in this period.

At the same time, there was no necessary connection between psychoanalysis and the social. David Eder, one of the most committed psychoanalysts to publish on "shell-shock", did not incorporate judgements based on rank into his theories of the war neuroses. Eder believed that early experiences were not particularly relevant in 'war shock', as it usually resulted from the strain of recent war experience.[59] But it is also possible that Eder's commitment to socialism and extensive experience working among the poor in the East End of London made him less liable to certain social prejudices than the Cambridge don Rivers or the independently wealthy MacCurdy.[60] The tendency towards theoretical elaboration within psychoanalysis, and possibly the encouragement this orientation provided towards consideration of early life and personality formation, led Rivers and MacCurdy to expand on pre-existent social biases where other doctors did not. Psychoanalysis did not create these biases, and Rivers' and MacCurdy's discussion of class/rank was an explicated but unreflexive position. For all Rivers' thoughtfulness in so many aspects of his work with "shell-shocked" men, he externalized the source of his relative failure with ranking patients rather than reflecting on whether he lacked the ability to understand these men on their own terms. In the early 1920s, Rivers still believed he had been unable to elicit accounts of complex dreams from private soldiers at Maghull Military Hospital because these men had a simpler mental life than the officers he dealt with at Craiglockhart, rather than because he was unable to relate to them, or because he lacked clinical skill in his early forays into psychoanalytic treatment.[61]

In the immediate post-war period, it was extremely rare for doctors to state that officers developed neurasthenia/anxiety neurosis and that ranking men developed hysteria.[62] These assertions are almost always directly traceable to Rivers and MacCurdy. The bare handful of

[59] Eder, *War-Shock*, p. 133. Although still a Freudian, Eder showed much sympathy for Jungian ideas at this time.
[60] M. Thomson, '"The Solution to His Own Enigma": Connecting the Life of Montague David Eder (1865–1936), Socialist, Psychoanalyst, Zionist and Modern Saint', *Medical History*, 55 (2011), 73.
[61] W.H.R. Rivers, *Conflict and Dream* (London: Kegan Paul, Trench, Trubner, 1923), pp. 6–7, 93–4.
[62] A. Carver, 'The Generation and Control of Emotion', *British Journal of Psychology*, 10:1 (November 1919), 60; S. Naccarati, 'Hormones and Emotions', *TMW*, 14 (January–June 1921), 1834.

references to the Rivers–MacCurdy thesis in the early 1920s includes statements by Henry Head, Rivers' friend and collaborator, and Walter Langdon Brown (1870–1946), who had known Rivers since his student days.[63] If we want to understand how the thesis became accepted in subsequent decades, no doubt it helped that Head was one of the foremost neurologists of his generation, and Langdon Brown one of the most influential physiologists. Likewise, until his death in 1922, Rivers took an active role in the institutions and organizations of psychological medicine and exerted great influence on opinion in this field.[64] By the mid-1920s, Rivers was firmly established as one the most important British psychologists, routinely listed alongside Freud, Jung, Adler, and McDougall as one of the 'outstanding names' in modern psychology.[65] In 1926, McDougall identified Rivers as the leader of the 'Psychological School', described as inspired by yet critical of Freud, and including William Brown, Millais Culpin, J.A. Hadfield, Bernard Hart, Hugh Crichton-Miller, T.W. Mitchell, E. Prideaux, Hugh Wingfield, and Henry Yellowlees.[66] Rivers' personal influence, as well as the explosion of interest in psychoanalysis at the end of the war, means it is likely that in the post-war era many doctors encountered "shell-shock" through his writings, and that the psychoanalytically influenced theories of Rivers and MacCurdy now seemed more plausible. It seems that few doctors referenced the thesis in print from the mid-1920s onwards, but those who did included some extremely influential adherents who presented the class dimensions of "shell-shock" as common knowledge. In his *Outline of Abnormal Psychology* (1926), McDougall claimed it was 'a matter of general agreement' that officers suffered from neurasthenia and privates from hysteria; in Henderson and Gillespie's massively successful textbook of psychiatry, which ran into several editions and became a standard work in the interwar period, this interpretation was

---

[63] H. Head, 'Observations on the Elements of the Psycho-Neuroses', *BMJ*, 20 March 1920, 389; W.L. Brown, 'A Presidential Address on Hunter, Gaskell, and the Evolution of the Nervous System', *Lancet*, 20 March 1920, 644; Anon., 'Endocrines and Psychoneuroses', *BMJ*, 24 March 1923, 514. James Crichton-Browne directly quoted Head's account of differential diagnosis in J. Crichton-Browne, 'The First Maudsley Lecture', *JMS*, 66:274 (July 1920), 215.

[64] Forrester, '1919: Psychology and Psychoanalysis, Cambridge and London'.

[65] R.M. Ladell, 'Correspondence: A French View of Freudism', *BMJ*, 3 October 1925, 769; J.A.M. Alcock, 'Review: W.A. White, Foundations of Psychiatry', Medical Section, *British Journal of Psychology*, 2:4 (1922), 339; H. Devine, 'Reviews: Psycho-Analysis', *BMJ*, 29 March 1924, 578–9; B. Hart, 'Review: T.W. Mitchell, Problems in Psychopathology', *British Journal of Medical Psychology*, 8:2 (1928), 162; J.R. Lord, 'Review: Psychopathology; A Survey of Modern Approaches', *JMS*, 77:316 (January 1931), 207.

[66] W. McDougall, *Outline of Abnormal Psychology* (New York: Charles Scribner's Sons, 1926), p. 23.

presented as the 'universally agreed' position.[67] By 1940, the Rivers–MacCurdy thesis had attained the status of established fact in surveys of literature on the war neuroses.[68]

It took two decades for the Rivers–MacCurdy thesis to embed itself within mainstream medical culture; but, as it *was* eventually accepted, it seems unlikely that medical men did not share, at least in some degree, the class prejudice at the heart of this interpretation. What requires elucidation is not the slow uptake of this thesis in the post-war period but the absence of comparable theories in wartime. One explanation is that the Rivers–MacCurdy thesis had several components. Many doctors observed some aspects of the clinical picture presented by Rivers and MacCurdy but disagreed with or did not actively subscribe to other parts. For example, doctors frequently diagnosed neurasthenia or anxiety neurosis in ranking men.[69] There is very little wartime support for this aspect of the differential diagnostic pattern claimed by Rivers and MacCurdy. However, doctors did often discuss the reasons for breakdown and peculiarities in symptom patterns among officers. Most agreed that the 'continual strain of heavy responsibilities' contributed to breakdown in officers.[70] This was a statement about military function, not social background – but it could easily feed into class prejudices. Less often, doctors claimed that officers rarely developed hysteria.[71] This observation sometimes reflected belief in the 'superior education and knowledge' of officers.[72] But other doctors maintained that hysterical symptoms did not appear in officers *or* senior non-commissioned officers, and instead

---

[67] Ibid., p. 2, fn; D.K. Henderson and R.D. Gillespie, *A Text-Book of Psychiatry for Students and Practitioners*, 3rd edn (London: Humphrey Milford/Oxford University Press, 1932), p. 486. See also E.S. Conklin, *Principles of Abnormal Psychology* (London: George Allen & Unwin, 1928), pp. 167–8.

[68] E. Wittkower and J.P. Spillane, 'A Survey of the Literature of Neuroses in War', in E. Miller (ed.), *The Neuroses in War* (London: Macmillan, 1940), p. 15.

[69] Anon., 'Special Hospitals for Officers', 1155; Anon., 'Lord Knutsford's Special Hospitals for Officers', 1201; McDowall, 'Functional Gastric Disturbance'; Armstrong-Jones, 'Mental and Nervous States in Connection with the War', 321–34; Eager, 'Record of Admissions', 277. See also the figures for 'nervous disease' in the Gallipoli Expeditionary Force in 1915, Macpherson *et al.* (eds.), *History of the Great War*, p. 2.

[70] Anon., 'War and Nervous Breakdown', 189; Smith, 'Shock and the Soldier. I', 817; Hale-White, 'Address on Some Applications of Experience', 228; Hurst, 'War Neuroses and the Neuroses of Civil Life', 146.

[71] Myers, 'Contributions to the Study of Shell Shock (IV)', 461; Mott, 'Lettsomian Lectures. II', 443; Mott, *War Neuroses and Shell Shock*, p. 95.

[72] Buzzard, 'Warfare on the Brain', 1097. However, the medical literature also includes several examples of diagnosis of hysteria in officers which passed without comment, suggesting that many doctors did not find this so unusual. See Scott, 'Hysterical "Paralysis"', 98–9; Eder, *War-Shock*, p. 28; R. Armstrong-Jones, 'Mental States and the War – The Psychological Effects of Fear. II', *Journal of State Medicine*, 25:10 (October 1917), 290–1.

suggested that youth, temperament, and rank were all important factors in the development of hysteria. This formulation has some similarities with the Rivers–MacCurdy thesis but makes no real comment on class.[73] Although some wartime medical observations aligned with some aspects of the Rivers–MacCurdy thesis, the slide into approbation of the whole did not occur until several years later. However, it seems that the central tenets of the thesis resonated with more widely held social prejudices not publicly expressed in wartime.

Such prejudices were rarely openly articulated in the medical literature on "shell-shock" but certainly existed. To take just two examples: in July 1916, Lieutenant-Colonel Frank Maxwell of the 12th Middlesex Regiment wrote to his wife that,

"Shell-shock" is a complaint which, to my mind, is too prevalent everywhere; and I have told my people that my name for it is fright, or something worse, and I am not going to have it. Of course, the average nerve system of this class is much lower than ours, and sights and sounds affect them much more. It means . . . that they haven't got our self-control, that's all.[74]

In the same year, a doctor speaking to a medical audience on 'the physiology of war' confidently asserted that just as 'savages' felt less pain than 'civilized' men, 'Tommies' could withstand more pain than officers. He was unsure whether this difference arose because educated men became more sensitive through the 'constant use and development of higher centres', or because 'the working man, like the savage has his sense dulled by a rougher life'.[75] Both commentators equated rank with class, assumed that "nervous" responses were differentiated along class lines, and situated these responses within the evolutionary framework of understanding. The dominant explanatory paradigms of pre-war medicine, which encouraged attention to heredity and often conflated social and biological weakness, continued to influence private or semi-private statements on "shell-shock".

The operation of the evolutionary framework of understanding, and its relation to social prejudice, was evident in many other spheres. These included discussions of neurosis in animals. In December 1917, the *Times* commented on equine trauma. The author praised the intelligence and courage of British horses, especially compared to weaker 'Argentine and

---

[73] Johnson, 'Hysterical Tremor', 627.
[74] Quoted in L. van Bergen, *Before My Helpless Sight: Suffering, Dying and Military Medicine on the Western Front, 1914–1918*, trans. Liz Waters (Farnham, Surrey, and Burlington, VT: Ashgate, 2009), p. 259.
[75] GHMSA: G/S6/13, Bennett, 'Physiology of War' (28 February 1916).

Canadian horses that lie down and flounder in any shell-hole that gives them excuse for rest'. He further noted that as with men, 'well-bred horses ... suffer more from shell shock than the low-bred ones'.[76] Similar assumptions informed the statement that nasal neuroses were 'much more common among the so-called "better" classes than among hospital patients' and therefore should be treated with serum derived from 'thoroughbred horses' rather than inferior specimens.[77] These comments, far more explicit in their prejudices than the medical literature on "shell-shock", illustrate the pervasiveness of judgements about "nervous" response and class, which could be applied to horses as well as to men.

It seems likely that the social prejudices expressed by Rivers and MacCurdy resonated with more doctors than those who chose to comment on these matters in wartime. Even if many doctors did believe that class or rank influenced breakdown, it is important that they avoided public comment on this fact during the war. The war did not dissolve social differences, but the emphasis on social unity in wartime limited the expression of such opinions, at least in relation to serving men. The angry reaction of the *British Medical Journal* to reports that 'the better mental equipment' of German officers rendered them less liable to the strains of warfare than rankers highlights this emphasis on national unity. The author's sarcastic retort that a more realistic explanation for these differences might be 'the greater comfort of [officers'] existence' is the most explicitly democratic (even socialistic) comment in the entire medical literature.[78] Patriotic sentiment temporarily wiped out articulations of explicit class prejudice in the upper echelons of the medical world, just as it led to demands for special privileges for soldiers, such as their admission to private squares in wealthy areas of London or priority access to first-class seating on commuter trains, placing them simultaneously at the top and outside of the usual hierarchies of class.[79]

The temporary retreat from explicitly hierarchical explanations for nervous breakdown, and the conscious effort to acknowledge parity of sacrifice, did not cause lasting changes to doctor–patient relations. Rather, this significant shift in wartime medical discourse, as compared to pre- and post-war medical opinion, indicates the belief that suffering transcended social class. However, this temporary retreat can also be seen as an exploitation of the ambivalences within the concept of

[76] Anon., 'Army Horses: Animal Sufferers from Shell Shock', *Times*, 28 December 1917.
[77] J.S. Fraser, 'The "Nasal" Neuroses, Regarded as Sensitisations of the Respiratory Tract: A Résumé of Recent Literature', *EMJ*, 19 (July–December 1917), 93.
[78] Anon., 'Shell Shock, Gas Poisoning, and War Neuroses', 656.
[79] Gregory, *Last Great War*, pp. 135–6.

traumatic neurosis rather than as a radical departure from it. This diagnostic category allowed doctors considerable latitude to decide whether neurosis originated in the weakness of the sufferer or the severity of the accident. In the pre-war period, the class prejudices of doctors trumped their theoretical commitment to the belief that traumatic neurosis could strike anyone. In wartime, the majority of "shell-shock" doctors refused to publicly comment on the class or rank of sufferers, instead implicitly highlighting the theoretical egalitarianism of the diagnosis of traumatic neurosis. After the war, their social prejudices re-emerged, albeit slowly, and in halting and piecemeal fashion. The ambiguities of pre-war medical approaches, together with the exceptional nature of war as the event precipitating neurosis, limited and contained the potentially radical implications of the insight that any man could break down under sufficient pressure. War was a great leveller, but only for the duration.

"Shell-Shock": The Making of a Masculine Diagnosis

There are many similarities in medical attitudes to gender and class in "shell-shock". As with class, doctors rarely explicitly discussed gender in their accounts of "shell-shock". They also adopted approaches familiar from pre-war medical discourse. The complexities and apparent contradictions of pre-war constructs of male hysteria carried over into wartime discourse. Doctors continued to employ evasive strategies which minimized the significance of male hysteria. However, the experience of "shell-shock" also sustained and extended distinctively masculine constructs of the disorder. Like male hysteria, "shell-shock" was complexly gendered; unlike hysteria, doctors implicitly defined "shell-shock" as an illness experienced *only* by men. This bolstered the masculine identity of the diagnosis. It could not make "shell-shocked" men into exemplars of the pre-war masculine ideal, but it did further displace and deny associations with the feminine.

Wartime medical discourse employed similar 'techniques of avoidance' to earlier writings on male hysteria. It seems that "shell-shock" doctors deliberately jettisoned the feminine heritage of hysteria. The silence is sometimes conspicuous. For example, in July 1916, the Australian surgeon Edward Milligan (1886–1972) described 'chloroform hypnosis' as a 'well-known method of treatment for hysteria' which could also be applied in "shell-shock".[80] As a gynaecologist pointed out in

---

[80] E.T.C. Milligan, 'A Method of Treatment of "Shell Shock"', *BMJ*, 15 July 1916, 73. Milligan's advocacy of this method influenced other doctors; see Myers, 'Contributions to the Study of Shell Shock (IV)', 463; Eder, *War-Shock*, p. 137.

subsequent correspondence regarding this article, chloroform usually provided pain relief for women in labour.[81] It is impossible that Milligan was not aware of the strong association between chloroform and childbirth, but he preferred to describe it as a treatment for hysteria rather than to compare soldiers to women in childbirth. A similar silence surrounded endocrine disorders. From 1917 onwards, doctors began to publish observations on physiological malfunction in "shell-shocked" soldiers. They did not mention that thyroid problems, usually much more common in women, were traditionally viewed as feminine disorders, even though pre-war and post-war discussions of thyroid-related illnesses often raised this point.[82]

For the most part, doctors avoided comparing "shell-shocked" men to hysterical women.[83] When doctors did confront similarities, they insisted that resemblances were more apparent than real or instituted new distinctions between the two groups. David Eder insisted that 'faradic current should not be used in hysterical mutism of soldiers, useful though it is in the common functional aphonia of girls and others' but did not explain why different treatment techniques were required.[84] Perhaps, like Grafton Elliot Smith and Thomas Pear, he believed that the 'intelligent, highly moral, over-worked' man was very different to 'the society lady suffering from lack of honest labour'.[85] Likewise, Arthur Hurst argued that the nervous exhaustion of the sorely tested soldier could not be compared to 'the quite abnormal nervous system of the young woman'.[86] Hurst had no qualms about acknowledging male hysteria but minimized its significance, even when this meant expanding the empire of the feminine disorder, as in his argument that if the persistent vomiting of gassed soldiers was

[81] Cooper, 'Correspondence: Treatment of "Shell Shock"', 242.
[82] R. Crawfurd, 'Graves' Disease: An Emotional Disorder', *KCHR*, 3 (1895–96), 45; R. Eager, 'An Investigation as to the Therapeutic Value of Thyroid Feeding in Mental Diseases', *JMS*, 58:242 (July 1912), 428; Naccarati, 'Hormones and Emotions', 1832; H. Crichton-Miller, 'The Psychic and Endocrine Factors of Functional Disorders, *BMJ*, 23 September 1922, 552; Anon., 'Ninetieth Annual Meeting of the British Medical Association: Section of Medicine: Discussion of Exophthalmic Goitre', *BMJ*, 11 November 1922, 913; W.L. Brown, 'A British Medical Association Lecture on Minor Endocrine Disturbances and Their Metabolic and Psychical Effects', *BMJ*, 8 December 1923, 1075.
[83] Rare exceptions are Campbell, 'War Neuroses', 502–3; Fearnsides, 'Essentials of Treatment', 46. Reports in nonmedical forums may have expressed more ambivalence towards "feminine" pursuits. See Reid, *Broken Men*, p. 93.
[84] Eder, *War-Shock*, pp. 122, 138.
[85] Smith and Pear, *Shell Shock and Its Lessons*, p. 102; see also pp. 31–4.
[86] Hurst, *Medical Diseases of the War* [1918], pp. 33–4.

hysterical, so must be sickness in pregnancy.[87] Men could not be *more* hysterical than women.[88]

The separation of "shell-shock" from female neurosis continued into the post-war period. In *Instinct and the Unconscious* (1920), Rivers argued that the psychoneuroses of civil life were caused mainly by disturbances of the sexual instinct, whereas war neuroses were caused by conflict between the instinct of self-preservation and the individual's sense of social duty. In civil life, women suffered from hysteria more often than men because they associated sex with dangers such as childbirth or unwanted pregnancy.[89] Rivers explained male and female hysteria as resulting from untenable demands on the danger instincts but conceptually separated female hysteria from male war neurosis twice over: once by relating it to the particularly civil and civil*ized* repression of the sexual instinct and again by tying it to female biological functions.

Medical writings on shell-shock therefore employed several 'techniques of avoidance', and set up many fine distinctions between male and female hysteria. But there is one very important difference between pre-war and wartime uses of such strategies: doctors did not overtly describe "shell-shocked" men as emasculated or effeminate.[90] In some cases, lack of comment seems to amount to a definite blind spot. One of W.H.R. Rivers' patients dreamt that his father-in-law waved 'a lady's corset' at him and shouted "I've a straight-waistcoat for him". Rivers saw this as evidence of the patient's antagonism towards his wife, rather than fears about his ability to fulfil the expected masculine role (an interpretation which fits just as well with the rest of the case history).[91] Wartime discussions of "shell-shock" rarely mentioned impotence, conventionally associated with homosexuality and loss of will.[92] Almost without

---

[87] A.F. Hurst, 'Hysteria in the Light of the Experience of War', *Archives of Neurology and Psychiatry (ANP)*, 2:5 (November 1919), 566–7.

[88] However, compare Hurst's position to the post-war comments of obstetrician Archibald Donald (1860–1937), querying whether women really were more liable to functional nervous disorders than men, as the war had shown the terrible effects of the 'nervous strain inseparable from life in the danger zone' on 'many of our bravest men, yet the great majority of married women go through the trials and discomforts of repeated pregnancy and the pain and dangers of several confinements with the nervous system undisturbed'; Anon., 'Section of Obstetrics and Gynaecology', *BMJ*, 29 October 1921, 699.

[89] Rivers, *Instinct and the Unconscious*, pp. 136–8; see also E.F. Buzzard's comments in Anon., 'Section of Obstetrics and Gynaecology', 703.

[90] Two notable exceptions, both referring to individual patients rather than to "shell-shocked" men in general, are R.A. Veale, 'Some Cases of So-Called Functional Paresis Arising out of the War and Their Treatment', *Journal of the RAMC*, 29:5 (November 1917), 608, 613, and Eder, *War-Shock*, pp. 98–9.

[91] Rivers, *Conflict and Dream*, pp. 22–8.

[92] A. McLaren, *Impotence: A Cultural History* (Chicago, IL and London: University of Chicago Press, 2007), pp. 107–14, 123.

exception, physicians mentioned impotence or homosexuality only if they directly employed psychoanalysis or were favourable towards it.[93] While it is possible that soldiers did not suffer from impotence or that doctors did not discuss sexual function with their patients, impotence was mentioned more often in post-war medical literature.[94] This may represent a deliberate wartime silence, or perhaps the later preoccupation of figures as diverse as Sigmund Freud and Marie Stopes with impotence as a symbol of masculinity in crisis.[95] The exclusion of potentially emasculating symptoms from wartime definitions of "shell-shock" contributed to medical constructions of the disorder as a masculine diagnosis.

However, exclusion of the feminine was even more important to the masculinization of "shell-shock". There were many levels to this exclusion. As female physicians were not permitted to join the RAMC, published wartime medical discourse on "shell-shock" was produced entirely by male doctors. Female nurses helped to care for "shell-shocked" men but did not publish on the disorder, and only one nurse was invited to give evidence to the War Office Committee of Enquiry into "Shell-Shock".[96] Nurses were usually mentioned in male medical accounts of the disorder only when doctors lamented that 'over-sympathetic' women hindered the recovery of nervous men.[97] According to this logic, women had no place in the therapeutic milieu. Most importantly, the published wartime medical literature defined "shell-shock" as a disease of men. Despite their experiences of grief, horror, and danger, women were not

[93] Forsyth, 'Functional Nerve Disease', 1401; C.S. Read, 'A Survey of War Neuro-Psychiatry', *Mental Hygiene*, 2:3 (July 1918), 376; Chambers, 'Mental Wards'; McDowall, 'The Genesis of Delusions', 189–90. The only exceptions I have found are G.H. Savage, 'Mental Disabilities for War Service', *JMS*, 62:259 (October 1916), 655, and F.W. Mott, 'Two Addresses on War Psycho-Neurosis. (II): The Psychology of Soldier's Dreams', *Lancet*, 2 February 1918, 169. Savage did not actually treat shell-shocked soldiers, and Mott referenced the claim that impotence was a common symptom to the psychoanalytically inclined John MacCurdy, backing up his statement with a few lines of Shakespeare rather than with clinical evidence.

[94] P. Bousfield, *"An Outline of Psychotherapy": A Lecture Delivered before the Deputy Commissioner of Medical Service* (London: Balliere, Tindall and Cox, 1919), p. 21; Hurst, 'War Neuroses and the Neuroses of Civil Life', 130; H. Somerville, 'The War-Anxiety Neurotic of the Present Day: A Clinical Sketch', *JMS*, 69:285 (April 1923), 173.

[95] McLaren, *Impotence*, pp. 151–9, 173; Carden-Coyne, *Reconstructing the Body*, pp. 174–7; Reid, *Broken Men*, p. 153.

[96] C. Hallett, *Containing Trauma: Nursing Work in the First World War* (Manchester: Manchester University Press, 2009), p. 158; Reid, *Broken Men*, p. 81.

[97] Hallett, *Containing Trauma*, p. 157; Hurst, 'War Neuroses and the Neuroses of Civil Life', p. 130. Reid, *Broken Men*, pp. 138–9, argues that female nurses were deliberately excluded from the care of "shell-shocked" men, partly because of male dominance in other forms of mental health nursing.

admitted to this community of suffering.[98] "Shell-shock" was a diagnosis produced by male physicians and applied to male soldiers. At the most basic definitional level, "shell-shock" was a masculine category of diagnosis. For the most part, historians have accepted this *de facto* definition and have neither noticed nor questioned the exclusion of women from claims to war neurosis.[99]

Although "shell-shock" was officially designated a masculine diagnosis, an order of being incommensurable with mere female suffering, fractures in this conceptualization were apparent even during the war. The feminine kept knocking at its edges or seeping back in. As it was believed that war regenerated corrupt masculinity, so it was argued it could turn "nervous" women into productive citizens.[100] As the war went on, the identification of the war neuroses with combat experience became crucial to the gendered construction of "shell-shock", but this did not sit easily with recognition that symptoms might manifest in men who had not seen active service.[101] Doctors realized that battlefield experience alone did not produce "shell-shock" and recognized the importance of grief, fear, danger, shock, and horror as causative factors in breakdown.[102] Under the conditions of total war, the experiences of non-combatants could encompass all these emotional reactions. Above all, there were important similarities between the conditions of service of frontline nurses and soldiers: both performed exhausting work in cramped conditions, underwent bombardment, and were continually exposed to death and mutilation.[103] The exclusion of frontline nurses from claims to "shell-shock",

---

[98] S. Das, *Touch and Intimacy in First World War Literature* (Cambridge and New York: Cambridge University Press, 2005), p. 195.

[99] For further discussion of the causes and consequences of this exclusion, see T. Loughran, 'A Crisis of Masculinity? Re-Writing the History of Shell-Shock and Gender in First World War Britain', *History Compass*, 11:9 (2013), 727–38. On nurses and "shell-shock", see D.J. Poynter, '"The Report on Her Transfer Was Shell-Shock": A Study of the Psychological Disorders of Nurses and Female Voluntary Aid Detachments Who Served Alongside the British and Allied Expeditionary Forces during the First World War, 1914–18', unpublished PhD thesis, University of Northampton (2008).

[100] Anon., 'Scotland', *BMJ*, 24 February 1917, 277; Weatherly, 'The War and Neurasthenia, Psychasthenia and Mild Mental Disorders. I'; T.A. Ross, 'Shell Shock', in H. Joules (ed.), *The Doctor's View of War* (London: George Allen and Unwin, 1938), p. 55. On war as a process of re-masculinization, see S.K. Kent, *Making Peace: The Reconstruction of Gender in Interwar Britain* (Princeton, NJ: Princeton University Press, 1993), pp. 13–30.

[101] Burton-Fanning, 'Neurasthenia in Soldiers'.

[102] Turner, 'Remarks on Cases of Nervous and Mental Shock'; Das, *Touch and Intimacy*, p. 195.

[103] Hallett, *Containing Trauma*, pp. 155–223; Das, *Touch and Intimacy*, pp. 176–203; M. Higgonet, 'Authenticity and Art in Trauma Narratives of WWI', *Modernism/Modernity*, 9:1 (2002), 91–107.

despite their potential equality of service, sacrifice, suffering, and danger, is the most powerful demonstration of its "official" construction as a masculine diagnosis.

Representations of war neurosis as originating in differently gendered forms of war experience reaffirmed ideas of "separate spheres". When doctors did mention women in published medical discourse, implicit claims to equality of sacrifice were undermined by explicit reassertions of traditional gender roles. In these rare acknowledgements of the potential war neurosis of women, doctors portrayed women as waiting, weeping, and hoping on the home front. Islay Muirhead (1857?–1948), a civilian practitioner, claimed that women were more prone to 'the war neuroses' because they were more affected by 'painful feelings, for example, anger, disgust, or anxiety'. He attributed this sensitivity to female 'instability and smaller control of feeling by intellect'.[104] The neurologist Wilfred Harris (1869–1960) believed that women developed war neurasthenia out of 'dread of injury to relatives or husbands fighting abroad'.[105] Advertisements for 'nerve remedies' reflected similar assumptions about female roles in wartime, portraying women as '[b]rooding in loneliness over the empty places that may never be filled again – dreading each letter, each paper lest unwelcome news is there'.[106] Doctors did not publicly relate female war neurosis to women's war service at home or abroad. Instead, women were portrayed as passive vessels of emotion, awaiting news from the battlefield.[107]

In medical discourse, as in war memorials or popular rhetoric about maternal sacrifice, the pain of women was publicly acknowledged and elaborated only when it took appropriately feminine forms.[108] Despite praise for women's willingness to take on "masculine" roles as part of the war effort, conceptions of sacrifice and suffering remained deeply gendered. In the careful construction of "shell-shock" as a masculine category of diagnosis, through the exclusion of the feminine and the writing out of potentially emasculating symptoms, doctors reaffirmed traditional gender roles. Nicoletta Gullace has argued that over the course of the war, reconfigurations of citizenship undercut the hegemony

[104] I.B. Muirhead, 'The Mental Factor', *TMW*, 11 (July–December 1918), 170–2; I.B. Muirhead, '"Shock" Psychology', *TMW*, 9 (July–December 1917), 309.
[105] Harris, *Nerve Injuries and Shock*, pp. 101–2.
[106] Advertisement for Sanatogen, *TMW*, 11 (July–December 1918), 215.
[107] T. Tate, *Modernism, History and the Great War* (Manchester and New York: Manchester University Press, 1998), pp. 11–12; Reid, *Broken Men*, p. 46; S.K. Kent, *Aftershocks: Politics and Trauma in Britain, 1918–1931* (Basingstoke: Palgrave Macmillan, 2009), pp. 19–20; Carden-Coyne, *Reconstructing the Body*, p.79.
[108] Carden-Coyne, *Reconstructing the Body*, pp. 143–50; Grayzel, *Women's Identities at War*, pp. 214, 233.

of sex and instead asserted the importance of sacrifice and service.[109] But the importance of sexual difference was retained in the medical sphere. The same impulses which led doctors to implicitly assert equality of suffering among men of different class and rank, and to temporarily write heredity out of their aetiologies of "shell-shock", also led them to ignore the potential existence of female war neurosis and to insist on the ultimate integrity – bruised but still intact – of the masculine identity of "shell-shock" patients. In wartime, psychiatric breakdown testified to the soldier's sacrifice. "Shell-shock" was another dubious privilege reserved for soldiers.

Men, Women, and Children in the Hierarchy of Evolutionary Development

So far, this chapter has focused on elisions, ellipses, and unexpected absences within medical discussions of "shell-shock" and has demonstrated complex alignments between pre-war and wartime medical discourse. The evasions of pre-war medical discourse on male hysteria, which reveal lurking fears of the feminine, are also found in wartime writings on "shell-shock". The gendering of "shell-shock" as male depended on an uneasy and incomplete exclusion of the feminine from the diagnosis and on the reassertion of traditional gender identities whenever the spectre of female war neurosis was raised. Yet in constructing "shell-shock" as a masculine diagnosis, doctors also drew on the concept of traumatic neurosis, with its origins in "modern", industrial, and male environments. Before the war, traumatic neurosis in men was most often associated with the working class. Most doctors refused to incorporate social prejudice into systematic theories of war neurosis, but these prejudices gradually gained more purchase in post-war discourse on "shell-shock". The apparent democratization of wartime did not fundamentally undermine conservative beliefs about class or gender, but this conscious drive towards recognition of the equality of (male) sacrifice nevertheless shaped wartime medical discourse on "shell-shock".

Although gender and class influenced diagnostic and therapeutic practices in myriad ways, doctors did not view "shell-shock" only in relation to these aspects of identity. Before the war, doctors viewed differential rates of traumatic neurosis in men and women as one symptom of

---

[109] N. Gullace, *"The Blood of Our Sons": Men, Women, and the Renegotiation of British Citizenship during the Great War* (New York and Basingstoke: Palgrave Macmillan, 2002), p. 2.

"modern" social pathologies which disrupted traditional relationships and patterns of life. In wartime, "shell-shock" generated a profusion of fears embracing the entire system of "civilized" biological and social relations. Concepts of gender and class formed only part of the wider constellation of medical ideas about human minds, bodies, and societies. Doctors placed "shell-shock" within the much broader matrix of evolutionary beliefs.

The application of evolutionary judgements is evident in the descriptions of "shell-shock" that doctors *did* apply to their patients as well as in the silences which pervaded wartime medical discourse. Although doctors rarely compared men under their care to hysterical women or explicitly commented on class or rank, they repeatedly and insistently likened "shell-shocked" men to children.[110] Sir John Collie (1860–1935), a pre-war expert on malingering who took this experience to the Ministry of Pensions in wartime, claimed that the mentality of sufferers was 'reduced more or less to the level of young children with their small powers of self-control, tendency to impulsive display of emotion, and marked suggestibility'.[111] Although more sympathetic to the plight of these men, Smith and Pear agreed that the nerve-shattered soldier behaved like a child and recommended that physicians adopt the same attitude 'which the sensible mother exhibits towards a child who exhibits sudden and unreasonable fear, anger, or any socially undesirable emotion'.[112] Rawdon Veale (1873–1954) emphasized that these men 'have become as little children and as little children they must be re-educated . . . as children they respond to encouragement, to censure, to praise or blame rightly bestowed'.[113] Because "shell-shocked" men behaved like children, doctors were forced to assume a strict maternal stance towards their charges.[114]

Doctors of all backgrounds and theoretical orientations compared "shell-shocked" men to children.[115] Charles Stanford Read, officer in

---

[110] On wider comparisons of soldiers to children, see S. Koven, 'Remembering and Dismemberment: Crippled Children, Wounded Soldiers and the Great War in Britain', *American Historical Review*, 99:4 (October 1994), 1167–1202; Hallett, *Containing Trauma*, pp. 164–7; Kent, *Making Peace*, p. 67. On soldiers' experiences of regression, see M. Roper, *The Secret Battle: Emotional Survival in the Great War* (Manchester and New York: Manchester University Press, 2009), especially pp. 243–75.

[111] Collie, 'Neurasthenia: What It Costs the State', 530.

[112] Smith and Pear, *Shell Shock and Its Lessons*, pp. 71–2, 92, 99.

[113] Veale, 'Some Cases of So-Called Functional Paresis', 613.

[114] On the maternal role of other army officers, see Roper, *Secret Battle*, pp. 165–6.

[115] See also Myers, *Shell Shock in France*, p. 55; L.R. Yealland, *Hysterical Disorders of Warfare* (London: Macmillan, 1918), p. 24; T.A. Ross, 'Anxiety Neuroses of War', in A.F. Hurst, *Medical Diseases of War* (London: Edward Arnold, 1944), pp. 153–4, 158; Herringham, *A Physician in France*, pp. 134–5; M. Nicoll, 'The Conception of Regression in Psychological Medicine,' *Lancet*, 8 June 1918, 797–8; Eder, *War-Shock*,

charge of 'D' Block, Netley, highlighted 'mental puerilism' as a form of hysteria characterized by 'childishness in speech and behaviour'.[116] Mott described cases of men emerging from stupor who behaved 'just as children do; they look at picture books, and they not only use the words which young children use, but the voice is modulated on the same juvenile standard'.[117] One of Hurst's amnesiac patients had regressed even further: he 'did not even know what his arms and legs were for, and had to be re-educated as you would teach a small baby'.[118] Some psychologists traced symptoms back to childhood and suggested that neurosis elided the passage of time and development of character separating boys from men. When explaining the origin of one soldier's claustrophobia in childhood experience, Rivers noted that 'the instinctive mode of reaction, which had had so great an effect upon the child of four as to make its suppression necessary, became powerless before the intelligence of the man of thirty'.[119] MacCurdy described the dreams of one patient as showing 'direct regression to childhood'. This soldier dreamt 'not that he was fighting against Germans, but that Indians were his foes'.[120]

These comparisons to children partially explain the lack of overt characterization of "shell-shocked" men as feminine. Historically, the 'obverse of manliness was often not so much femininity as childishness'.[121] "Shell-shock" was depicted as a challenge to masculine identity but also located within accepted understandings of masculinity and maturity which emphasized the potential curability of war neurosis through attainment of self-control.[122] However, conceptualizations of war neurosis as regression also gestured towards deeper, darker threats. In the evolutionary model of mind, the behaviour of women and of children were conceptually aligned. But emotion and lack of volition – the hallmarks of hysteria – were

---

pp. 55–6; A.J. Brock, 'The Re-Education of the Adult. 1: The Neurasthenic in War and Peace', *Sociological Review*, 10:1 (Summer 1918), 28; Culpin, *Psychoneuroses of War and Peace*, p. 13; Somerville, 'War-Anxiety Neurotic of the Present Day', 171, 174–5. Paul Lerner discusses examples of regression in "shell-shocked" soldiers recorded by Austro-Hungarian and German psychoanalysts; see Lerner, *Hysterical Men*, pp. 167, 189–92.

[116] Read, 'A Survey of War Neuro-Psychiatry', 369–70.

[117] Mott, 'War Psychoses and Psychoneuroses', 232–3. There are extended accounts of such cases in Mott, *War Neuroses and Shell Shock*, pp. 80–4.

[118] Hurst in *RWOCESS*, p. 25.

[119] W.H.R. Rivers, 'Why Is the "Unconscious" Unconscious? II', *British Journal of Psychology*, 9:2 (October 1918), 244.

[120] MacCurdy, *War Neuroses*, p. 44. See also p. 28.

[121] L. Davidoff, *Worlds Between: Historical Perspectives on Gender and Class* (Cambridge: Polity, 1995), p. 233.

[122] J. Meyer, 'Separating the Men from the Boys: Masculinity and Maturity in Understandings of Shell Shock in Britain', *Twentieth Century British History*, 20:1 (2009), 3, 20–1.

also perceived as characteristics of children, "primitive" races, and animals. Simple or exclusive binary oppositions of male and female did not apply within the evolutionary model of mind. Indeed, the female was perhaps the least relevant point of reference for understanding the male mind. "Civilized" children recapitulated racial development, but at puberty, the sexes took different developmental paths.[123] Women stopped short of the level of evolution potentially achievable by men but also developed distinctive sexual characteristics which were entirely their own. At various stages of development, man was animal, "savage", and child, but never woman.

The "civilized" masculine mind was viewed as the apex of evolutionary development. "Shell-shocked" soldiers fell short of the ideal standard not only of masculinity but also "civilized" humanity. More than this, because individual development recapitulated racial and evolutionary development, loss of "higher" control meant the resurgence of characteristics associated with earlier stages of evolution. The childlike "shell-shocked" soldier was dangerously close to the animal and the "primitive". The epidemic of male hysteria threatened to fracture "civilization" itself.

Conclusion

When historians try to explain why men choose (or not) to fight, how they endured (or did not) the conditions of industrialized warfare, or what the war meant for individual and social relations, they necessarily invoke even larger questions, which for the most part remain unarticulated, about the capacity for meaningful action in the face of powerful structural constraints. Gender and class are both formative elements of individual subjectivity, and are always and necessarily social. Histories which make no claims to speak about gender or class are nevertheless unavoidably saturated with assumptions about the operation of both aspects of identity in everyday life.[124] The same is true of medical discourse on "shell-shock". In wartime, doctors rarely explicitly discussed class or gender, but these silences speak volumes about doctors' own position of power over patients, their unwitting attempts to bolster the masculine identity of "shell-shock", their belief in the equality of

[123] Shaw, 'Lecture on the Special Psychology of Women', 1264.
[124] For example, even when the analysis does not use these terms, historical explanations of the success of recruitment propaganda in stimulating voluntary enlistment implicitly draw on ideas of the hegemony of bourgeois models of masculinity. See W.J. Reader, *At Duty's Call: A Study in Obsolete Patriotism* (Manchester and New York: Manchester University Press, 1988); M. Eksteins, *Rites of Spring: The Great War and the Birth of the Modern Age* (London: Papermac, 2000), pp. 175–91.

sacrifice of serving soldiers, and their subscription to the values and aims embodied in ideals of the warrior hero.

After the war, social prejudices around class, gender, and psychological breakdown gradually crept back into medical descriptions of "shell-shock". The absences of wartime medical discourse were less radical than they seemed. Wartime silence on the class and gender profile of sufferers of "shell-shock" can be viewed as an extension of the ambivalence within pre-war conceptualizations of traumatic neurosis, in which doctors had considerable freedom to decide whether illness resulted from the patient's own weakness or the horror of the precipitating event. Under the conditions of war, doctors temporarily adopted a public stance which did not link breakdown to social origins. However, this position was predicated on the utterly exceptional nature of wartime conditions, and manifested as silence rather than as positive statements about equality. This meant that after the war, it was all too easy to assume that the lessons of "shell-shock" did not apply to civilian life and to slide back into old habits of thought.

Ultimately, the experience of "shell-shock" reinforced existing medical attitudes towards gender and class. This is perhaps most evident in psychoanalytically inspired theories of "shell-shock". The social prejudice at the heart of the Rivers–MacCurdy thesis shows that class bias could facilitate the remoulding of radical psychological theories to express conservative social attitudes. In wartime, psychoanalytically oriented doctors were perhaps more inclined than non-"analytic" doctors to devote attention to character formation in early life. In the decades after the war, when doctors were freed from the compulsion to implicitly assert equality of sacrifice among their patients, this social conservatism resonated with mainstream medical opinion and was retrospectively enshrined in theories of "shell-shock". The war therefore simultaneously provoked, limited, and contained radical explorations of the nature of individual and social identity.

Nevertheless, while the war lasted, doctors' public loyalty to "shell-shocked" patients not only undercut some of the most entrenched medical beliefs about the lesser worth of those who suffered from psychiatric illness, but also hinted at continued anxieties about the direction and future of "civilization". In early 1916, Frederick Mott ended his Lettsomian lectures on "shell-shock" with a quotation from the now-forgotten wartime novel *Aunt Sarah and the War* (1915):

Lord, if they could listen to the unceasing shells that drive some men deaf, some men blind, some men dumb, and other men crazy, and these all of them MEN, with a newly earned meaning in the word; for there's a new meaning now in many an old word. We shall want a brand-new Dictionary, and its [sic] deuced hard work on old Murray, that just at the end of his great work he shall need to begin it all again.[125]

This statement emphatically defended the manliness of "shell-shocked" men in the face of unbearable strain. The claim that the dictionary needs to be rewritten to accommodate new meanings of masculinity was intended to underline the extent of wartime heroism. But it ended up underscoring the devastation of war and its disruption of all the old certainties, including language itself. The war threatened the established structures of "civilized" life. Because pre-war approaches to nervous and mental disorder, especially the evolutionary framework of understanding, continued to influence medical attitudes, "shell-shock" was embedded within a constellation of anxieties about identity which extended beyond gender and class and encompassed the history of the human race and the foundations of human "civilization". It embodied a profound and unsettling threat. Doctors acknowledged this threat but also sought ways to contain it, not least through their continued commitment to will as the core of "civilized" British manliness and character.

[125] Mott, 'Lettsomian Lectures. III', 553.

5   Re-Making Men
Will in Medical Approaches to "Shell-Shock"

In 1914, Britain was the only major European power without a system of conscription. Over the next two years, the second-largest volunteer army in the history of the nation was raised.[1] The possibility of introducing conscription had been debated in the opening decades of the twentieth century, but the British government retained its commitment to voluntarism for both pragmatic and ideological reasons. As Britain did not intend to field a large-scale army comparable to those of continental Europe in any future war, conscription seemed costly and unnecessary. The outbreak of war put conscription back on the political agenda, but most politicians desperately clung to the hope that the necessary expansion of the army could be achieved within the voluntary system. A broadly liberal paradigm, which regarded free will as crucial to the constitution of a patriotic citizenry, cut across traditional political divisions. This tradition viewed liberty as integral to the British national character. Voluntarism therefore symbolized all the values which Prussian militarism threatened. Only in May 1916, long after it became evident that the voluntary system could not provide the manpower needed for total war, was universal conscription introduced.[2] The reluctance to take this step demonstrates how tightly bound the principle of voluntarism was to cherished beliefs about national character, manhood, and citizenship. In the end, compulsion became acceptable only as part of the 'working-out of an economy of sacrifice', in which the population imbued the state with the responsibility to ensure, insofar as possible, equality of suffering. Even so, the ethics of voluntary service continued to dominate public life.[3]

---

[1] Gregory, *Last Great War*, p. 73.

[2] H. Strachan, 'Liberalism and Conscription, 1789–1919', in H. Strachan (ed.), *The British Army: Manpower and Society into the Twenty-First Century* (London: Frank Cass, 2000), pp. 10, 12–13; Gullace, *"Blood of Our Sons"*, pp. 103–4, 108; I. Bet-El, *Conscripts: Lost Legions of the Great War* (Stroud: Sutton, 1999), p. 5.

[3] The continued influence of the ethics of voluntary service can be seen in the smooth(ish) working of the tribunal system set up to assess claims for exemption from military service staffed by volunteers. Gregory, *Last Great War*, pp. 71–111, quotation p. 111.

At the heart of debates on conscription were the issues of free will and the rights of the individual citizen when the safety of the state or nation was threatened. These debates drew on established discourses of national character and manliness, which yoked free will to other positive attributes including self-restraint, perseverance, strenuous effort, courage in the face of adversity, and adherence to duty.[4] British traditions of martial heroism exemplified this view of ideal national manhood, emphasizing the transcendental potential of inner control over external might: one elementary school reader published in 1900 reminded students that Nelson's 'strength was in his heart and in his will, not in his body'.[5] This emphasis on will carried over into public discourse on recruitment. In Britain, the decision to enlist was portrayed as evidence of the moral conviction of the soldier, and the stimulus to profound inner transformation. Even after conscription was introduced, the sacred aura of the volunteer still haloed popular images of the British soldier.[6] The culture of voluntarism shaped assumptions about the motivation and moral worth of British soldiers until the end of the war and beyond.

As painfully evidenced by the introduction of conscription, in wartime the operation of will ceased to be a matter for abstract speculation and instead became woven into the urgent question of what the state could legitimately demand of its male citizens. This question applied not only to how men were delivered to the battlefield but also to what happened to their minds and bodies on arrival. Consequently, debates on "shell-shock" inevitably pushed up against deep-seated cultural beliefs about will, masculinity, and citizenship. Historians do not agree on how the experience of war affected views of character and manliness.[7] Some emphasize the prevalence of harsh moral judgements against "shell-shocked" men and see this condemnation as an extension of pre-war attitudes towards male nervous illness.[8] Other historians argue that the experience of "shell-shock" fundamentally challenged and transformed

---

[4] S. Collini, *Public Moralists: Political Thought and Intellectual Life in Britain, 1850–1930* (Oxford: Clarendon Press, 1991), pp. 92–94, 100, 113; M. Collins, 'The Fall of the English Gentleman: The National Character in Decline, c. 1918–1970', *Historical Research*, 75:187 (February 2000), 94; Micale, *Hysterical Men*, pp. 55–8; Smith, *Free Will and the Human Sciences*, p. 27.

[5] S. Heathorn, 'Representations of War and Martial Heroes in English Elementary School Reading and Rituals, 1885–1914', in J. Marten (ed.), *Children and War: A Historical Anthology* (New York and London: New York University Press, 2002), pp. 108–9.

[6] Gullace, *"Blood of Our Sons"*, p. 102; I. Bet-El, 'Men and Soldiers: British Conscripts, Concepts of Masculinity, and the Great War', in B. Melman (ed.), *Borderlines: Genders and Identities in War and Peace, 1870–1930* (London: Routledge, 1998), pp. 81–3; Bet-El, *Conscripts*, p. 209.

[7] Fiona Reid emphasizes ambivalence and the coexistence of condemnation with care and sympathy among different sections of the population. Reid, *Broken Men*, p. 25.

[8] Oppenheim, *"Shattered Nerves"*, pp. 150–2; Bourke, *Dismembering the Male*, pp. 115–18.

these beliefs. For Chris Feudtner, the acknowledgement that any man could break down under sufficient stress 'forced western society to take note and modify its views on mental illness, human motivation, and other issues far beyond the immediate problems of disabled soldiers'.[9] From this perspective, "shell-shock" revealed the ultimate fragility of the human psyche, undermined the bombastic stoicism applied to so many areas of social life, and fostered more sympathetic attitudes towards damaged or nervous individuals.

In this view, the dethroning of will was a necessary condition of the broader positive cultural changes stimulated by the war. The realization that self-control could not be maintained under all conditions irreparably damaged the belief in strong will which typified Victorian notions of character. However, medical discourse reveals a different, more complicated movement. The experience of trench warfare *did* provoke reassessments of the notion of courage, and the partial normalization of fear as a response to warfare: but, perhaps perversely, will remained central to the theorization and treatment of "shell-shock" and to the conceptions of "civilized" human nature and social life on which psychological medicine rested. A certain conceptualization of will, shaped by the evolutionary framework of understanding, was deeply embedded in discourses of masculinity and national character. It was loss of will, as the most recently acquired and most distinctively human faculty, which made "shell-shock" such a disturbing phenomenon. The implications of this loss were so disastrous that the ultimate aim of treatment always had to be restoration of self-control, the critical signifier of "civilized" British manhood. Although "shell-shock" held the latent potential to radically disrupt established sensibilities, the strength of existing cultural discourses around will and nervous breakdown constrained this potential. The war did not force a fundamental reimagining of human nature.

Will, Emotion, and the War Neuroses

In March 1915, John Herbert Parsons, a distinguished ophthalmologist acting as a specialist consultant to the home troops, delivered a paper on 'the psychology of traumatic amblyopia following explosion of shells' to the neurological section of the Royal Society of Medicine.[10] Parsons argued that under certain conditions, any soldier would inevitably

---

[9] Feudtner,'"Minds the Dead Have Ravished"', 409; see also Bogacz, 'War Neurosis and Cultural Change'; Stone, 'Shellshock and the Psychologists', pp. 265–6.

[10] Parsons, 'Psychology of Traumatic Amblyopia'. Amblyopia is a disorder of the visual system causing poor or blurry vision. Parsons' account of "shell-shock" was strongly influenced by the psychologist William McDougall's social psychology, discussed in Chapter 6.

develop "shell-shock", but the manner of recovery proved the worth of the man. Doctors could read character, conduct, and social feeling from the soldier's attempts to regain self-control and could correlate each stage of "shell-shock", from initial unconsciousness through to complete mastery of the self, to different levels of evolutionary development. This account anticipated several recurring themes in the medical literature, further elaborated as the war went on: the view of war neurosis as an imbalance of emotion and will; the depiction of emotion as "primitive" and will as "civilized"; the condemnation of men dominated by emotion; the elision of self-control with the 'will to recover'; the close association between restoration of self-control and return to health; and the ultimate reaffirmation of will as the measure of the man.[11]

In Parsons' view, soldiers must use will and character to fight against the unremitting, intense fear which characterized trench warfare. Because fatigue, terror, and excitement simultaneously impaired the normal powers of restraint and judgement and incited powerful instinctual and emotional reactions, soldiers must exert continual effort to control emotion, drawing on all their reserves of 'positive self-feeling', patriotism, and honour. This control was hard-won but tenuous and easily shattered if a shell explosion knocked a man unconscious. Such a blow reduced the soldier to 'an emotional animal' dominated by fear, 'the most potent of the primeval instincts', who lacked the 'volitional control' necessary to coordinate 'all those complex factors which make up the character of the man'. However, as the soldier gradually regained full consciousness, his capacity for self-control revived. At this stage, the essential character of the man revealed itself. The 'naturally mean-spirited man' sought to hide the shameful emotion of fear and to avoid renewed exposure to danger, but the man of 'fine character' strove to suppress fear as he became 'more and more conscious of the ideals of conduct which have shaped his character'. The soldier could only achieve full recovery through this painful and hard-won suppression of fear.[12]

In this theory of "shell-shock", the fact of breakdown implied no moral failure, but the soldier's ability to recover laid bare his innermost nature. Doctors could even infer from the manner of recuperation why men had really enlisted. Men who joined up because of peer pressure were likely to remain 'partial wrecks, too fearful of a renewal of their terrifying

---

[11] See Sharif Ismail's discussion of this article as 'the earliest manifestation of the psycho-physical synthesis' in wartime medical literature. S. Ismail, 'A "Creative Tension": The Royal Army Medical Corps and the Interplay of Psychological and Physiological in the Rise of a Psychoanalytic Synthesis, 1915–22', *Psychoanalysis and History*, 7:2 (2005), 193–4.

[12] Parsons, 'Psychology of Traumatic Amblyopia', 61–4.

experience to be of any use in the fighting line'. The man 'impelled by a noble ideal', on the other hand, not only made a full recovery but also emerged regenerated 'by the sense of a moral victory won'.[13] This mode of reasoning excused the doctor for failure to cure "shell-shocked" patients and displaced responsibility for breakdown from the war to the individual. It also left the supremacy of will within notions of character unchallenged. The partial normalization of fear as an emotion inescapable under specific circumstances deferred rather than dissolved the stigma attached to breakdown. Men who collapsed might be morally blameless: but *confirmed* war neurotics were inherently flawed human beings, lacking in both will power and patriotism.

This account demonstrates how the concept of will formed a conduit between medical and cultural discourses of masculinity, character, and patriotism. Similar slippage between perceptions of lack of self-control as behavioural trait and as pathological symptom is evident in discussions of malingering. Military and medical experts identified loss of control as the most important factor separating genuine "shell-shock" victims from shirkers. For this reason if no other, the problem of volition was always at the heart of the war neuroses: lack of will, above all other manifestations, defined "shell-shock" as an illness. However, most doctors perceived a continuum which stretched from 'uncontrollable functional disorder' to 'sheer purposeful malingering'.[14] The question of will was therefore central to the implementation of military discipline, which depended on the degree to which individuals could be held responsible for their actions. As the Committee of Enquiry concluded, if a soldier was capable of exercising self-control but nevertheless refused to 'face the situation', he was guilty of cowardice, a crime which carried the death penalty. In cases of "shell-shock", difficulties arose from the delicate decision as to 'whether the individual has or has not crossed that indefinite line which divides normal emotional reaction from neurosis with impairment of volitional control'.[15]

The will was always at fault in "shell-shock", but it was not a disorder of will alone.[16] As discussed in Chapter 1, within the evolutionary

---

[13] Ibid., 63–4.

[14] Myers, 'Contributions to the Study of Shell Shock (IV)', 466–7; Jones, 'War Shock and Freud's Theory of the Neuroses', 29–30; see also R. Cooter, 'Malingering in Modernity: Psychological Scripts and Adversarial Encounters during the First World War', in R. Cooter, M. Harrison, and S. Sturdy (eds.), *War, Medicine and Modernity* (Stroud: Sutton, 1999).

[15] Summary of findings, *RWOCESS*, p. 139.

[16] Charles Myers argued that "shell-shock" was caused by the pathological disorder of inhibition, not 'derangement of the will'. 'Will' and 'inhibition' were closely linked in pre-war psychological medicine, so this is an extremely fine distinction but nevertheless

framework of understanding which dominated psychological medicine, mind was defined as a unified and integrated structure made up of the three basic faculties of emotion, thought, and will. Healthy mental functioning depended on the correct operation of these faculties and maintenance of the proper relations between them. All mental disorders were potentially explainable in terms of the faulty working of individual faculties and as the result of imbalance between them. Most often, medical theories portrayed "shell-shock" as an imbalance of emotion and will.[17] The symbiotic relation between emotion and will meant that abundance in one direction necessarily entailed loss in the other: emotion could expand its empire only by encroaching on the territory of the will.[18] The war neuroses were consistently described in terms of struggle between the two faculties: a condition in which 'emotions have taken the place of a forceful will-power'; 'a state of persistent or recurring fear, which overrides the self-control of the individual'; or 'the sapping of a man's morale by sudden or prolonged fear which subordinates a man's power of will to his instinct of self-preservation and ultimately reduces him to a state wherein he cannot control his emotions'.[19]

These battles of emotion and will were conceived as clashes between the "primitive" and "civilized" constituents of human identity. In an unusually explicit statement on the evolutionary significance of emotion and will, Robert Armstrong-Jones described war neurosis as a condition in which fear, 'the oldest as well as the most intense of the emotions', overrode the action of the will, 'the highest and essentially the most human characteristic of the mind'.[20] In his view, the struggle of the individual soldier retold the story of human evolution itself. Man had 'experienced and recognized' fear 'from his earliest stages', but he had also 'tried to avoid and control' it, 'lest it should seize his whole

telling in its rejection of the language of character. Myers, 'Contributions to the Study of Shell Shock (IV)', 467.

[17] Theories of "shell-shock" usually minimized the role of the intellectual faculties, perhaps because thought disorders were associated with psychosis rather than neurosis. It is also possible that nervous or mental collapse did not seem an irrational response to the physical and emotional demands of trench warfare.

[18] Mott, 'Chadwick Lecture', 39; A.F. Hurst, 'Nerves and the Men (The Mental Factor in the Disabled Soldier)', *Reveille*, 2 (November 1918), 260.

[19] Quotations, Veale, 'Some Cases of So-Called Functional Paresis', 608; T.R. Elliott and J.F.C Fuller in *RWOCESS*, pp. 29, 71. See also Wolfsohn, 'Predisposing Factors of War Psycho-Neuroses', 179; G.H. Savage, 'Mental War Cripples', *Practitioner*, 100:1 (January 1918), 4; P.D. Hunter, 'Neurasthenia and Emotion', *Practitioner*, 103:5 (November 1919), 349.

[20] Armstrong-Jones, 'Psychology of Fear', 349, 351; R. Armstrong-Jones, 'Dreams and Their Interpretation', *Practitioner*, 98:3 (March 1917), 201; R. Armstrong-Jones, 'Correspondence', *JMS*, 64:267 (October 1918), 407–8.

personality'.[21] Because faultless command of the will represented the apogee of human development, states in which the will was held in abeyance – such as sleep and dreaming – were fundamentally regressive, associated with women, children, and the insane.[22] Many other doctors instituted evolutionary hierarchies in their discussions of "shell-shock". Walter Duncanson Chambers, an asylum psychiatrist serving in France with the Royal Inniskilling Fusiliers, viewed 'hysterical' men who lost control as on a par with 'mental defectives' and 'negroes'.[23] In an article on 'the wear and tear of flying', Thomas Rippon, a captain in the Royal Air Force Medical Services (RAFMS), claimed rigid self-control as a 'marked characteristic' of the average British man, in contrast to 'the more emotional Latin type'.[24] The "primitive" status of emotion meant that loss of self-control threatened the masculine, social, and human ideal: will promoted man to "civilization", and its absence demoted him to a lower realm.

Because emotion and will were aligned with different stages of individual, social, and racial development, when doctors defined "shell-shock" as a surfeit of emotion or a shortfall of will, they also implied normative judgements of sufferers. Although all cases of war neurosis involved impairment of emotion and will, different doctors allocated diverse parts to these faculties as they plotted trajectories of breakdown. The prominence afforded to emotion or to will varied across the medical literature. Theories emphasizing the role of "primitive" emotion in the development of "shell-shock" assigned sufferers to a lower order of being. Theories stressing the role of will – even in the context of failed struggles to exert control over emotion – placed "shell-shocked" soldiers on a higher level, from which they had temporarily slipped but could regain through renewed exercise of self-control.

Comparison of two accounts demonstrates the different effects achieved by an emphasis on emotion rather than will or vice versa. In one widely reported lecture, Sir John Collie, medical director of the Ministry of Pensions, persistently accentuated the role of emotion in war neurasthenia. He listed the physical conditions of trench warfare

---

[21] Armstrong-Jones, 'Psychology of Fear', 350, 357.

[22] Anon., 'Discussion on the Nervous Child', *BMJ*, 1923 (2), 969; Armstrong-Jones, 'Dreams and Their Interpretation', 205, 210–11, 213.

[23] Chambers, 'Mental Wards', 154, 173. James Crichton-Browne, in contrast, claimed that 'North-American Indians and negroes have a control over the reactions of painful and disagreeable stimuli which Europeans do not possess', and so 'the coloured races engaged in the war have suffered less from shell-shock than our men'. Crichton-Browne, 'First Maudsley Lecture', 214.

[24] T.S. Rippon, 'The Wear and Tear of Flying', *TMW*, 12 (July–December 1919), 326–7.

among the predisposing causes of war neurosis but placed much greater stress on 'fear, fear of being afraid, [and] terrifying experiences'. Collie argued that neurasthenic soldiers became trapped in a 'vicious circle' in which ever more 'intense emotion' accumulated until they eventually lost 'self-control'. He acknowledged the courage of many "shell-shocked" men, but Collie also built up a picture of war neurasthenia as based on selfish fear and self-obsession.[25] The evidence of William Tyrrell (1885–1968), a squadron leader in the RAFMS, to the Committee of Enquiry offered a virtual mirror image of Collie's approach. Tyrrell defined "shell-shock" as 'exhaustion of the nervous energy which controls will-power and self-control, with the resultant loss of control' resembling 'a paralysis of the inhibitory nervous system'. This description linked the physiology of emotion to the human attribute of will through the dual meaning of 'nerves', and effectively de-emotionalized the war neuroses.[26] Even when Tyrrell argued that attempts to hide fear contributed to nervous collapse, this emphasis on concealment further screened the emotions.[27] In accentuating will rather than emotion, Tyrrell depicted the erosion of control as the sad end to a noble struggle, whereas Collie portrayed it as the unavoidable outcome of temperamental egocentrism.

The subtle differences of emphasis in these two accounts almost amount to different theories of causation or different types of "shell-shock" – one caused by intense fear, the other by persistent and accumulated demands on the moral and nervous reserves of the individual. Across the medical literature, doctors made similar distinctions between patterns of breakdown according to the relative roles of will and emotion.[28] The official medical history of the war set out two aetiological models of "shell-shock". In the first, exhaustion and

---

[25] Collie, 'Management of Neurasthenia'; Anon., 'Neurasthenia in Soldiers', *Lancet*, 23 June 1917, 962; Anon., 'The Management of Neurasthenia and Allied Disorders in the Army', *TMW*, 8 (January–June 1917), 642; Anon., 'Cure of Shell-Shock', *Times*, 14 June 1917.

[26] William Tyrrell in *RWOCESS*, p. 30.

[27] Tyrrell's sympathetic analysis was undoubtedly informed by his own experience of near breakdown. Tyrrell told the Committee of Enquiry that he had suffered from "shell-shock" and provided anonymous testimony on this aspect of his experience. The quotations above are from the section of the *RWOCESS* in which he is named and speaks purely as a medical officer. For further details of Tyrrell's "shell-shock" and his post-war experiences, see M. Barrett, *Casualty Figures: How Five Men Survived the First World War* (London: Verso, 2007), pp. 92–121.

[28] In another account which drew explicitly on evolutionary theory, Robert Armstrong-Jones explained different patterns of breakdown as the result of activity at different evolutionary levels of the central nervous system. Armstrong-Jones, 'Mental States and the War – The Psychological Effects of Fear. II', 290–1; Armstrong-Jones, 'Psychology of Fear', 358, 389; R. Armstrong-Jones, 'Psychological Medicine', *Nature*, 99 (March–August 1917), 301.

successive painful or terrible incidents gradually eroded self-control; in the second, it broke down suddenly through horror or fear. The authors concluded that the 'circumstances of war' influenced breakdown but maintained that 'the temperament of the individual soldier' also 'played a large part'. It is not clear whether these authors used 'temperament' to describe biologically inscribed attributes, but later references to the rapidity of breakdown in 'the physical degenerate and the neuropath' suggest that this reading cannot be ruled out.[29] Similar assumptions informed the distinction that Charles Myers made, decades after the end of the war, between the 'good' and 'bad' nervous subject: the former was 'often a highly intelligent person, keeping full control over his unduly sensitive nervous system; the latter, usually of feebler intellect, having little hold over his instinctive acts to escape danger, the emotions which impel him to them, and the resulting conflicts'.[30] The application of normative judgements to individual soldiers according to the perceived mode of breakdown displaced responsibility for psychological suffering from the war onto the soldier and repeated the conclusion of pre-war debates on traumatic neurosis: that 'the intensity of the "shock" is not measured in terms of trauma but of individual sensitiveness'.[31] In this way, and despite the evident and acknowledged horrors of modern warfare, doctors upheld traditional standards of self-control in wartime.

Treatment by "I Will": Lewis Yealland and the Electrical Cure

The continued resonance of will within conceptions of character and manliness is also evident across therapeutic approaches to "shell-shock". As discussed in Chapter 3, doctors employed eclectic treatments for the nervous and mental disorders of war, from conservative regimes based on diet and rest to the "miracle cures" achieved at Seale Hayne. However, this apparent diversity masks the correspondence between different therapeutic techniques. Because doctors saw "shell-shock" as characterized by loss of self-control, the fundamental aim of any treatment aspiring to more than amelioration or removal of symptoms was repair and renewal of the will. Echoing John Herbert Parsons' assertion that recovery proved the measure of the man, many doctors identified absence of the 'will to recover' as the main reason for failures of

---

[29] Macpherson et al., History of the Great War, pp. 17–18.
[30] Myers, Shell Shock in France, p. 38.
[31] Wolfsohn, 'Predisposing Factors of War Psycho-Neuroses', 180.

cure.[32] In their depictions of *wilful* lack of will, as when Collie stated that patients remained ill because of 'stubbornness, lack of will-power, or refusal of further treatment', some of these claims also recalled pre-war medical discourse on hysteria.[33] Even when doctors accepted the patient's sincere desire for recovery, they still identified 'self-control' as both the prerequisite for, and emblem of, his return to health.[34] If the essence of the patient's illness was loss of self-control, then the doctor must strengthen the will and thus lead the patient to independence. This emphasis on the reinstatement of the will united therapies which shared no other common features.

This is most evident when we compare "disciplinary" and "analytic" therapies.[35] Most historians place at opposite ends of the therapeutic spectrum the electrical cure employed by Lewis Yealland at the National Hospital for the Paralysed and Epileptic, Queen Square, London, and the modified analytic therapies associated with Maghull Military Hospital near Liverpool and with W.H.R. River's practice at Craiglockhart War Hospital, Edinburgh. As briefly discussed in Chapter 4, Eric Leed's influential account of these treatments argued that doctors punished hysterical rankers with "disciplinary" therapies designed to make maintenance of the symptom more painful than return to combat, but treated neurasthenic officers sympathetically with 'talking cures' aimed at uncovering repressed complexes and furthering self-knowledge.[36] Elaine Showalter extended this interpretation to argue that while "disciplinary" treatments punished hysterical men for their perceived femininity, neurasthenic officers were treated with compassion because their behaviour came 'much closer to an acceptable, even heroic male ideal'.[37] A long historiographical tradition depicts these treatments as polar opposites.

---

[32] On the 'will to recover' in "shell-shock", see D. Drummond, 'Correspondence: War Psycho-Neurosis', *Lancet*, 2 March 1918, 349. The will to recover was also central in approaches to physical injury and disability: rehabilitation programmes and medical textbooks portrayed the mastery of prostheses as a masculine achievement of will over the self. See Carden-Coyne, *Reconstructing the Body*, pp. 184–5, and W.J. Gagen, 'Remastering the Body, Renegotiating Gender: Physical Disability and Masculinity during the First World War, the Case of J. B. Middlebrook', *European Review of History*, 14:4 (2007), 525–41.

[33] Collie, 'Management of Neurasthenia', 9. See also Bramwell, 'Recent Advances in Medical Science: Neurology', 437; Culpin, 'Practical Hints on Functional Disorders'.

[34] White, 'Observations on Shell Shock', 422.

[35] These terms are in double quotation marks because the practitioners involved did not describe themselves as distinct schools in this way.

[36] Leed, *No Man's Land*, pp. 169–80; B. Shephard, 'Shell-Shock', in H. Freeman (ed.), *A Century of Psychiatry*, 2 vols. (London: Mosby-Wolfe Medical Communications, 1999), vol. 2, pp. 35–6.

[37] Showalter, *Female Malady*, pp. 167–94; E. Showalter, 'Rivers and Sassoon: The Inscription of Male Gender Anxieties', in M. Higgonet *et al.* (eds.), *Behind the Lines:*

To the soldier on the receiving end of treatment, whether he was treated using analysis or painful doses of electricity undoubtedly made an enormous difference. Likewise, an individual doctor's willingness to induce physical pain tells us much about his view of the clinical relationship. Nevertheless, "analytic" and electrical therapies display important similarities. Both forms of treatment drew on similar conceptualizations of will and afforded the same importance to its role in breakdown and recovery. The centrality of will in different therapeutic approaches to "shell-shock" demonstrates both the influence of assumptions about human nature inherited from pre-war psychological medicine, and the extent to which these beliefs contained and neutralized the potentially radical challenge of "shell-shock" to Edwardian masculine ideals. War-time doctors saw the exercise of will as essential to mental health and appropriate masculine behaviour.

Yealland, a Canadian neurologist who served as resident medical officer and then registrar at the National Hospital during the war, described his technique as suggestion followed by rapid re-education.[38] As previously discussed, doctors commonly used suggestion to treat the hysterical symptoms of "shell-shock", and at least some contemporaries saw no real difference between Yealland's methods and those developed by doctors such as Arthur Hurst.[39] According to Yealland, the most powerful weapon in the physician's arsenal was his personality, particularly his adoption of 'an air of authority which will brook no denial'.[40] Yealland envisaged therapy as a titanic battle of wills in which the physician used every means at his disposal to ensure ultimate dominance. Again, this emphasis on medical authority was not unusual. All suggestive treatments were perceived to work through 'the dominance of a strong mind over a weak one', and to boil down to 'a contest between the physician's personality and that of the hysterical patient'.[41]

Gender and the Two World Wars (New Haven, CT, and London: Yale University Press, 1987), pp. 61–9; E. Showalter, 'Hysteria, Feminism and Gender', in S. Gilman *et al.* (eds.), *Hysteria beyond Freud* (Berkeley, Los Angeles, and London: University of California Press, 1993); E. Showalter, *Hystories: Hysterical Epidemics and Modern Culture* (London and Basingstoke: Picador, 1997), pp. 30–112.

[38] Yealland developed the method with the physiologist Edgar Adrian (1889–1977), who was later awarded the Nobel Prize with Charles Sherrington for research on neuromuscular coordination. Adrian parted company with Yealland because he became convinced that the method did not prevent relapse. Shephard, *War of Nerves*, p. 80.

[39] J.S. Bury, 'The Physical Element in the Psycho-Neuroses', *Lancet*, 10 July 1920, 66.

[40] Adrian and Yealland, 'Treatment of Some Common War Neuroses', 871.

[41] Anon., 'Medical Societies: Royal Society of Medicine', 438; J.P. Stewart, 'The Treatment of War Neuroses', *ANP*, 1:1 (January 1919), 20.

As an adjunct to the power embodied in his person, Yealland used electricity. Use of electricity was not unusual in itself. Physical therapies often included mild electrical massage; some doctors applied electrical current to kick-start 'lost' functions and prove to patients that no organic injury existed; and physicians employing suggestive therapies often displayed electrical apparatus as part of the theatrics of cure.[42] There are also some second-hand accounts of the use of faradization to flush out malingerers in the belief that painful electrical treatment would "encourage" men to stop pretending to be ill.[43] When Yealland explained his preference for electricity as the vehicle of suggestion, he offered two fairly conventional reasons: it was 'mysterious' enough to convince the patient of its efficacy, and strong currents could break down 'unconscious barriers to sensation'. Yealland only departed from common practice with his third reason: that treatment could be made 'extremely painful ... if the patient is one of those who prefer not to recover'. In Yealland's view, 'the hysterical type of mind' was characterized by 'weakness of the will and of the intellect, hypersuggestibility and negativism'. He believed that the patient's will, feeble in every other respect, baulked all attempts to break down fixed belief in his disability. The "disciplinary" element of the treatment therefore had to tackle 'the fixed idea which is giving rise to the functional symptom' and break down 'the unconscious resistance of the patient to the idea of recovery'.[44]

What did this mean in practice? 'Case A1' was a private who had participated in the retreat from Mons and taken part in most of the major battles of the war (including the Marne, First and Second Ypres, Hill 60, Neuve Chapelle, and Armentières) before collapsing on active service in Salonika in July 1916. He could not speak when he awoke, and remained mute until he came under Yealland's care nine months later. Case A1 was not typical of Yealland's patients.[45] His mutism had persisted for an unusually long time and had proved impervious to many different "treatments" – including hypnotism, strong electricity to the neck and throat,

---

[42] See, for example, Hewat, 'Clinical Cases from Medical Division', 211–22; Fraser, 'War Injuries of the Ear', 118–19; Fearnsides, 'Essentials of Treatment of Soldiers', 48; Stopford, 'So-Called Functional Symptoms'; Anon., 'Functional Anosmia', *BMJ*, 25 January 1919, 110; Anon., 'British Medical Association Special Clinical Meeting', 710; Dillon, 'Neuroses among Combatant Troops', 65.

[43] Eder, *War-Shock*, p. 138.

[44] Adrian and Yealland, 'Treatment of Some Common War Neuroses', 868–9.

[45] Ismail rightly points out that Case A1 was not typical of Yealland's patients and that Yealland dealt mainly with extremely severe cases of hysteria: Ismail, '"Creative Tension"', 190. However, Yealland did exploit the atypical aspects of the case for rhetorical purposes, and the discussion in *Hysterical Disorders of Warfare* therefore provides an excellent guide to Yealland's own conception of the essential aspects of the treatment.

placing 'hot plates' at the back of his mouth, and applying lighted cigarettes to the tip of his tongue – before he was sent to Yealland.[46] Yealland spent longer on the treatment and discussion of this patient than any other individual case in his published writings on the war neuroses. Case A1's treatment is the set piece of Yealland's *Hysterical Disorders of Warfare* (1918): he opened the book with this case to show readers what he could achieve with even the most difficult patient and how far he was prepared to push the conventionally accepted limits of the doctor's role in pursuit of "cure". This case was not typical, but Yealland deployed it as the exemplar of his methods.

The treatment is extremely distressing to read about.[47] Yealland locked the soldier in a darkened electrical room and attached electrodes to his pharynx. An initial application of strong electricity knocked the patient 'backwards, detaching the wires from the battery'. Yealland continued to apply electricity until the soldier could whisper. When Case A1 grew tired, Yealland walked up and down the room with him to keep him awake. Each whisper was hard-won, 'accompanied by an almost superhuman effort, manifested by spasmodic contraction of the muscles of the neck, the head being raised by jerks'. Twice the patient tried to escape but could not force the door open; at another moment, he broke down in tears. Yealland continued to apply electricity until the soldier could repeat all the vowels, then all the letters of the alphabet, and then the days of the week, months of the year, and numbers. Even after Case A1 could produce coherent speech, Yealland continued to apply electricity until he no longer stammered or spasmed. However, as the spasms disappeared from the patient's neck and jaw, his right arm developed a tremor. Yealland again applied electricity to the arm until the tremor ceased, but it then reappeared in the soldier's other arm. He explained that 'before it disappeared altogether [the tremor] had to be chased from the left arm, right arm, then from the left leg, and finally from the right leg'. This treatment lasted four hours in all.

For all its abstract similarities to other suggestive therapies, there is nothing else in the British medical literature remotely like Yealland's systematic treatment concept, which combined the performance of extreme medical authority with faradization.[48] Studies of case notes from Queen Square and other hospitals suggest that Yealland was almost

---

[46] Yealland, *Hysterical Disorders of Warfare*, pp. 7–8.
[47] The discussion of the treatment in this paragraph is from Ibid., pp. 7–15.
[48] Linden, Jones, and Lees argue that other physicians at Queen Square also used faradism, isolation, and physical therapies. Linden, Jones, and Lees, 'Shell Shock at Queen Square', 1987. However, while other doctors used similar therapeutic tools, Yealland's systematic treatment concept seems to have been unique in Britain.

certainly the only doctor in the United Kingdom to practise this form of treatment.[49] This was not because other doctors opposed the method. Yealland's method attracted no criticism at all in the wartime or immediately post-war period. In fact, *Hysterical Disorders of Warfare* was favourably reviewed in the medical press and praised for its 'insight into the mind of the sufferer' and 'immediate and practical usefulness'.[50] It is likely that Yealland had 'more admirers than rivals in his methods', as one reviewer put it, because the success of the treatment depended so much on his own personality that it could not easily be copied.[51] Moreover, Yealland avoided the charge, often levelled at other suggestive techniques, that his treatment did no more than remove the symptom and thus left the patient vulnerable to relapse.[52] Why did contemporaries sanction this painful and aggressive method while objecting to apparently innocuous forms of suggestion?

It is likely that Yealland's method met with the approval of other doctors because it combined high rates of success in the removal of symptoms, even in apparently intractable cases, with due attention to stiffening the patient's moral backbone. From this point of view, the important aspect of his treatment was 're-education' following removal of the symptom. Wartime writers rarely explicitly defined re-education, and the term could be applied to very different techniques, as will be seen in my later discussion of "analytic" methods. However, Bernard Hart stated that re-education could indicate two different psychotherapeutic processes: first, 'a process of training whereby it is sought to modify a symptom' and second, 'the process whereby causal factors, which have been elicited by analysis, are modified or re-arranged, so that they no longer produce morbid effects'.[53] Yealland's use of re-education fell into the first camp. He aimed to bring 'the disordered function back to the

---

[49] Leese, "'Why Are They Not Cured?'"; Humphries and Kurchinski, 'Rest, Relax and Get Well', 108; K. Fitzpatrick, 'Primum non nocere: War-Related Functional Nervous Disorders, Treatment and Diagnosis at the Royal London Hospital 1914–1918', unpublished Master's dissertation, Institute of Historical Research London (2009), p. 45. Yealland's obituary passed over his war work in one sentence, suggesting that his treatment was not remembered as a particularly significant episode in the development of approaches to "shell-shock", and was no longer notorious by the 1950s. Anon., 'Obituary: Lewis Ralph Yealland', *Lancet*, 13 March 1954, 577–8.

[50] Anon., 'Review: Hysterical Disorders of Warfare', *Lancet*, 24 August 1918, 242.

[51] Anon., 'Hysterical Disorders of Warfare', *BMJ*, 10 August 1918, 134.

[52] Yealland did not systematically collect figures charting relapse and recovery. However, in 1919, he claimed he was still in touch with about one hundred patients, and cure (including subsequent 'freedom from anxiety') had proved permanent for about 90 per cent of these men. Anon., 'British Medical Association Special Clinical Meeting', 710.

[53] B. Hart, *Psychopathology: Its Development and Its Place in Medicine* (London: Cambridge University Press, 1927), p. 125.

normal by re-directing until the bad habit is lost'. The re-educative process, consisting of rapid and 'authoritative' orders to carry out the lost function, should start as soon as 'the least sign of recovery has appeared'.[54] The painful "disciplinary" element ensured that patients would be receptive to re-education. Yealland inflicted pain in order to break down resistance to recovery and so that re-education could be carried out: the patient's suffering was another tool of treatment, not its ultimate end.[55]

The process of re-education obviated conventional critiques of suggestion because it aimed to make the patient participate in cure through his own efforts. When treating Case A1, Yealland told him, "Remember, there is no way out, except by the return of the proper voice and the door. You have one key, I have the other; when you talk properly I shall open the door so that you can go back to bed".[56] He told another patient, "I am treating you with, 'I will' . . . You must give up that subconscious 'I will not'; now make every attempt to walk alone, you will not fall".[57] The 'I will' perhaps referred to the will Yealland himself put behind the treatment, but it also referred to the will of the patient, which required re-direction.[58] Yealland's explanation of the ethos underlying treatment could have been his manifesto: 'If there is no alternative between walking and falling down the patient will usually find himself able to walk'.[59] Suggestion removed the symptom, but ultimately the patient must rely on his own efforts to perform the function. The logic behind the brutality of the treatment was not punishment but that the weak-willed hysteric needed a strong and even painful spur to return to normal health.

Yealland also emphasized the positive aspects of re-education. He saw the instillation of self-reliance and control as essential to restore both the patient's lost function and his lost identity. When treating Case A1,

---

[54] Adrian and Yealland, 'Treatment of Some Common War Neuroses', 868, 870.

[55] Yealland did not always use pain as a therapeutic tool and did not always use strong currents: see *Hysterical Disorders of Warfare*, pp. 39–41. It is likely that Yealland justified the disciplinary elements of treatment as a response to urgent war conditions and that these did not form part of his usual treatment of hysteria. In 1923, he suggested that many physicians inflicted pain in order to end an hysterical fit but did not explicitly refer to disciplinary or punitive aspects of treatment. Other aspects of his approach (use of suggestion and the aim of removing symptoms) remained the same. L.R. Yealland, 'Hysterical Fits: With Some Reference to Their Treatment', *Lancet*, 15 September 1923, 551.

[56] Yealland, *Hysterical Disorders of Warfare*, p. 13.   [57] Ibid., p. 151.

[58] Henry Smurthwaite viewed treatment by suggestion and persuasion as the transference of his own will to the patient: 'The patient has lost his will power and confidence, which we must restore by force of our own energy and influence . . . We instil that necessary power into him'. Smurthwaite, 'War Neuroses', 183.

[59] Adrian and Yealland, 'Treatment of Some Common War Neuroses', 871.

Yealland began by reminding the patient of his status as a soldier and a man: "Remember, you must behave as becomes the hero I expect you to be ... A man who has gone through so many battles should have better control of himself". When the patient began to cry and attempted to leave the room, Yealland reminded him that he was "a noble fellow": "these ideas which come into your mind and make you want to leave me before you are cured do not represent your true self ... you must make every effort to think in the manner characteristic of your true self – a hero of Mons". From this point on, Case A1's attitude 'changed considerably, and from that time he made every attempt to recover'. At the end of the treatment, when all physical disabilities had been vanquished, Yealland again told the soldier, "You are a hero". This statement might now read as the final embellishment on the straitjacket of idealized masculinity which Yealland had so brutally reimposed; but in Yealland's account, Case A1 is gratified by praise, thrilled by the success of the treatment, and exclaims at its end, "Doctor, doctor, I am champion!"[60]

In Yealland's reports, patients were often grateful to him, and occasionally offered effusive thanks for his help.[61] Of course, the testimony of a self-appointed medical saviour should be approached with caution. But even if these depictions of patients' gratitude are entirely fictional, they are still crucial for understanding the image Yealland wanted to project. There is evidence that the prospect of treatment by Yealland provoked severe anxiety in some patients, and that some even discharged themselves from hospital against medical advice rather than undergo further treatment.[62] It is also possible, however, that Yealland told the (partial) truth. Men trained to view self-control as the foundation of self-respect might have found "cure" an almost unbearable relief, and a reprieve – even if it involved an experience very like torture, and meant their return to war. This interpretation amplifies, rather than diminishes, the peculiar awfulness of this form of treatment.

"Analytic" Therapies

A common thread runs through Yealland's electrical treatment and eclectic "analytic" therapies: the emphasis on self-control, self-reliance, and strength of character. At the level of the patient's experience, there can be no meaningful comparison between "analytic" treatments and those which bordered on torture. However, drawing out shared

---

[60] Yealland, *Hysterical Disorders of Warfare*, pp. 7–14.
[61] Ibid., pp. 17, 30, 43, 111, 114, 129–30, 138, 143, 153–4, 184, 192.
[62] Linden, Jones, and Lees, 'Shell Shock at Queen Square', 1984.

concepts, beliefs, and approaches helps us to understand the collective context within which doctors devised theories and therapies, and to measure the extent to which "shell-shock" forced changes in the medical worldview. Comparison of "analytic" and "disciplinary" treatments shows that similar ideas about character and willpower underpinned radically different therapies. Core beliefs about gender, identity, and human nature remained intact despite the experience of "shell-shock".

"Analytic" is not a synonym for "psychoanalytic". Military doctors did not employ psychoanalysis proper as a treatment for "shell-shock". Here, "analytic" describes the approaches of doctors who were keenly interested in psychodynamic theories and used modified psychological techniques to treat "shell-shocked" soldiers. This group included Grafton Elliot Smith, T.H. Pear, W.H.R. Rivers, William Brown, and Montague David Eder. With the exception of Eder, these doctors all spent time attached to Maghull Military Hospital.[63] Under the aegis of Richard Rows (d. 1925), Maghull became a hub for wartime exploration of psychological approaches.[64] Although different from each other in several respects, these "Maghull" doctors all favoured forms of treatment based on re-education (sometimes described as persuasion and re-education, or analysis and re-education) for war cases. This reflects the enthusiasm at Maghull for Déjerine's psychotherapeutic techniques.[65] All "analytic" therapists, including those who did not serve at Maghull, understood war neurosis primarily as a form of psychological illness, and believed that effective treatment rested on understanding the particular elements of past experience that had led symptoms to develop, while also acknowledging that ideal treatments were not always possible under war conditions.

Like other physicians, most "analytic" doctors portrayed "shell-shock" as an imbalance of emotion and will. However, they also believed that patients suffered because they did not 'appreciate the real value' of their

---

[63] Throughout this chapter, I refer to doctors who served at Maghull, although not necessarily at the same times, as "Maghull" doctors. I bracket these doctors together to emphasize similarities in their approaches, but the double quotation marks indicate that publications cited may have been produced either during or after the period of service at the institution.

[64] On Maghull, see Shephard, '"The Early Treatment of Mental Disorders"'; Jones, 'Shell Shock at Maghull and the Maudsley'.

[65] T.H. Pear, 'The War and Psychology', *Nature*, 102:2253 (3 October 1918), 88; Shephard, 'The Early Treatment of Mental Disorders', p. 444. In turn, Déjerine drew on the writings of the Swiss physician Paul Charles Dubois. For descriptions of both approaches, see Raitt, 'Early British Psychoanalysis', 73. For an account of persuasion, see Bramwell, 'Recent Advances in Medical Science: Neurology', 437–8.

war experiences.[66] Richard Rows argued that the prolonged strain of war service exhausted patients and lowered their self-control, leading to fixation on the emotional elements of war experience. In Rows' view, over-emotion, lack of control, and the inability to place troubling aspects of war experience in their proper perspective characterized "shell-shock".[67] The doctor's role was to help patients understand the 'true significance' of their history and condition through the therapeutic process of re-education (here used in Hart's second sense).[68] As patients gained insight into 'the nature and mode of origin' of their 'mental illness', the 'excessive emotional tone' of memories and outlook dissipated, and 'rapid improvement' in general condition followed.[69] All "analytic" doctors who served at Maghull agreed with the basic elements of this approach to "shell-shock", although some discussed aetiology in more detail than others, or adopted other forms of treatment when circumstances made alternative therapies desirable on grounds of efficiency or speed.

The method of re-education practised by most "Maghull" doctors depended on the active (will-ful) cooperation of intelligent patients as well as on the doctor's skill and tact. It involved conducting extended 'interviews' with patients to ascertain the exact nature of the incident(s) leading to breakdown. The doctor should elicit the patient's history, explain 'the reason and the mechanism' of the illness, and show the patient 'how he can educate himself to regain that which was lost'. The patient was induced 'to face the trouble, to reason about it, and to recognize it simply as a memory of the past instead of allowing it to dominate him'.[70] William Brown called this method 'autognosis' (self-knowledge) because through it, 'the patient learns to understand himself'. For Brown, this knowledge was inseparable from the exercise of will: the therapeutic value of autognosis lay in the truth that '[s]elf-knowledge brings with it self-control in the psychic domain'.[71] To achieve lasting results, the patient 'must be convinced that it was he himself who worked the "cure," or he cannot hope in future to "cure"

---

[66] McDowall, 'Functional Gastric Disturbance', 88; Rivers, *Instinct and the Unconscious*, p. 149; Brown, 'Hypnosis, Suggestion, and Dissociation', 734; Forsyth, 'Functional Nerve Disease', 1403.

[67] Rows, 'Mental Conditions'; Rivers, 'War-Neurosis and Military Training', 525–6; Rivers, 'Address on the Repression of War Experience', 177.

[68] Smith and Pear, *Shell Shock and Its Lessons*, pp. 41, 53–4.

[69] Rows, 'Mental Conditions'; Smith and Pear, *Shell Shock and Its Lessons*, p. 72.

[70] Rows, 'Mental Conditions'.

[71] W. Brown, 'The Treatment of Cases of Shell Shock in an Advanced Neurological Centre', *Lancet*, 17 August 1918, 198.

himself'.[72] Millais Culpin varied the usual method by enlisting 'an intelligent patient who has been through the "cure"' to convince the next patient of its effectiveness, joining practical demonstration of results to medical exhortations.[73] Indeed, in all such treatments, the doctor's role was conceived as minimal. "Analytic" doctors directly correlated the extent of medical intervention required to the patient's intelligence and willpower. A sharp, determined patient would quickly grasp the nature of treatment and effectively re-educate himself.[74] Doctors repeatedly emphasized that the success of "analytic" therapy depended on active patient participation and 'effort of will'.[75]

Like other "analytic" doctors, W.H.R. Rivers favoured re-education and stressed the patient's active contribution to treatment.[76] However, Rivers' theory of repression nuanced his account of the operation of will in recovery. Rivers argued that many symptoms of war neurosis originated in unsuccessful attempts to repress memories of war experience rather than in the nature of the experience itself.[77] Like other "Maghull" doctors, Rivers believed that patients suffered from lack of self-understanding and from distorted perspectives on their war experience. Rivers added to this formula the argument that unsuccessful efforts to thrust unpleasant memories out of consciousness compounded these other problems.[78] Attempts at repression were conscious, intelligent,

[72] Ross, 'Prevention of Relapse of Hysterical Manifestations'; see also KCHMSA: KHU/C1/M9, R. Dansie, 'The Psychology of the Voice' (15 January 1919).
[73] Culpin, 'Dreams and Their Value in Treatment', 156.
[74] Smith, 'Shock and the Soldier. II', 855, 857; Smith and Pear, Shell Shock and Its Lessons, p. 67; McDowall, 'Functional Gastric Disturbance', 78; McDowall, 'Mutism in the Soldier', 58.
[75] Eder, 'Address on the Psycho-Pathology of the War Neuroses', 268; Myers, Present-Day Applications of Psychology, p. 43.
[76] There is a good short summary of this approach in W.H.R. Rivers, 'Freud's Psychology of the Unconscious', Lancet, 16 June 1917, 914; see also Rivers, Instinct and the Unconscious, p. 125.
[77] The role of repression in producing neurosis is unclear in Rivers' writings, although it seems that over time, he attributed more importance to repression. In most writings, he did not clearly distinguish between repression in the production and in the maintenance of neurosis. Rivers did not explicitly discuss the role of repression in producing war neurosis in his classic 1918 article on the subject, but in the post-war period did propose renaming anxiety neurosis 'repression-neurosis' to better reflect the aetiology of the disorder. Rivers, 'Address on the Repression of War Experience', especially 173; Rivers, Instinct and the Unconscious, p. 124.
[78] Michael Roper argues that Rivers' 'emphasis on the secondary mechanism of repression reflected the tension that military doctors sometimes experienced between humane impulses and military duty: Rivers could do something about how the memory of the event was handled, but not about the way the war itself was waged'. Roper, Secret Battle, p. 248.

and most definitely *willed*.[79] For Rivers, therapeutic intervention must involve specific attention to what the patient was trying to avoid or forget.[80] Because of this emphasis on repression, Rivers did not view re-education as the doctor's sharp spur to a latent or sluggish willpower so much as the bipartite process of the patient's deliberate and willed surrender of an unsuccessful course of action and the re-direction of an already active will.[81] This positive appraisal of the patient's capacity for willed action may explain why Rivers took a more collaborative and patient-centred approach than most "shell-shock" doctors.

Among prominent "analytic" doctors, there were two partial exceptions to the general preference for treatment by re-education. William Brown used light hypnosis to produce abreaction (the cathartic reliving of emotional experiences) in hysterical patients, and David Eder practised suggestion on war cases. Both developed these techniques on active service and administered them to large numbers of patients with relative speed. Brown identified abreaction of the emotional affect caused by traumatic incidents as the crucial component in treatment. His ideal method of treatment was mental analysis, but he used the 'short cut' of light hypnosis to produce abreaction in early cases of hysteria.[82] Although he did not explicitly discuss abreaction, when on active service, Charles Myers similarly valued hypnosis as a method to revive lost memories, stating that the 'restoration of past emotional scenes constitutes a first step towards obtaining that volitional control over them which the individual must finally acquire if he is to be healed'.[83] Brown emphasized that he used hypnosis only to produce abreaction and reiterated the usual criticisms of hypnotic suggestion: it treated the symptom, not the cause; it did not require the patient to take an active part in treatment; it increased suggestibility; and repeated hypnosis caused dissociation.[84]

---

[79] Rivers, 'Address on the Repression of War Experience', 177; Rivers, *Instinct and the Unconscious*, pp. 124–5.

[80] It is perhaps partly because Rivers attributed such importance to the willed process of repression that he valued methods such as dream analysis and free association, which probed patients' psyches when they had temporarily relinquished control. Rivers, 'A Case of Claustrophobia', 239; Rivers, 'Address on the Repression of War Experience', 176; Rivers, *Instinct and the Unconscious*, p. 123.

[81] Rivers, 'Address on the Repression of War Experience', 175.

[82] Brown, 'Treatment of Cases of Shell Shock in an Advanced Neurological Centre', 199–200; Brown, 'Hypnosis, Suggestion, and Dissociation', 736; W. Brown, 'War Neurosis: A Comparison of Early Cases Seen in the Field with Those Seen at the Base', *Lancet*, 17 May 1919, 836.

[83] Myers, 'Contributions to the Study of Shell Shock (II)', 69.

[84] Brown, 'Hypnosis, Suggestion, and Dissociation', 735.

Eder was the only "analytic" doctor to fully endorse suggestive therapies for war neurosis. He insisted that psychoanalysis was the only method to truly deal with underlying causes rather than symptoms but compared its use in war cases to taking up 'a Nasmyth hammer to crack a nut'. Because war neurotics had only broken down under severe stress, Eder reasoned, they were not susceptible to increased suggestibility, mental weakness, or relapse in the same way as civilians who had collapsed under lighter strain.[85] Under war conditions, suggestion was the most appropriate treatment as it 'most rapidly relieves the patient and sends him back to the army most quickly'. Eder therefore used psychoanalysis for diagnostic purposes only, reasoning that suggestive treatment was more effective when it targeted the underlying cause of the problem and that the war-shocked man required only the 'temporary reinforcement of his own will-power' supplied by suggestion.[86] Perversely, Eder's deep commitment to psychoanalysis led him to view suggestion as suitable for war cases. If psychoanalysis was the *only* method of treatment in which 'the patient learns for himself the real significance of his disease, a privilege only acquired by a bitter self-realization', then all other forms of treatment were more or less equal.[87]

In fact, Eder's definition of suggestion as 'all methods which depend upon the physician's directing and governing the patient' incorporated the "Maghull" style of re-education.[88] "Maghull" doctors doubtless would have protested that their methods strengthened the patient, but several examples hint at the dictatorial undertones to their approaches.[89] Most obviously, patients were consistently portrayed as unable to grasp the true import of what had happened to them, while the doctor's lofty detachment enabled him 'to see both the past and the present experiences [of patients] in their right proportions'.[90] Unspoken but

---

[85] Eder, *War-Shock*, pp. 132–4; see also p. 11.

[86] Quotations Eder, 'Address on the Psycho-Pathology of the War Neuroses', 268; Eder, *War-Shock*, pp. 130, 133; see also pp. 99, 132, 134, 140.

[87] Ibid., pp. 132–3.

[88] Ibid., p. 139. Eder himself sometimes adopted similar authority over the patient. He did not always share diagnostic conclusions or reveal the nature of suggestions made under hypnosis, deeming this unnecessary when analysis was undertaken for diagnostic rather than therapeutic purposes. He was also equivocal about apparent medical mistreatment of some patients, a stance resulting either from the attempt to maintain a balanced view, tact, or professional loyalty. See Eder, *War-Shock*, pp. 63–4, 99–100, 121.

[89] Jessica Meyer points out that all treatments for "shell-shock" involved doctors assuming authority over the patient, albeit to different degrees, and that this authority depended on rank, professional status, and age as well as specific therapeutic methods. Meyer, 'Separating the Men from the Boys', 13–14.

[90] Brown, 'War Neurosis', 836; Rivers, 'Address on the Repression of War Experience', 177.

ever-present behind this assumption was the view of patients' emotional reactions as incommensurate with the facts of their experience. This kind of implicit reasoning is evident in a paper on functional gastric disorders by Maghull doctor Colin McDowall. He discussed a patient who had fought in some of the major battles of the war, suffered facial injuries from a shell explosion, and then endured the loss of a child. McDowall paid little attention to the nature of the man's war experience but diagnosed his tendency to 'take things too much to heart' as one of the main causative factors in his condition.[91]

It is now difficult not to feel that sometimes psychological breakdown was an entirely proportionate response to the war, but "shell-shock" doctors rarely came to this conclusion, even if they sometimes skirted quite close to it. Grafton Elliot Smith and T.H. Pear insisted that the "shell-shocked" patient's reason was not 'ineffective or impaired': if anything, it operated hyper-efficiently to tell him 'quite correctly, and far too often for his personal comfort' that his own actions had contributed to some 'disastrous and memory-haunting' event. The patient's 'reason, rather than the lack of it' proved his worst enemy.[92] This argument implied that the war, rather than the individual, was to blame for breakdown – a conclusion that doctors shied away from in the later years of the war. However, Smith and Pear did not follow their argument through to this conclusion. Instead, like other "analytic" doctors, they asserted the physician's superior ability to rationalize war experience and to place it in the 'correct' perspective for patients. Indeed, they saw the patient's refusal to accept medical 'arguments and persuasions' as 'resistances' caused by 'auto-suggestion and false beliefs'. While recommending that hypnosis should be avoided whenever possible, Smith and Pear nevertheless believed that it was legitimate to hypnotize patients in order to make them receptive to the doctor's point of view.[93] This assumption of medical dominance was of a piece with their use of the analogy of the sensible mother and unreasonable child to describe the relationship between doctor and patient.[94]

Faint traces of a similarly authoritarian stance infuse W.H.R. Rivers' descriptions of re-education as well as his characterization of anxiety neurosis as a 'regressive' reaction involving childish modes of expression.[95] Nevertheless, elsewhere Rivers exhibited an empathy which

---

[91] McDowall, 'Functional Gastric Disturbance', 83–4.
[92] Smith and Pear, *Shell Shock and Its Lessons*, p. 3.   [93] Ibid., p. 39.
[94] Ibid., pp. 71–2.
[95] Rivers, *Instinct and the Unconscious*, pp. 149–50; Rivers, 'Address on the Repression of War Experience', 177.

implicitly validated the patient's extreme reaction to his war experience. Rivers insisted that attempts to repress memories often stemmed from 'excess rather than defect in certain good qualities'.[96] This was a radical reassessment of the moral motives behind repression: compare Rivers' statement with the psychologist Carveth Read's (1848–1931) description of the repression of unpleasant memories as an 'unhealthy' form of 'mental self-mutilation', typically practised by 'children, weak-minded people, unstable, fastidious, and morbidly sensitive people'. In Read's view, repression connoted at worst 'moral cowardice', and at best 'weakness and unfitness for life in this world'.[97] Rivers, on the other hand, sought to help patients see what had been 'good or even ... noble' in their conduct.[98] This sympathetic attitude led Rivers to adopt more collaborative approaches to treatment than many other "analytic" doctors. Other doctors set out their techniques using words such as 'show', 'explain', and 'tell'; Rivers spoke of 'conversation', 'discussion', and 'encouragement', and described attempts to make dream analysis 'a matter in which the patient and I are partners'.[99] Rivers' emotional identification with patients could even lead treatment to fail. One of his patients had been thrown headfirst by a shell explosion into the abdomen of a German corpse, leaving the young officer sickened by the memory of rotting flesh and noxious gases filling his mouth and nose. Rivers could find no redeeming feature of this experience to enable the patient to cope with what had happened and as a result could not confidently advise giving up attempts at repression.[100] In this case at least, Rivers felt the horror of the patient's experience and was therefore unable to intellectualize it.

Yet despite his empathy with patients, Rivers did not waver from his belief that the war must be fought to the finish and that "shell-shocked" men must, if possible, be returned to service.[101] He did not see this as imposing an ethos of patriotic duty and military honour on men whose breakdown had proved their unconscious rejection of these values, but rather as helping them to fulfil the most deeply held desires of the adult

---

[96] Rivers, 'War-Neurosis and Military Training', 533.
[97] C. Read, 'The Unconscious', *British Journal of Psychology*, 9:3 (May 1919), 291, 298.
[98] Rivers, 'Freud's Psychology of the Unconscious', 914.
[99] Rivers, *Conflict and Dream*, p. 59; Rivers, 'Freud's Psychology of the Unconscious', 914.
[100] Rivers, 'Address on the Repression of War Experience', 174.
[101] Using Rivers' descriptions of his dreams as evidence, Elaine Showalter argues that his support for the war wavered from early in 1917. Rivers himself explained wartime dreams that suggested less than total support for the war as originating in his 'egoistic' tendencies: he wanted the war to end so that he could return to research work, but this desire conflicted with his conscious political belief that Britain should fight to the finish. See Showalter, *Female Malady*, pp. 187–8; Rivers, *Conflict and Dream*, pp. 118–36, 165–80.

personality. Rivers not only denied that repression was a pathological process in itself but also maintained that it was a 'necessary element in education and in all social progress'. In his view, the patients he treated suffered not because they attempted to repress memories of their war experience, but because these attempts were unsuccessful.[102] The basic premise of Rivers' theorization of the production and maintenance of anxiety neurosis was that men desperately wanted to carry out their duty, and fought to do so, even against the ineradicable instinctual forces which clamoured within, shrieking for survival. The fact of anxiety neurosis could almost be taken as an index of character, of the patient's 'excess' of 'certain good qualities'.[103] Rivers validated the truth of the patient's emotional response to war because he endorsed the values which he believed led men to break down.

"Analytic" doctors did not reappraise the central tenets of the Victorian and Edwardian ideal of masculine character, but instead reinforced the importance of living up to the values it embodied.[104] Eder described a case in which hypnotism had failed, and he reverted to persuasion: his exhortations prompted 'a flood of tears' in the patient, who 'lay awake all that night making up his mind that he would walk, and the next day the sticks were relinquished, he was cured of the paraplegia'.[105] It is difficult to conceive of a more literal demonstration of the belief that the patient must learn to 'stand on his own feet and rely on his own strength'.[106] "Analytic" doctors consistently described re-education in the language of a militarized, masculine ethos of honour, stoicism, and self-control.[107]

---

[102] Rivers, 'Address on the Repression of War Experience', 173. See also Stoddart, 'Morison Lectures on the New Psychiatry. Lecture I', 587, 590. Another "Maghull" doctor, Percy Hunter, similarly described the desire to repress memories as 'perfectly proper, and [making] for strength of character'. Hunter, 'Neurasthenia and Emotion', 356.

[103] Rivers, 'Freud's Psychology of the Unconscious', 914; Rivers, 'War-Neurosis and Military Training', 533.

[104] Paul Lerner argues that in Germany, psychoanalysts, like other doctors, 'subscribed to hierarchies of patient value, and many submerged individual health to a concern with the needs of the national community'. Lerner, *Hysterical Men*, p. 171.

[105] Eder, *War-Shock*, pp. 72–3.

[106] Rivers, *Conflict and Dream*, pp. 35–6. See also Stoddart, 'Morison Lectures on the New Psychiatry. Lecture II', 643.

[107] The definition of re-education in the Report of the War Office Committee of Enquiry into "Shell-Shock" underlined the moral imperatives driving this form of treatment: 'Having cleared away the symptoms, it was found necessary to submit the patient to a course of graduated experiences which should prepare him for taking on his duty again, and accompanying this it was necessary to implant a raised moral view very often with a widening of the intelligent conception of the military and social necessities, so that the patient should have sufficient stability and moral support to again face the stresses of his service'. *RWOCESS*, pp. 129–30.

The patient's effort to gain 'proper' understanding of his war experience was depicted as a confrontation in which he squared up to his past and mastered it. The patient must 'face the trouble', 'face the situation', 'face the music of his emotional experiences', 'face life's difficulties', and realize that 'life is relentless'.[108] The war neurotic's mind was 'likened to a government at war with the government of a neighbouring country and at the same time carrying on a civil war within its own borders': but cowardice in the face of the enemy could not be permitted even when the foe lurked within the patient's own psyche.[109] Doctors had to make patients see the impossibility of 'running away' from troubling memories.[110] There was no separation of the medical and the moral in this form of treatment: it aimed at nothing less than the reassertion of courage in the domain of the self.

The Naturalization of Fear and the Maintenance of Will

The concept of will occupied a central place in theories of "shell-shock" across the full spectrum of medical opinion. The continued importance of will within psychological medicine is implicitly denied by historians who view "shell-shock" as the catalyst for fundamental reimaginings of human nature, and interpreted as evidence of medical callousness and insensitivity by those who recognize the tenacity of pre-war notions of self-control and character. Neither approach captures the complexity of doctors' attitudes towards "shell-shocked" patients or their views on the potential implications of "shell-shock" for what they saw as "civilized" social life. In war, the needs of the army were also the needs of the country. The soldier's symptoms were perceived as a struggle between 'selfish and social tendencies', and the doctor had to 'throw his weight into the scale on behalf of the latter'.[111] The war made the exercise of will into a matter of life or death for the individual soldier and the army he served, and the doctor in military uniform had a professional duty to uphold military standards of discipline and control. For some, loss of self-control in "shell-shock" became a totem of the dangers war posed to

---

[108] Rows, 'Mental Conditions'; Smith and Pear, *Shell Shock and Its Lessons*, p. 54; Rivers, 'Freud's Psychology of the Unconscious', 914; Rivers, 'Address on the Repression of War Experience', 175; Hunter, 'Neurasthenia and Emotion'; Eder, *War-Shock*, pp. 106, 111–13. Christine Hallett shows that nurses used the same language of 'facing it' as they tried to help men come to terms with their traumatic injuries and to retain their self-respect and masculine identity. Hallett, *Containing Trauma*, p. 165.

[109] C.H.L. Rixon and D. Matthew, *Anxiety Hysteria: Modern Views on Some Neuroses* (London: H.K. Lewis, 1920), p. 26; Culpin, *Psychoneuroses of Peace and War*, p. 50.

[110] Rivers, 'Address on the Repression of War Experience', 174.

[111] *RWOCESS*, p. 130.

"civilization" itself. The exercise of will was imperative to maintain the society that soldiers represented and defended: "civilization" was built on the repression of instinct and emotion.[112] Loss of self-control struck at the core of what it meant to be a "civilized" human and underlined the tenuousness of this identity.

The experience of "shell-shock" did lead many doctors to conclude that 'a psychoneurosis may be produced in almost anyone if only his environment be made "difficult" enough for him', a statement officially sanctioned by the War Office Committee of Enquiry into "Shell-Shock".[113] This acknowledgement that any man could break down under sufficient stress has often been viewed as irreversibly damaging pre-war notions of masculine character as built on strong will, helping to usher in more humane attitudes towards mental illness, and forcing reconsideration of what constituted individual and social weakness. Yet this reassessment of the limits of human endurance did not diminish the place of will in idealized views of character or perceptions of acceptable behaviour in everyday life. In fact, and perhaps paradoxically, the naturalization of fear and emotion under wartime conditions entailed heightened emphasis on willpower. Awareness of human vulnerability to breakdown could lead to conclusions as depressing as they were shocking: if 'all human beings are hysterical to a certain extent, in that they are human', then it was even more necessary to take preventive action against hysteria.[114] The realization of actual human frailty reinforced belief in individual will as the safest guard against potential disintegration and made control of external conduct seem even more integral to the maintenance of "civilized" social life. At the end of the war, self-control was perceived as more important than ever to individual identity, military functioning, and "civilization".

This did not mean that doctors denied the existence of intense emotion in warfare, or its contribution to breakdown. Most doctors accepted that every soldier felt fear. Even conservative commentators insisted that

---

[112] Armstrong-Jones, 'Dreams and Their Interpretation', 204; see also GHMSA: G/S6/15, J.R. Hill, 'Social Physiology' (27 October 1921); J.A. Berry, 'A Plea for a National Laboratory for the Study of Mental Abnormality', *BMJ*, 14 January 1928, 46.

[113] Smith and Pear, *Shell Shock and Its Lessons*, pp. 87–8; Culpin, *Psychoneuroses of Peace and War*, p. 40; *RWOCESS*, p. 92. However, witnesses to the Committee of Enquiry insisted that breakdown was not inevitable and that some men were more liable than others to mental collapse. Simon Wessely describes these views as reflecting Edwardian values of courage and moral fibre. Wessely, 'Twentieth-Century Theories on Combat Motivation', 271.

[114] D.E. Core, 'Correspondence: Hypnosis in Hysteria', *Lancet*, 5 October 1918, 471. Core later claimed that 'hysterical people in their psychology approach the non-human type closer in comparison than people who are not obtrusively hysterical'. D.E. Core, 'Some Clinical Aspects of Certain Emotions', *British Journal of Medical Psychology*, 5:4 (1925), 322.

an 'attack of neurasthenia is no more a reflection on a man's courage than is the presence of a bullet. Both bear witness to the fact that he has probably been in the thick of the fight'.[115] However, the mere acknowledgement of fear among soldiers did not represent a significant departure from earlier views. Even early recruitment propaganda had accepted that the soldier felt fear and had drawn the same line between courage and cowardice, emphasizing the ability of military discipline to teach a man that he 'can master fear, can still be afraid in the sense of realizing danger, and yet by an exercise of will power can say to himself, "Yes, I see it and in a sense fear it, but please God; 'funk' it I never will!" for fear and funk are far apart'.[116] In 1939, the medical psychologist Frederick Dillon drew on Victorian adventure fiction to explain the 'epitome of the therapeutic aim' at the advanced treatment centre where he had worked in 1918: quoting from Robert Louis Stevenson's *Kidnapped* (1886), he claimed that, 'To be feared of a thing and yet to do it is what makes the prettiest kind of a man.'[117]

Changing attitudes are better demonstrated through the redefinition of courage to incorporate the experience of fear. As the war went on, it became more common for medical commentators not only to acknowledge that all soldiers felt some degree of fear but also to present fear as a necessary constituent of courage.[118] Armstrong-Jones emphasized that 'it is not the man who is incapable of fear that has the highest form of courage'. There were people 'like children with fire, that are not afraid, because they have never experienced fear, and there are others who are too stolid, too obtuse, or too unimaginative to feel fear'.[119] Smith and Pear went further, claiming that men who did not feel fear could not be described as 'brave'. The only truly brave man was 'one who, feeling fear, either overcomes it or refuses to allow its effects to prevent the execution of his duty'.[120] A speaker to the Guy's Hospital Physiological Society vividly underlined this point, telling his audience, 'I bet no man wins the V.C., who hasn't a trace of sugar in his urine' (referring to the effect of strong emotion on the production of blood glucose).[121] Alan Grimbly, a recently qualified physician serving in the

[115] Collie, 'Management of Neurasthenia', 5

[116] J.C. Kernahan, *The Experiences of a Recruiting Officer* (London: Hodder and Stoughton, 1915), p. 72.

[117] Dillon, 'Neuroses among Combatant Troops', 66.

[118] Hurst, *Medical Diseases of the War* [1918], p. 1; C. Bird, 'From Home to the Charge: A Psychological Study of the Soldier', *American Journal of Psychology*, 28:3 (July 1917), 335.

[119] Armstrong-Jones, 'Psychology of Fear', 357.

[120] Smith and Pear, *Shell Shock and Its Lessons*, p. 9.

[121] GHMSA: G/S6/14, R. Hodgkinson, 'Fear – The Major Emotion in War' (28 February 1919), p. 30.

Royal Navy, even argued that fear 'forms the foundation of the fighting efficiency of our Navy'. However, he also insisted on the definite line between courage and cowardice. Fear was only one part of courage. The other was self-control. In cowardice, fear had triumphed 'over the will'.[122]

The naturalization of fear in warfare did not lessen the requirement for self-control but rather heightened the need for emotion to be controlled by 'strong will power'.[123] The military machine demanded rigid control. In its recommendations on training, the Committee of Enquiry advised that soldiers be instructed that 'every man feels fear at some time ... and that to feel afraid is a natural thing and nothing to be ashamed of', but also 'that no good soldier ever allows this feeling to influence him, that to give way to fear is reprehensible, and that no properly-trained soldier will have difficulty in carrying out his duty whatever the circumstances'.[124] These instructions underlined the importance of individual and collective willpower. Any man would be 'rattled' by the experience of battle, 'but discipline and self-control will steady him'. Like muscles, discipline and willpower could be strengthened through exercise, and the aim of training must be to teach soldiers to 'endure the hardship of war ... and make the superhuman effort which battle demands'. In the final analysis, 'the army with the greatest intensity of purpose' would triumph, and purpose was only willpower in another form. An army depended 'upon the will-power of the individuals' composing it; the most important part of the military machine, the oil keeping its wheels turning, was the self-control of the individual. Ultimately, warfare was 'based upon and limited by the human factor', and individual loss of control disrupted the smooth working of the entire apparatus.[125]

Medical insistence on self-control coalesced with and supported military views of willpower. Yet doctors were not simply agents of military power, charged with enforcing an externalized code of masculine behaviour on unwilling subjects. It is sometimes argued that doctors in different combatant nations refused to admit fear as a legitimate response to combat because they did not want to 'turn the male gaze inwards' and acknowledge their own vulnerability as men at severe cost to their own masculine power.[126] In this view, doctors adopted harsh attitudes

---

[122] Grimbly, 'Neuroses and Psycho-Neuroses of the Sea', 248.
[123] Marr, *Psychoses of the War*, p. 47; Hunter, 'Neurasthenia and Emotion', 352; N. Raw, 'Fear and Worry', *JMS*, 75:311 (October 1929), 578, 582–3.
[124] Recommendations of *RWOCESS*, p. 155.   [125] Ibid., pp. 203–6.
[126] M. Humphries, 'War's Long Shadow: Masculinity, Medicine, and the Gendered Politics of Trauma, 1914–1939', *Canadian Historical Review*, 91:3 (September 2010), 529–31. This interpretation draws on Mark Micale's arguments about medical ambivalence towards male hysteria.

towards "shell-shocked" men to safeguard their authority and to bulwark the normative codes of gendered behaviour which ensured their domination. However, British medical discourse on "shell-shock" for the most part recognized, even if it did not fully validate, extreme emotional responses to war in "normal" men. Moreover, when "analytic" doctors asserted that the strain of war could erode any man's resilience, this was not put forward as an abstract fact about patients but as a truth about human nature which applied to themselves as well as to others. Charles Myers' choice of words is telling: 'beyond a certain limit, even in the strongest of *us*, self-control is no longer possible'.[127] Nevertheless, doctors were enmeshed in the matrix of values and beliefs making up contemporary notions of masculine character. As a consequence, they saw loss of control as the loss of all that was most valued in the self, and as terrible to contemplate in the self as in others.[128] It was because, rather than in spite of, their awareness of each man's ultimate defencelessness against the onslaught of modern war that doctors upheld the inviolability of will.

Conclusion

As a diagnostic category, "shell-shock" was a response to the awful novelties of industrial warfare but was nevertheless constructed out of existing knowledges. This dual origin constrained the radical possibilities of "shell-shock" within the boundaries of existing modes of understanding body and mind. The operation of will in theories of "shell-shock" demonstrates the complex interplay of pre-war and wartime factors in shaping both the diagnosis and its potential to generate medical and cultural change. Before 1914, the diagnosis of traumatic neurosis had created a model of male breakdown as grounded in masculine environments, and this category therefore contained the potential to destabilize conventional attitudes to male nervous illness. This potential remained undeveloped before the war, as sufferers were deemed emotional, suggestible, and constitutionally weak. The radical potential of the diagnosis of "shell-shock" to overturn these attitudes similarly went unrealized.

---

[127] Myers, *Present-Day Applications of Psychology*, p. 42. My italics. See also Roper, *Secret Battle*, p. 302.

[128] A 1918 report on the treatment of mental illness suggested that 'to lose control of oneself' was 'to become something that is not oneself'. M.N., 'Dr. Weatherly's Offensive', *TMW*, 11 (July–December 1918), 202. This was echoed by an anonymous review in the *King's College Hospital Gazette* which portrayed 'collapse of individuality and the debasement of will' as part of the same process. Anon., 'Review: The English Review', *King's College Hospital Gazette*, 3:1 (February 1924), 366.

"Shell-shock" opened up space for greater sympathy and understanding of soldiers who broke down, but the absolute horror of war meant that this insight was not readily applied to normal social life. It was clear why men might break down in response to trench warfare, but the view of mental and nervous collapse as a loss of will persisted alongside acceptance of mental disintegration under extreme conditions. Although some soldiers were partially or completely absolved of responsibility for breakdown, their illnesses were still perceived as failures of self-control, and the task of doctors was always to repair the malfunctioning will.

The concept of self-control retained its hold on medical culture during the war. If anything, the experience of "shell-shock" strengthened the belief of British doctors in strong will as requisite for effective individual and social action. In this respect, wartime medical discourse reflected deeper currents in social life and culture. Samuel Smiles' *Self-Help* (1859), that much maligned symbol of Victorian notions of character, was reprinted several times during the war. Clearly, its message continued to resonate with some audiences.[129] Official and semi-official languages of reconstruction took up the Smilesian rhetoric of self-improvement, portraying the stoic recoveries of injured men as examples of the power of self-transformation and the 'triumph of the individual over the anonymity of mass warfare'.[130] These narratives did not constitute a form of top-down rhetoric blasted at hapless citizens; people sought out memoirs and fiction asserting the ability of active agents to control their worlds. This was not a denial of the chaos and suffering of war but a way of managing it. As Alison Light points out, 'Trauma provokes conservative as well as radical responses'.[131]

It is even possible that in the interwar period, the ideal of a strong, emotionally independent masculinity exercised a powerful imaginative hold precisely because it had been thrown into crisis by the war.[132] Although new forms of psychological reflexivity are evident in the memoirs and fiction of many veterans, these did not entirely displace older models of character and conduct. As Michael Roper states, these authors 'were always engaged in a process of continuing identification with, as well as distancing from, the social codes of "manliness"'. The 'tradition of stoic manliness' was modified rather than abandoned as a result of the war.[133]

---

[129] C. Tylee, *The Great War and Women's Consciousness: Images of Militarism and Womanhood in Women's Writings, 1914–64* (Basingstoke: Macmillan, 1990), p. 71; Rutherford, *Forever England*, p. 97.

[130] Carden-Coyne, *Reconstructing the Body*, p. 313.   [131] Light, *Forever England*, p. 200.

[132] Ibid., p. 171.

[133] M. Roper, 'Between Manliness and Masculinity: The "War Generation" and the Psychology of Fear in Britain, 1914–1950', *Journal of British Studies*, 44:2 (April 2005), 360, 356.

Overlap and interaction between different forms of self-understanding, and the continuing appeal of older forms of manly stoicism, is evident in the cult around T.E. Lawrence (1888–1935). Graham Dawson views Lawrence as a new kind of adventure hero who offered an imaginary resolution to the contradiction between contemplative and active strands within dominant concepts of masculinity. Dawson emphasizes the importance of continual assertions of self-control and willpower to Lawrence's heroic persona and the appeal of this self-willed masculine agency to contemporary audiences.[134] The myth of Lawrence of Arabia drew on many elements of the Victorian and Edwardian warrior ideal, an ideal which perhaps reached its logical apotheosis in the post-war era in the forms of masculinity extemporized by the British Union of Fascists.[135]

All this shows that will retained its central place in the social imaginary as it did in medical culture. The concept of will was too deeply embedded in British culture to be rooted out in such a short space of time. As the attribute raising the British above their flighty European neighbours and imperial subjects, will was essential to the maintenance of "civilized" British power and prestige. But perhaps even more importantly, will was an integral and valued aspect of the self-perception of citizens. The valorization of self-control is often perceived as a negative feature of early twentieth-century British culture, and historians have portrayed the apparent crumbling of the stoic ideal of character as one of the positive consequences of the First World War. However, the stiff upper lip did not necessarily harm those who held it. As Christine Hallett argues, it is not easy to draw the line between containment and repression, and extreme self-control should not automatically be viewed as a 'pathology of war'. Containment may have helped men to cope with emotions and to release them in a socially sanctioned way. It was certainly viewed by medical personnel as essential to their own work healing broken men.[136]

The continued belief in will as an essential part of national character and manly behaviour also provides a clue as to how we might explain one of the puzzling differences between British therapeutic techniques for "shell-shock", and those developed in France and Germany. Although Lewis Yealland used "disciplinary" treatment, this approach was not

---

[134] G. Dawson, *Soldier Heroes: British Adventure, Empire and the Imagining of Masculinities* (London and New York: Routledge, 1994), pp. 171–2, 187, 198–9, 228. See also Rutherford, *Forever England*, p. 96.

[135] T. Collins, 'Return to Manhood: The Cult of Masculinity and the British Union of Fascists', *International Journal of the History of Sport*, 16:4 (2000), 159.

[136] Hallett, *Containing Trauma*, pp. 175–6, 201–2, 226.

adopted on a wider scale within Britain.[137] "Disciplinary" treatments attracted many more adherents in France and Germany and were employed and publicized at a much earlier stage of the war.[138] In both countries, accounts of these therapies invoked the language of will. War hysteria was associated with lack of will or misplaced will.[139] Both countries also had historic traditions of compulsory military service entirely absent in Britain.[140] As a result, conscription did not provoke the agonized ethical and political soul-searching so much in evidence in Britain. However, the view of conscription as a morally neutral system had implications for opinions of the conscript. He was not perceived as morally inferior to the volunteer, but nor had he taken any positive action to demonstrate his superior worth as a soldier and a citizen. In France and Germany, the soldier had to prove his merit through his conduct in war rather than through the mere fact of service.

When conscription was introduced to Britain in 1916, it was only tolerated as a measure "for the duration". The tradition of voluntarism continued to shape ideas of martial valour throughout the war. Ilana Bet-El argues that voluntarism – and by extension, free will – became endowed with even greater significance during the first years of the war. In recruitment campaigns, the traditional masculine role of soldier-as-warrior came to be redefined as soldier-as-volunteer. Enlistment constituted an act of will superseding battle itself in the public mind. Although half the men who served in the British armed forces between 1914 and 1918 were conscripts, the enduring myth of the First World War as a war of volunteers testifies to the intensified power of ideas of will in wartime and their effect on the cultural memory of the war.[141]

[137] I refer here to a systematic concept of "disciplinary" treatment, such as that practised by Yealland, rather than to forms of treatment which inflicted pain purely as a form of punishment. There is some evidence of the latter approach in Britain, but much of it is anecdotal, suggesting that punitive tactics were not systematically employed or generally condoned.
[138] Before the First World War, electrical therapies were far more popular in Germany than in Britain: see Linden, Jones, and Lees, 'Shell Shock at Queen Square', 1979. This may have encouraged German doctors to adopt electrical treatments, but it does not explain why they did not take off in Britain, especially given the high level of wartime experimentation with other allegedly novel approaches such as hypnosis.
[139] M. Roudebush, 'A Patient Fights Back: Neurology in the Court of Public Opinion in France during the First World War', *Journal of Contemporary History*, 35:1 (2000), 36; Roudebush, 'Battle of Nerves', 267; Lerner, *Hysterical Men*, pp. 37–8, 50–2, 102–14, 203–4.
[140] Strachan, 'Liberalism and Conscription', pp. 6, 8.
[141] Bet-El refers to voluntarism, and to the perceived moral significance of enlistment as a transformative act, rather than explicitly referring to 'will'. However, the importance of free will in debates on conscription justifies this reading of her argument to emphasize the power of will. Bet-El, 'Men and Soldiers', pp. 81–3; Bet-El, *Conscripts*, p. 209.

Throughout the war, acceptance of military service as a necessary duty remained extraordinarily high, and there is little to suggest that conscripts were less motivated than their volunteer predecessors.[142] The belief in free will and the superior status of the volunteer survived despite the introduction of compulsion.

The lingering influence of the voluntary principle can also be glimpsed in wartime medical discourse on "shell-shock", which played down the difference between volunteers and conscripts.[143] Although not entirely absent, there was relatively little discussion on the differences between conscripted men and volunteers while the war lasted.[144] Given the firm belief in the moral superiority of volunteers before 1916, this dearth of comment is remarkable. After 1919, it became slightly more common for doctors to comment on the physical and psychological inferiority of conscripts.[145] However, while the war lasted, British "shell-shock" doctors wrote about their patients as men who had already proved their will to fight, and for whom breakdown was an unfortunate consequence of war, rather than as men who had been compelled to fight and needed further compulsion. This positive view of the soldier's will to fight may explain both the rarity of "disciplinary" therapies in Britain and the absence of affirmations of heroic identity (of the kind Yealland sometimes expressed) in French and German reports of "disciplinary" treatment. A lasting legacy of voluntarism was the tendency of British doctors to perceive the aim of their therapies as restoration of will rather than as the attempt to implant self-control where none previously existed. British doctors did not see themselves as machine guns driving men back to the front, as in Freud's famous formulation, but as aides who helped the "shell-shocked" soldier relocate his will and, with it, his desired self.

---

[142] In the two years after the introduction of conscription, 208,430 men volunteered. Watson, *Enduring the Great War*, pp. 54, 62.

[143] G. Corrigan, *Mud, Blood and Poppycock: Britain and the Great War* (London: Cassell Military Paperbacks, 2004), p. 74.

[144] Rare examples of wartime comment are Mott, 'Two Addresses on War Psycho-Neurosis. (I)', 128, and J. Keay, 'The Presidential Address on the War and the Burden of Insanity', *JMS*, 64:267 (October 1918), 326.

[145] Abrahams, 'Medical Officer in Charge of a Division'; Chambers, 'Mental Wards', 171; Davy, 'Address on Some War Diseases', 837; Ross, 'Shell Shock', p. 53; Mott, in Anon., 'British Medical Association Special Clinical Meeting', 709.

6   Animal Bodies and Minds
Instinct and Regression in "Shell-Shock"

In February 1919, the Guy's Hospital Physiological Society heard a paper on 'Fear – The Major Emotion in War'. The speaker, recorded only as R. Hodgkinson, vividly recounted the evolutionary history of fear as revealed through the physiological effects of emotion. Any severe threat provoked the instinct of self-preservation ('the fundamental instinct innate in every living thing and creature – as it is the most primitive, so it is the most potent, and is always with us') into definite action, and set off a chain of physiological responses.[1] These reactions, evolved to equip the organism for fight or flight, constituted 'as complete a mobilisation, as a Continental Power at war'.[2] After detailing these physiological effects, Hodgkinson came to the crux of his problem: why flight did not always follow fear. What raised man 'above the lower animals, which when confronted with danger, merge their emotion and motor action together into headlong flight?'[3] His answer was 'the will'.[4] The soldier in a front line trench under bombardment understood the threat he faced, felt 'the call of self preservative instinct innate in every living thing', and experienced the mobilization of his sympathetic nervous system. But his will, provoked by duty or fear of accusations of cowardice, overrode the instinct for flight.[5] The soldier suffered for this resolve. A body mobilized for flight but forced to stay still trembled, perspired, and became exhausted through the accumulation of unspent adrenalin and the continuous effort of will. Under these conditions, it was only a matter of time before the soldier 'crack[ed] up'.[6]

Hodgkinson's definition of courage acknowledged the power of fear and its physiological effects but also reinforced the importance of will. He described a brave man as 'one who under whatever conditions has enough will power left at his command to make his body carry out his

---

[1] GHMSA: G/S6/14, R. Hodgkinson, 'Fear – The Major Emotion in War' (28 February 1919), p. 3.
[2] Ibid., p. 5   [3] Ibid., p. 21.   [4] Ibid., p. 22.   [5] Ibid., pp. 22–3.
[6] Ibid., pp. 24–7.

wishes and to inhibit any self preservative tendencies': a courageous man 'must know fear', and 'must have a strong will'.[7] Yet there was 'a limit to the endurance of all men'. The struggle against flight ('this repression, as psychologists call it') could not be maintained indefinitely. The 'constant mobilisation from fear, without time for recuperation' would eventually 'beat nerve and tissue'. After breakdown, it took years for a man to 'build up his system and brain power again'.[8] These sentiments were common enough in medical literature on "shell-shock", but more unusually, Hodgkinson closely identified with the soldier's fear. After several pages of dry description, Hodgkinson outlined the bodily reactions of the man who felt fear but nevertheless fulfilled his duty: 'knocking heart, rapid pulse, laboured respiration, [and] trembling muscles and limbs', sometimes so severe that 'his arms may vibrate so that he cannot light a cigarette, and his knees knock together'. Quite casually, Hodgkinson then told his audience that he could 'speak of the latter from experience'.[9] At this moment, the paper moved from detached scientific description to first-hand account: this was not a prescription for how warrior heroes should act but the testimony of a soldier who had laboured under fear and fire.

Hodgkinson's paper demonstrates medical commitment to the values of duty and self-control, mustered by a doctor who admitted his own fear in the face of enemy shellfire. It also shows how easily physiological theories of emotion fitted into medical conceptualizations of "shell-shock" as an imbalance of emotion and will. From 1917 onwards, more and more doctors incorporated physiological elements into their explanations of the war neuroses. Because physiological theories emphasized powerful instinctual responses, these explanations appealed to doctors whose views of emotion and instinct derived from Darwin as well as those influenced by Freud. As it became more common for doctors to describe "shell-shock" as the outcome of instinctual conflicts, they also invoked concepts of the herd instinct and group mind ('social physiology') familiar from pre-war British psychological medicine and social thought.[10] Instinctual theories of "shell-shock" often borrowed from psychoanalysis but also replicated the ambivalence of native pre-war approaches to instinct and social behaviour. "Analytic" doctors shared the hierarchical understandings of instinct/volition, animal/human, and "primitive"/"civilized" dominant in evolutionary approaches to mind. Within mainstream medicine, wartime engagement with psychoanalysis depended on how far these theories of mind could be expressed in the

---

[7] Ibid., p. 30.   [8] Ibid., pp. 33–4.   [9] Ibid., pp. 24–5.
[10] GHMSA: G/S6/15, J.R. Hill, 'Social Physiology' (27 October 1921), p. 1.

vernacular of British psychological medicine. This "translation" simultaneously inspired further interest in psychoanalysis and restricted the reach of its more radical implications.

"Shell-Shock" and the Physiology of Emotion

In February 1918, the *Lancet* reported on the trial of a milk dealer accused of selling impure produce. The defendant claimed that the milk had been drawn during an air raid, and the cows were 'suffering from shell shock'. Although the bench did not accept the defence, the *Lancet*'s reporter pointed out that 'restlessness or nervousness' might well disturb the bovine metabolism and affect mammary secretions, just as the same emotions affected lactating women.[11] The notion of "shell-shock" in cows now seems faintly ludicrous, but physiological conceptions of the disorder were common in the later years of the war. As the war went on and more soldiers displayed symptoms of physical and mental exhaustion, physiological theories seemed to explain symptoms which resisted most established forms of cure.[12] Because these theories made the instinct of self-preservation central, and associated fear with the animal body and instinct, they were easily integrated with other approaches built on the evolutionary assumptions of psychological medicine. Furthermore, in physiological theories, body and mind were conceived as complexly and irreducibly connected, and so these theories could be adapted by doctors with quite different interests. Physiological theories provided a vital point of contact for doctors interested in the potential bodily causes of "shell-shock", and those more concerned with psychological aspects of the disorder. Although many historians portray wartime medical discourse as characterized by rigid divisions between physical and psychological approaches, the popularity of physiological theories underlines that this assumption is mistaken.

The researches of Harvard physiologist Walter B. Cannon (1871–1945), especially his *Bodily Changes in Pain, Hunger, Fear and Rage* (1915), sparked wartime interest in physiological theories of emotion.[13] Arguing explicitly from the precepts of Darwinian evolutionary

[11] Anon., 'Shell Shock in Cows', *Lancet*, 2 February 1918, 187–8. In one of the more unusual attempts to exploit the commercial possibilities of war, manufacturers of powdered formula also pointed to the effects of 'strife and worry' on mothers' milk; in this context, the milk dealer's defence seems less far-fetched. See Grayzel, *Women's Identities at War*, p. 117.

[12] Shephard, 'Shell-Shock', p. 37.

[13] "Shell-shock" doctors most often cited Cannon, but they also drew on the American surgeon George W. Crile's (1864–1943) pioneering work on the physiological effects of

theory, Cannon described human behaviour as motivated by instinct and emotion rather than reason and conscience. The 'primitive experiences' of major emotions and their accompanying bodily responses were common to humans and the lower animals.[14] Cannon demonstrated that the effects of intense emotion equipped organisms for fight or flight through the secretion of adrenin (adrenalin), which increased the level of sugar in the blood, circulated blood to the major organs more efficiently, reduced the effects of muscular fatigue, and aided blood coagulation.[15] These reflex responses arose out of the 'primary and essential' instinct of self-preservation. They overrode all the other activities of the body, could not be reproduced even by the most 'supreme act of volition', and were often 'distressingly beyond the control of the will'.[16] Cannon did not linger on the possible pathological effects of intense emotion but noted that these bodily changes could depress or paralyze organisms if they were unable to take action after mobilization for fight or flight.[17] "Shell-shock" doctors explored this prospect.

Cannon's physiology of the emotions replicated the evolutionary hierarchies of pre-war psychological medicine. In his view, the "primitive" and all-powerful emotions of fear and rage gave no quarter to will or to normal bodily functions. Happy and unaware organisms nonetheless existed in a perpetual state of preparation for intense struggle, primed for even the most superficially benign environment to unleash hostile forces at any second. Nature red in tooth and claw lurked beneath the façade of "civilization". Under threat, the animal inheritance would resurface and trample over the most recent and most human acquisitions of evolution. Emotion wreaked this destruction in the cause of animal survival. Cannon's physiological research, formulated within the same evolutionary framework which shaped the worldview of all "shell-shock" doctors, was easily assimilated into manifold explanations for war neurosis, from somatic interpretations to psychoanalytic theories of the unconscious as a storehouse of instinctual tendencies and their emotional accompaniments.

From 1917 until well into the post-war period, the physiological effects of emotion formed an important part of the clinical picture of "shell-shock".[18]

---

emotion and on the Russian physiologist Ivan Pavlov's (1849–1936) research on involuntary reflex actions.

[14] W.B. Cannon, *Bodily Changes in Pain, Hunger, Fear and Rage: An Account of Recent Researches into the Function of Emotional Excitement* (New York and London: D. Appleton, 1920) [1915], pp. vii, 1–3.

[15] Ibid., pp. 184–218.   [16] Ibid., pp. 185, 218, 267–75, 281–2.   [17] Ibid., p. 189, fn.

[18] See particularly the summary of evidence in *RWOCESS*, p. 100.

Doctors sometimes directly cited Cannon.[19] More often, they simply observed enlarged thyroids, symptoms of Graves' disease, and general metabolic and endocrine disturbances among invalided soldiers.[20] These signs of physiological malfunction supported divergent interpretations of war neurosis. Most obviously, emphasis on these symptoms corroborated the view that "shell-shock", in at least some of its manifestations, was a somatic disorder.[21] This approach was prominent among doctors who had served in France, as in the neurologist William Johnson's (1885–1949) study of cases of hyperthyroidism at the NYDN centre he commanded. Johnson concluded that a 'large number of so-called psychoneuroses are cases in which the symptoms are due to a state of disordered internal secretion the result largely of emotional exhaustion, and, to a less degree, of physical exhaustion'. He classed this group as 'exhaustion syndrome' and recommended the conservative therapies used for other somatic disorders: rest, diet, tonics, and an occasional dose of Dove's powder.[22] The description of neurasthenia in the official medical history of the war published in 1923 was modelled on this account of exhaustion syndrome.[23]

Psychologists, psychiatrists, and neurologists attempting to synthesize physical and psychological approaches also employed physiological theories of emotion. Edith Green, a Medical Research Committee scholar employed as assistant to Frederick Mott at the Maudsley Hospital, investigated 'blood pressure and surface temperature in 110 cases of shell shock', but also considered the relationship between hypotension

---

[19] Armstrong-Jones, 'Psychology of Fear', 347, 365–6; R. Armstrong-Jones, 'Mental States and the War – The Psychological Effects of Fear. I', *Journal of State Medicine*, 25:8 (August 1917), 243–4; Read, 'Survey of War Neuro-Psychiatry', 366; R.H. Steen in 'Discussion: Functional Gastric Disturbance in the Soldier', 144.

[20] Garton, 'Shell Shock and Its Treatment', 584–5; Ballard, 'Psychoneurotic Temperament', 370–1; MacCurdy, *War Neuroses*, pp. 21, 23; Eder, *War-Shock*, pp. 77–8, 85; Tombleson, 'Account of Twenty Cases'; Burton-Fanning, 'Neurasthenia in Soldiers', 910; Chambers, 'Mental Wards', 173; Campbell, 'War Neuroses', 503; Williamson, 'Remarks on the Treatment of Neurasthenia and Psychasthenia', 714; Tooth, 'Neurasthenia and Psychasthenia', 328; Eager, 'War Psychoses', 424.

[21] See Hurst, 'Observations on the Etiology and Treatment of War Neuroses', 413; Hurst, *Medical Diseases of the War* [1918], pp. 35–40; Hurst, 'War Neuroses and the Neuroses of Civil Life', 128, 148–52; Mott, 'Two Addresses on War Psycho-Neurosis. (I)', 127, 129; F.W. Mott, 'Application of Physiology and Pathology to the Study of the Mind in Health and Disease', Section of Psychiatry, *PRSM*, 8:3 (1914–15), 15; Mott, *War Neuroses and Shell Shock*, pp. 19–22; F.W. Mott, 'Neurological Aspects of Shock', *Lancet*, 12 March 1921, 520.

[22] W. Johnson, 'Symptoms of Hyperthyroidism Observed in Exhausted Soldiers', *BMJ*, 22 March 1919, 336–7. A similar explanation was developed by Dudley Carmalt-Jones (1874–1957), commanding officer of the medical division of a military hospital in France: D.W. Carmalt-Jones, 'War-Neurasthenia, Acute and Chronic', *Brain*, 42:3 (October 1919), 210–12.

[23] Macpherson *et al.*, *History of the Great War*, pp. 21, 19.

and terrifying dreams.[24] Percy Hunter, an asylum psychiatrist in civilian life, theorized that neurasthenic exhaustion resulted from prolonged repression of emotion. Once mobilized, if not released through muscular activity, emotion devoured energy 'like a parasite' and exhausted 'the cell' (the patient). To regain equilibrium, the muscular system through which emotion was normally expressed had to be activated. Hunter believed this should be achieved by the patient talking about his war experience.[25] This approach was similar to William Brown's 1919 revision of the theoretical basis for his therapeutic use of abreaction. Brown had earlier argued that physical symptoms were the equivalents of repressed emotional memories and that abreaction neutralized the psychological effects of strong emotion. He now argued that shock caused "psychical" *and* physiological dissociation and that abreaction worked by 'overcoming synaptic resistances in specific parts of the nervous system, and so put the nervous system into normal working order again'.[26]

If physiological theories of emotion could be used to integrate different approaches to "shell-shock", they were also invoked to avoid or resolve conflict. Grafton Elliot Smith and Thomas Pear cited Cannon's research in the first edition of *Shell Shock and Its Lessons* (1917), but did not make much of it.[27] However, when Robert Armstrong-Jones criticized their apparent assumption that "shell-shock" was 'entirely of psychic origin', Smith and Pear used these references to Cannon to demonstrate their awareness of the bodily components of the disorder.[28] In the preface to the second edition, they explicitly reminded readers of the importance of Cannon's work for understanding "shell-shock".[29] Although this might be seen as an attempt to deflect criticism, those sympathetic to medical holism saw in physiological theories the opportunity to build bridges between different medical specialties and to create a universal theory of war neurosis.[30] This research seemed to reveal that boundaries between

[24] E. Green, 'Blood Pressure and Surface Temperature in 110 Cases of Shell Shock', *Lancet*, 22 September 1917, 456.

[25] Hunter, 'Neurasthenia and Emotion', 350. For a similar theory foregrounding instinctual responses, see E.F. Ballard, *An Epitome of Mental Disorders: A Practical Guide to Aetiology, Diagnosis, and Treatment for Practitioners, Asylum and R.A.M.C. Medical Officers* (London: J. & A. Churchill, 1917), p. 143.

[26] Brown, 'War Neurosis', 835; Brown, 'Hypnosis, Suggestion, and Dissociation', 735. In the former article, Brown also supported Mott's theories on the role of the endocrine glands in war neurosis.

[27] Smith and Pear, *Shell Shock and Its Lessons*, p. 8; Smith, 'Shock and the Soldier. I', 816.

[28] R. Armstrong-Jones, 'The Psychopathy of the Barbed Wire', *Nature*, 100 (September 1917–February 1918), 1–3; Smith and Pear, 'Letters to the Editor', 65.

[29] Smith and Pear, *Shell Shock and Its Lessons*, p. x.

[30] On the appeal of endocrinological research as a counter to the apparent mechanism of specialization, see Cantor, 'Diseased Body', pp. 354–5.

the functional and organic were illusory. Doctors of all schools called on physiological theories to show the reciprocal relations between body and mind.[31] Synthesis appealed to "analytic" doctors as much as to their non-"analytic" counterparts. "Analytic" doctors investigated the relation between sympathetic and nervous disorders, urged further investigation of the physiological aspects of mental disorder, and called for greater cooperation between physiology and psychology.[32]

The physiological view of intense emotion as a primitive animal response which worked through the body to overwhelm every other function of the organism complemented existing interpretations of breakdown as the outcome of struggle between emotion and volition.[33] Consequently, physiological theories appealed to doctors from across the entire spectrum of medical opinion. They were perfectly compatible with crude "psychic" theories which claimed that in "shell-shock" the "primitive" emotion of fear 'gain[ed] dominion' and weakened the 'controlling power' of the mind, carrying the protective mechanism of fear 'out of the normal into the abnormal'.[34] They coalesced with "analytic" interpretations of war neurosis as the outcome of conflict between the instinct of self-preservation and 'certain social standards of thought and conduct, according to which fear and its expression are regarded as reprehensible'.[35] They were easily synthesized with neurological explanations which contended that war neurosis developed when 'primitive instincts and emotions cease to be corrected or controlled by higher mental activities which, from the individual and the racial point of view, are of

---

[31] J.I. France, 'Nervous and Mental Symptoms of Heart Disease', *TMW*, 4 (January–June 1915), 355–7; Armstrong-Jones, 'Mental States and the War – The Psychological Effects of Fear. II', 290–1; Anon., 'The Interdependence of the Sympathetic and Central Nervous Systems', *BMJ*, 26 October 1918, 471; W.L. Brown, 'The Croonian Lectures on the Role of the Sympathetic Nervous System in Disease. IV', *Lancet*, 7 June 1919, 970; Carver, 'Generation and Control of Emotion', 61; Bury, 'Physical Element in the Psycho-Neuroses', 68.

[32] D. Orr and R.G. Rows, 'The Interdependence of the Sympathetic and Central Nervous Systems', *Brain*, 41:1 (June 1918), 15–21; C.S. Myers, 'A Final Contribution to the Study of Shell Shock: Being a Consideration of Unsettled Points Needing Investigation', *Lancet*, 11 January 1919, 53; W.H.R. Rivers, 'Psychology and Medicine', *British Journal of Psychology*, 10:2 (March 1920), 193.

[33] For example, the physiologist Walter Langdon Brown emphasized that the sympathetic system was 'for ever beyond the control of the will'. Although the 'highest organism is the most self-controlled … the sympathetic cannot be thus controlled'. Nothing could 'prevent the response to an emotion once evoked'. W.L. Brown, 'The Croonian Lectures on the Role of the Sympathetic Nervous System in Disease. I', *Lancet*, 17 May 1919, 833.

[34] Anon., 'The Mental Factor in Modern War: Shell Shock and Nervous Injuries', in *The Times History of the War* (London: The Times, 1916), pp. 321–2, 324–5.

[35] Rivers, 'War-Neurosis and Military Training', 514.

later development'.[36] The trend towards physiological and instinctual theories of "shell-shock" demonstrates the continued influence of evolutionary modes of thought, which united doctors working in otherwise distinct theoretical and clinical traditions. The evolutionary framework of understanding did not erase differences between physicians, but it did provide points of contact which enabled conversation, synthesis, and avoidance of conflict. In this fashion, evolutionism helped to diffuse and make acceptable diverse approaches, and also encouraged the piecemeal adoption of new theories and practices in ways that were not fundamentally opposed to the existing approaches of psychological medicine.

"Shell-Shock", Instinct, and Regression

In May 1919, W.H.R. Rivers delivered the inaugural address of the medical section of the British Psychological Society, on the theme of 'Psychology and Medicine'. Six months after the armistice, assessing the significance of recent advances in psychological medicine, Rivers believed that the most important development was the turn towards the exploration of instinct, emotion, and the unconscious.[37] He claimed the 'outstanding fact' revealed by recent experience was that mental disorders were caused by 'the re-entrance into activity of instinctive tendencies' conflicting with 'the needs of social life'. In modern "civilized" societies, psychoneurosis arose from incomplete suppression of instinctive tendencies 'incompatible with the needs of society, and with the ultimate happiness of the individual as a member of society'. As a state in which suppressed instinctive tendencies regained 'the predominance they once held, both in the history of the race and in the infancy of the individual', psychoneurosis constituted a regression. For Rivers, the future development of psychological medicine depended on greater understanding of instinct, psychoneurosis, and the processes of individual, racial, and social evolution; and so he urged doctors and psychologists to examine all "primitive" forms, from 'the animal, the child, the savage, [and] the subject of regression', to the 'simpler and

---

[36] E.F. Buzzard in *RWOCESS*, pp. 74–5.

[37] Rivers, 'Psychology and Medicine', 184. Other prominent doctors, psychologists, and social scientists made similar assessments. See C.S. Myers, 'Psychology and Industry', *British Journal of Psychology*, 10:2 (March 1920), 178; W. McDougall, 'Presidential Address: The Present Position in Clinical Psychiatry', *JMS*, 65:270 (July 1919), 148; Parsons, *Mind and the Nation*, p. 6; A. Farquharson, 'The Oxford Conference on the Correlation of the Social Sciences', *Sociological Review*, 15:1 (January 1923), 49.

cruder' societies of the past, and 'those of the savage and barbarous peoples who still occupy the less comfortable regions of the earth'.[38]

Rivers' account of psychoneurosis as regression was caught between the evolutionary approaches of late nineteenth-century psychological medicine and the Freudian psychoanalytical perspectives diffused throughout British medicine and culture in the interwar period. Rivers achieved such success as a popularizer of modified psychoanalytic approaches because he was able to recast and carve up psychoanalytic ideas and practices to suit the self-conscious eclecticism of the native tradition. This process was incredibly important in the dissemination of psychoanalysis in Britain. In debates on "shell-shock", instinct, emotion, and the unconscious were explored from several medical viewpoints, including the physiological. Although not all doctors accepted the psychoanalytical definition of the unconscious, they were familiar with the notion of the bodily unconscious, a repository of ancestral (most prominently instinctive) experience that determined individual behaviour under certain circumstances.[39] Cannon's researches demonstrated the effects of emotion on the bodily unconscious. When "analytic" doctors pointed out correspondences between the 'psychic unconscious' and the 'physiological unconscious', or psychological repression and physiological inhibition, they revealed the influence of this shared heritage, and the convergence between psychoanalytic and other approaches in their own theorizations of "shell-shock".[40]

Different strands of psychological medicine merged in instinctual theories. In the bitter correspondence on psychoanalysis which scarred the correspondence columns of the *British Medical Journal* throughout January 1917, correspondents agreed on one point: that the foundation of human behaviour was instinct.[41] The primacy of the instinct of self-preservation in physiological theories of emotion corresponded both to "analytic" theories of "shell-shock" as resulting from the conflict between instinct and social standards, and to older modes of understanding human behaviour as the struggle between "primitive" and "civilized"

[38] Rivers, 'Psychology and Medicine,' 187; W.H.R. Rivers, 'Sociology and Psychology', *Sociological Review*, 9:1 (Autumn 1916), 1–13.
[39] Taylor, 'Obscure Recesses'; Otis, 'Organic Memory and Psychoanalysis'.
[40] Orr and Rows, 'Interdependence of the Sympathetic and Central Nervous Systems', 18; Rivers, 'Why Is the "Unconscious" Unconscious? II', 243; G.H. Fitzgerald, 'Some Aspects of the War Neurosis', Medical Section, *British Journal of Psychology*, 2:2 (January 1922), 120. For non-"analytical" comparisons of physiological inhibition and "psychic" self-control, see Herringham, *Physician in France*, p. 141; Brown, 'Presidential Address', 642–3.
[41] Thomson, 'Correspondence: Psycho-Analysis'; Armstrong-Jones, 'Correspondence: Psycho-Analysis'; C.A. Mercier, 'Correspondence: Psycho-Analysis', BMJ, 13 January 1917, 65.

elements of mind. Ernest Jones described 'the conflict between the unconscious and consciousness' as 'the conflict between the animal and the human in man, or between the primitive and the civilised': this was the conventional language of mainstream psychological medicine, familiar to his audience and second nature to any doctor trained in Britain within the previous forty years.[42] This language of emotion and will permeated "analytic" and non-"analytic" accounts of war neurosis alike. Even David Forsyth, a more orthodox Freudian than most "analytic" doctors, adopted familiar forms of expression to argue that the 'powerful' and 'ineradicable' emotion of fear, prompted by the instinct of self-preservation, could be 'coerced only by a still more powerful effort of will'.[43]

Doctors from different medical specialties shared the view of "shellshock" as regression or as a struggle between "higher" and "lower" aspects of the self. Oscar Pearn, an asylum psychiatrist in peacetime, described the symptoms of his soldier patients as examples of 'regression' because they represented 'an attempt at adaptation on lower psychic levels when the superior functions are in abeyance'.[44] For the neurologist Donald Core (1882–1934), such adaptations were 'inherited physiological reaction[s]', the counterpart of auto-amputation of a wounded limb by crabs, newts, and lizards, or loss of appetite in a brooding bird waiting for eggs to hatch. These actions, like hysterical symptoms, dissociated the individual from painful impressions to ensure 'the welfare of the race'.[45] In the concept of the 'archaic and primitive' unconscious, "analytic" doctors found a similar connection between 'us, the heirs of all ages' and 'primitive man'.[46] It is no surprise to find the psychoanalyst David Eder using the anthropological research of Sir James Frazer (1854–1941) to interpret the unconscious symbolism of "shell-shock".[47] "Analytic" doctors viewed the domination of the unconscious as a regressive state. Their discussions of soldiers' dreams lingered on symbols of individual and racial reversion: fights with Indians rather than Germans, fears of 'blood-thirsty and savage' black

---

[42] E. Jones, 'Why Is the "Unconscious" Unconscious? II', *British Journal of Psychology*, 9:2 (October 1918), 250.

[43] Forsyth, 'Functional Nerve Disease', 1401–2.

[44] Pearn, 'Psychoses in the Expeditionary Forces', 108. See also Maurice Nicoll in 'Discussion: The Repression of War Experience', 18.

[45] Core, 'Some Mechanisms at Work in the Evolution of Hysteria', 366.

[46] Eder, *War-Shock*, pp. 60, 65; E. Jones, 'War and Individual Psychology', *Sociological Review*, 8:3 (July 1915), 169; Stoddart, 'Morison Lectures on the New Psychiatry. Lecture I', 587, 590; Rivers, 'Freud's Psychology of the Unconscious', 912.

[47] Eder, *War-Shock*, pp. 65, 70, 82.

men, 'terrifying animals', images of Chinamen, and the appearance of an ichthyosaurus at Paddington Station.[48]

The shared evolutionary framework of understanding explains broad similarities between theories of "shell-shock" as regression, but specific influences also stretched across different medical specialties. Many doctors turned to the neurologist John Hughlings Jackson's theory of dissolution, discussed in Chapter 1.[49] In Jackson's view, pathological nervous and mental conditions developed when the "primitive" levels of the nervous system escaped the control of the higher and more recently evolved planes. The influence of Jacksonian dissolution permeated neurology and psychiatry and is evident in theories representing "shell-shock" as the manifestation of lower levels of nervous function.[50] As Freud also incorporated Jacksonian principles into his theories of neurosis, "analytic" doctors were exposed to Jackson's influence from three directions: Jackson's own writings, the teachings of the British medical psychologists he influenced, and Freud's appropriations.[51] Jackson's work provided another point of convergence between psychoanalytic approaches and native traditions. In March 1915, W.H.B. Stoddart's discussion of cutting-edge psychodynamic approaches dealt with Freud at great length but ended with the assertion that the 'fundamental principles of our new psychiatry' had all been foreseen back in the 1890s by 'the great man' – Jackson.[52] Undoubtedly, this claim sweetened an audience potentially unsympathetic to psychoanalysis and likely to disdain theories emanating from

[48] MacCurdy, *War Neuroses*, p. 44; J. Young, 'Two Cases of War Neurosis', Medical Section, *British Journal of Psychology*, 2:3 (April 1922), 232–3; Rivers, *Instinct and the Unconscious*, pp. 74–5, 98. See also Mott, 'Two Addresses on War Psycho-Neurosis. (II)', 172. Although not concerned with dreams, Myers' discussion of a case of narcolepsy combines several images of the "primitive": C.S. Myers, 'Treatment of a Case of Narcolepsy', *Lancet*, 28 February 1920, 491–3.

[49] Interest in Jackson revived during the war, mainly through the activities of neurologist Henry Head. See H. Head, 'Some Principles of Neurology', *Brain*, 41:3-4 (November 1918), 349.

[50] See, for example, Savage, 'Mental War Cripples', 1.

[51] Thomas Claye Shaw, the psychiatrist discussed in Chapter 1 as a potential influence on St Bartholomew's medical students, explained mental disorder in obviously Jacksonian terms. See Shaw, 'On Degradation of Type in the Insane', 169, 171; Shaw, 'On the Forecast of Destructive Impulses', 11. On the influence of Jackson on "shell-shock" doctors, see Nicoll, 'Conception of Regression', 798; Anon., 'Review: H. Crichton-Miller (ed.), *Functional Nerve Disease*', *British Journal of Psychology*, 10:4 (July 1920), 351; Rivers, *Instinct and the Unconscious*, pp. 148–52; Young, 'W.H.R. Rivers and the War Neuroses'; Young, *Harmony of Illusions*, pp. 42–85. On Freud and Jackson, see F.G. Sulloway, *Freud, Biologist of the Mind: Beyond the Psychoanalytic Legend* (London: Fontana Paperbacks, 1980), pp. 252–8, 270–1.

[52] Stoddart, 'Morison Lectures on the New Psychiatry. Lecture I', 590; Carver, 'Generation and Control of Emotion', 60; Anon., 'A Psychiatrist's Review', *BMJ*, 12 March 1921, 394.

the Austro-Hungarian empire, but it also reflected the influence of Jackson on British medicine and psychiatry.[53]

From several standpoints – physiology, biology, neurology, psychology, and "analytic" perspectives – "shell-shock" was conceived as a triumph of the body, the animal, and the "primitive" over the highest accoutrements of human "civilization". Despite the important differences between physiologists, psychiatrists, and psychoanalytically inclined doctors, all viewed "shell-shock" as regression to a lower level of individual or racial development. Similarities in these conceptualizations of "shell-shock" derived from the common evolutionary framework of understanding. The war exposed many doctors to problems of mind, brain, and nerves that they had not previously encountered. As a result, several experimented with new theories and clinical practices. But their understandings of war neurosis and of the psychodynamic theories they read about were refracted through the lens of British medical culture. This helps to explain both the radicalism of wartime engagement with psychoanalysis and the conservatism of certain aspects of British "analytic" approaches.

British Social Psychology and "Shell-Shock"

The most important "analytic" modification to Freudian theory was the rejection of an exclusively sexual aetiology for neurosis.[54] This rejection is most often depicted as a negative movement: the removal of an aspect of psychoanalytic theory that strait-laced British doctors found distasteful. But "analytic" doctors did more than take the sex out of Freud. They formulated an alternative explanation of war neurosis as the result of conflict between the instinct of self-preservation and the demands of social life (variously conceived as duty, conscience, the 'social impulse', or herd instinct). This emphasis on instinctual conflict made use of existing modes of thought within psychological medicine. Of course, such explanations emerged out of the circumstances of war: for soldiers, threats to self-preservation were more immediately apparent than the potential sexual

---

[53] If mention of Jackson was designed to normalize Freud for British audiences, it worked. Mott argued there was no essential difference between the concept of the censor and 'inhibition exercised by the highest centres of control', and therefore Freud's ideas were not so alien (or revolutionary) after all. Mott, 'Two Addresses on War Psycho-Neurosis (II)', 169.

[54] J.L. Birley, 'Goulstonian Lectures on the Principles of Medical Science as Applied to Military Aviation', *Lancet*, 29 May 1920, 1150; W. Calwell, 'An Address on Elementary Psychology in General Hospital Teaching', *BMJ*, 21 May 1921, 737; Anon., 'Reports of Societies: Psychotherapy', *BMJ*, 24 February 1923, 327.

basis of neurosis. But "analytic" theories also took this form in Britain because existing traditions accentuated the role of the instinct of self-preservation and emotions such as fear in breakdown, and emphasized the social dimensions of individual psychology.[55] Both "analytic" and non-"analytic" instinctual theories drew on this legacy and made 'the great primordial instinct of self-preservation', with its accompanying emotion of fear, central to the causation of "shell-shock".[56] This mode of invoking instinct provides another example of the (partial) normalization of radical theories of mind through "translation" into the native idiom.

This influence can be seen in ambivalent conceptualizations of the role of herd instinct and/or other social forces in the development of "shell-shock". The crowd psychologies of French theorists such as Gustave Le Bon (1841–1931) and Gabriel Tarde (1843–1904) emphasized the irrational, suggestible, and "primitive" nature of the group mind.[57] In Britain, theorists did not make such clear evaluative contrasts between individual and collective conduct, and quite often extrapolated from individual character to collective behaviour.[58] In British social psychology, characterizations of the crowd as imitative, impulsive, and emotional sat alongside influential home-grown theories of the social instinct or impulse as the source of valuable attributes such as altruism and conscience on which "civilization" itself was built.[59] As a consequence, British concepts of the herd instinct or social impulse exhibited tension between its status as both "lower" attribute and source of "higher" forms of individual conduct. These tensions carried over into theories of "shell-shock" as resulting from conflict between the instinct of self-preservation and duty or herd instinct, and were further inflected by the powerful urges towards military cohesion and national unity colouring all aspects of wartime life.

Before the war, surgeon Wilfred Trotter (1872–1939) and psychologist William McDougall were the most influential English theorists of social behaviour.[60] Their social psychologies responded to the perceived

---

[55] Shaw, 'Suicide and Sanity', 1067; KCHMSA: KHU/C1/M8, W. Brown, 'Freud's Theory and Its Uses in Diagnosis' (21 January 1913). On the relation of anthropology to social psychology in pre-war Britain, see Thomson, '"Savage Civilisation"'.

[56] Chambers, 'Mental Wards', 158; Mott, 'Two Addresses on War Psycho-Neurosis. (I)', 127–8; Ballard, 'Psychoneurotic Temperament', 374; Rivers, Conflict and Dream, p. 151.

[57] R. Smith, The Fontana History of the Human Sciences (London: Fontana Press, 1997), pp. 749–55.

[58] Smith, Free Will and the Human Sciences, pp. 39–41.

[59] H.C. Greisman, 'Herd Instinct and the Foundations of Biosociology', Journal of the History of the Behavioral Sciences, 15 (1979), 360.

[60] On social psychology and ideas of national character, see R. Romani, National Character and Public Spirit in Britain and France, 1750–1914 (Cambridge: Cambridge University Press, 2002), pp. 251–60.

challenges of democratic mass society but were presented as 'objective biological account[s] of social evolution'.[61] Of the two, Trotter was more often directly cited by "shell-shock" doctors, but McDougall's conception of the social sources of character and conduct corresponded more closely to the influential theories of W.H.R. Rivers (both men were veterans of the 1898 Torres Straits anthropological expedition). In different ways, both theorists encapsulated the ambivalence at the heart of British social psychologies, and both attempted to resolve what Thomas Dixon identifies as the main 'moral questions' arising from Darwin's account of the social instincts and conscience: 'not whether or not human beings were animals, but whether and in what respect their intelligence and morality was any different from that of lower animals'.[62] Trotter struggled to provide a positive answer to this question, but McDougall managed to construct a theory of social conduct as both grounded in instinct *and* distinctively human. In adaptations of these theories, "shell-shock" doctors similarly managed to find a place for noble qualities of self-sacrifice and duty within models of human behaviour as motivated by instinct and emotion.

Trotter is now most often encountered as a footnote to Freud, who included his theory of the herd instinct in a short survey of previous works on the group mind in 'Group Psychology and the Analysis of the Ego' (1921).[63] This is perhaps appropriate: although not a psychoanalyst himself, as the person who introduced Ernest Jones to Freud's work, Trotter was an important backstage figure in the history of British psychoanalysis.[64] Trotter first elaborated his theory of the herd instinct in the *Sociological Review* in 1908 and 1909. These articles were quickly taken up by proponents of the 'new psychology'.[65] Bernard Hart listed the herd instinct among 'the great primary instincts' in his *The Psychology of Insanity* (1912).[66] In his 1915 Morison lectures on the 'new psychiatry', W.H.B. Stoddart devoted much attention to the 'controlling force' of the herd instinct, 'perpetually ... in antagonism' to the other three

---

[61] R. Soffer, 'New Elitism: Social Psychology in Prewar England', *Journal of British Studies*, 8:2 (May 1969), 111–12.

[62] Dixon, *Invention of Altruism*, p. 174.

[63] S. Freud, 'Group Psychology and the Analysis of the Ego' [1921], *SE*, vol. 18, pp. 118–21. Freud criticized Trotter's theory because it left 'no room at all for the leader'.

[64] Jones, *Free Associations*, p. 159.

[65] On the 'new psychology', see N. Rose, *The Psychological Complex: Psychology, Politics and Society in England 1869–1939* (London: Routledge Kegan & Paul, 1985), pp. 182–90.

[66] B. Hart, *The Psychology of Insanity* (Cambridge: Cambridge University Press, 1912), pp. 133–7, 167; B. Hart, 'The Psychology of Freud and His School', *JMS*, 56:234 (July 1910), 444.

instincts of self-preservation, nutrition, and sex.[67] One reviewer claimed that the *Sociological Review* had 'constantly received enquiries' about these articles from the moment of first publication up until their book-length elaboration in Trotter's *Instincts of the Herd in Peace and War* (1916).[68]

In the immediate pre-war period, Trotter's theory provided ways of thinking about character, motivation, society, and politics which simultaneously acknowledged the instinctual basis of mental life, and reserved an important place for qualities combining individual and social goods, such as altruism and conscience – even though Trotter denied the "individual" nature of these characteristics and redefined them as outgrowths of instinct. Trotter viewed the herd instinct as fundamental to human evolution and psychology. The herd was 'not only the source of [man's] opinions, his credulities, his disbeliefs, and his weaknesses, but of his altruism, his charity, his enthusiasms, and his power'.[69] Because the most important factor governing the structure of the mind was sensitivity to the herd, only suggestions deriving from the herd were acceptable to the mind. This made humans both suggestible and insensitive to experience. For Trotter, suggestibility and irrationality, which crowd psychologists saw as features of the mob, were qualities always latent in the normal human mind. Humans were not 'suggestible by fits and starts, not merely in panics and in mobs, under hypnosis, and so forth, but always, everywhere, and under any circumstances'.[70]

At the same time, the most valuable aspects of individual and social conduct originated in herd instinct. Individuals sought to avoid the disapproval of the herd at all costs and so felt the emotions of guilt and duty, which developed into conscience and altruism. Altruism, depicted as a form of 'expansive egoism' based in the gregarious animal's sense that other members of the herd were to 'a certain extent identical with himself and part of his own personality', was therefore stripped of its intrinsic moral worth.[71] Likewise, the description of herd instinct as 'a controlling power from without', forcing individuals to obey the promptings of the herd even against their own judgement, undermined conceptions of conscience as a virtue based in reason and autonomous

---

[67] Stoddart, 'Morison Lectures on the New Psychiatry. Lecture I', especially 583–4.

[68] M.E.R., 'Dr Trotter on the Herd Instinct', *Sociological Review*, 9:1 (Autumn 1916), 60.

[69] W. Trotter, 'Herd Instinct and Its Bearing on the Psychology of Civilised Man', *Sociological Review*, 1:3 (July 1908), 227, 231–5.

[70] Ibid., 237–9, 242–3.

[71] W. Trotter, 'Sociological Application of the Psychology of the Herd Instinct', *Sociological Review*, 2:1 (January 1909), 36–9, 52–3; W. Trotter, *Instincts of the Herd in Peace and War* (London: Ernest Benn, 1919), pp. 122–5.

action.[72] Nonetheless, Trotter's theory also represented socially motivated acts of self-sacrifice as essential to social cohesion, and so it could be coerced into uneasy coexistence with existing discourses of character.[73] This is how most "shell-shock" doctors deployed concepts of the herd instinct, despite William McDougall's protestation that the wartime medical literature invoked 'herd instinct' simply as a 'fashionable substitute' for 'conscience'.[74]

McDougall's own work drew heavily on traditional conceptions of character and viewed social conduct as a development out of herd instinct rather than as synonymous with it. McDougall had co-founded the British Psychological Society in 1901 and was one of the most influential early twentieth-century British psychologists. In his *Introduction to Social Psychology* (1908), McDougall put instinct at the centre of human psychology and provided a platform which could accommodate both behaviourist and psychoanalytical approaches.[75] This account of the instinctual basis of experience and conduct aimed at 'a philosophy of the place of humans in nature, an ethics and a social science', and became one of the best-selling English-language psychological texts of the interwar years.[76] Like Trotter, McDougall viewed the gregarious instinct as prompting feelings of 'uneasiness in isolation and satisfaction in being one of the herd' and therefore as driving individuals towards conformity with public opinion.[77] But the gregarious instinct alone could not explain the highest forms of social conduct. These originated in the social genesis of the idea of the self and in the 'self-regarding sentiment', a combination of pride and self-respect developing out of the individual's view of himself in relation to others. All higher forms of conduct depended on the voluntary control of instinctive impulses and the motive for positive action provided by the self-regarding sentiment. These powers were inculcated by systems of reward and punishment which taught the habit of submission to authority, as well as by impulses derived from the gregarious instinct towards harmony with one's peers.[78]

---

[72] Trotter, 'Sociological Application of the Psychology of the Herd Instinct', 39–43.

[73] For examples, see D.A. Thom, 'War Neuroses: Experiences of 1914–1918', *Journal of Laboratory and Clinical Medicine*, 28:1 (1942–43), 502; Read, 'A Survey of War Neuro-Psychiatry', 372, 380; Brown, 'Presidential Address', 644.

[74] W. McDougall, 'Instinct and the Unconscious. VI', *British Journal of Psychology*, 10:1 (November 1919), 42.

[75] Thomson, *Psychological Subjects*, pp. 55–70.

[76] R. Smith, *Between Mind and Nature: A History of Psychology* (London: Reaktion Books, 2013), p. 215.

[77] McDougall, *An Introduction to Social Psychology*, pp. 84, 188–9.

[78] Ibid., pp. 174–5, 200–1.

The self-regarding sentiment grew out of concern with public opinion, but in its highest form, it enabled a man 'to apply his adopted principles of action, the results of his deliberate decisions, in spite of the opposition of all other motives'.[79] McDougall equated the highest development of the self-regarding sentiment with conscience, the power to do what was right 'regardless of the approval or disapproval of the social environment'.[80] The self-regarding sentiment extended beyond the individual's immediate environment to incorporate any group which the individual identified with the self, including family, community, and nation.[81] As such, it was an essential part of the individual's moral equipment, leading individuals to subjugate personal desires to the needs of 'social co-operation', even if this meant self-sacrifice, 'as when the patriot soldier in giving his life in battle brings glory upon himself as well as upon his country'.[82] For McDougall, then, the gregarious instinct provided the drive towards social conduct, especially as the source of the non-rational and emotional force individuals attached to public opinion; but to achieve the highest forms of conduct, synonymous with conventional notions of character, the man must rise above the promptings of the herd, exercise his own judgement, and 'substitute himself, as it were, for his social environment'.[83] In this formulation, McDougall retained the features of reason, autonomy, and conscience which defined traditional notions of character despite his insistence on the unbroken continuum between the individual and social. Instinctual theories of "shell-shock" replicated this ambivalence around the individual, the social, and the extent to which instinct could be resisted or redirected.

"Shell-Shock" as a Conflict between Instinct and Duty

In the later years of the war, it became more common for doctors to explain "shell-shock" as the result of conflict between the instinct of self-preservation and 'social standards', duty, or herd instinct. "Analytic" and non-"analytic" doctors put forward theories of instinctual conflict. "Analytic" doctors, who often extended themes developed by the 'new psychology' before the war, owed a clear debt to Freud as well as to British social theory. For non-"analytic" doctors, the social psychologies developed by McDougall and Trotter were more influential. Instinctual theories of "shell-shock" contributed to the dissemination of psychoanalytic ideas, but the forms these theories took in the British medical literature were determined by distinct traditions within native social thought.

[79] Ibid., pp. 253–4.   [80] Ibid., pp. 201, 180–1.   [81] Ibid., p. 206.   [82] Ibid., p. 208.
[83] Ibid., pp. 253–4.

A silence at the heart of W.H.R. Rivers' theories reveals this influence. In his theory of anxiety neurosis, Rivers raised the "shell-shocked" officer to almost heroic status. The officer's breakdown testified to honourable attempts to repress fear, the valiant struggle for self-control, and commitment to abstract ideals of honour and duty. In this view, "shell-shock" was a battle between the "primitive" instinctual forces of the organism and the social values internalized as character. However, Rivers did not explain *how* the imperative to meet 'certain social standards' achieved sufficient force to withstand the instinctual urge towards self-preservation. He pointed to the 'acquired experience' of education, training, and social roles but never showed how these factors attained enough power to combat instinct.[84] He transposed McDougall's analysis of the highest forms of social conduct to the battlefield but fudged the origin of this conduct in instinct. This silence reinscribed and deepened tensions within British social psychologies between the "lower" status of herd instinct and the "higher" forms of conduct it generated.

Rivers did not only fail to satisfactorily explain how social standards acquired the force of instinct. He conceptually separated instinct from social values. Modern "civilized" societies were built on the repression of instinct; social organization depended on the control of 'instinctive tendencies'.[85] In formulations such as 'conflict between the instinct of self-preservation and certain social standards of thought and conduct, according to which fear and its expression are regarded as reprehensible', he deliberately avoided making duty the analogue of herd instinct.[86] In Rivers' writings, the gregarious instinct was always "lower": it was the source of suggestion and 'the mass-reactions of the crowd', it provoked hysterical responses to danger, and it dominated social behaviour in "primitive" societies.[87] He divorced the definitely regressive 'instinctive tendencies' from 'the forces by which they are controlled'. The latter

---

[84] Rivers, 'War-Neurosis and Military Training', 523–6. Addressing a similar problem, Millais Culpin argued that education was 'largely a matter of the control of desires, and so early does this control begin that the controlling force – Authority, Social Suggestion, or whatever we may call it – is uncritically accepted and tends to acquire as much strength as those desires to which it is opposed': Culpin, *Psychoneuroses of Peace and War*, p. 20. This explanation grounded resistance to instinct in processes of suggestion or obedience rather than responsibility and duty, and broke down Rivers' distinction between "higher" and "lower" forms of conduct and of breakdown.
[85] Rivers, 'Psychology and Medicine', 187.
[86] Rivers, 'War-Neurosis and Military Training', 514. Bernard Hart's reference to 'a group of forces compounded of self-respect, duty, discipline, patriotism' is another good example of the combination of clumsiness and precision in British attempts to define exactly *what* came into conflict with the instinct of self-preservation. *RWOCESS*, p. 77.
[87] Rivers, *Instinct and the Unconscious*, pp. 41, 90, 94–8, 106, 132–3, 149; Rivers, 'Psychology and Medicine', 187.

could be more or less "primitive", childish, or mature responses to mental conflict or environmental danger.[88] Indeed, his own commitment to 'social standards' as the motivating force of "civilized" behaviour led to some strange conclusions. Rivers recounted a patient's dream: the man was about to commit suicide when he heard his son's voice saying, "Don't do it, daddy, you'll hurt me too." In Rivers' analysis, the child's voice 'represented the element in the conflict arising out of the social sentiment whereby a suicide inflicts a stigma upon those he leaves behind him'.[89] The failure to consider the man's love for his son and his grief at the idea of leaving and hurting him is an odd blind spot but fits with Rivers' general tendency to emphasize social over individual (selfish) tendencies in the mental conflicts of educated patients.

Ambivalence within conceptions of the herd instinct is evident elsewhere. Frederick Mott saw the herd instinct as enabling the sacrifice of 'individual interest and even life in the interests of the herd', and as essential to the progress of "civilization". The herd instinct controlled "lower" instincts and impulses, and generated feelings of duty and patriotism.[90] However, it was also the source of suggestibility and imitation. This quality of the herd instinct could be turned to good use in the creation of group cohesion, but unmanaged, might initiate an epidemic of "shell-shock". The challenge of mental hygiene was to balance the individual and the social spirit 'by encouraging all those factors and conditions in education which support moral [sic], discipline, self-sacrifice, and *esprit de corps*' without 'repressing or destroying that individual self-control and independent originality in thought and purposive action which is essential for national progress'.[91] Military training increased suggestibility so that soldiers would respond automatically to commands, but the military authorities and "shell-shock" doctors also feared the consequences of pathological suggestibility in the group mind. The medico-military attitude was that "shell-shock", 'like measles, [is] so infectious that you cannot afford to run risks with it at all': the 'infectious character of loss of control' could not be ignored.[92] Neither theories of "shell-shock" nor programmes of

---

[88] Rivers, *Instinct and the Unconscious*, pp. 119–20, 5.

[89] Rivers, *Conflict and Dream*, pp. 25, 72.

[90] Mott, 'Body and Mind', 3; Mott, 'Psychopathology of Puberty and Adolescence', 288–90; Mott, 'Two Addresses on War Psycho-Neurosis. (I)', 129.

[91] F.W. Mott, 'A British Medical Association Lecture on Psychology and Medicine', *BMJ*, 10 March 1923, 407; Anon., 'British Medical Association Special Clinical Meeting', 709.

[92] Anon., 'Mental Factor in Modern War', pp. 325–6; Lord Gort in *RWOCESS*, p. 50; see also pp. 28–9, 38–9, 66, 121; Myers, *Shell Shock in France*, p. 95; Smith, 'Shock and the Soldier. I', 813.

military training could resolve the status of herd instinct as the ultimate source of both suggestibility and the 'social ideal self'.[93]

This distinction between instinct and social conduct reformulated the opposition between theories of "shell-shock" that emphasized the causative role of over-abundant emotion and those that accentuated the battle for self-control. Mental breakdown could be viewed either as the individual's unwitting assertion of the self against the needs of the army and the nation or as the end result of an individual's noble struggle to live up to social ideals despite powerful instinctual urges. The theme of "shell-shock" as antisocial disorder was anticipated early in the war in bombastic paeans to the benefits of military life. The army was seen as a remedy for social ills: the *British Medical Journal* extemporized that pursuit of 'the common weal' would cure the self-indulgence of 'the podgy shopkeeper', the alcoholic, and the neurasthenic, and predicted that only weaklings would 'go to the wall'.[94] Later on, it was not difficult to perceive some symptoms of war neurosis as a repudiation of social relationships. Charles Myers described mutism and deafness as attempts to cut off 'the two main channels of intercourse with others'.[95] More than this, E.W. Scripture claimed that 'the stutterer at the bottom of his soul objects to human society'.[96] Arthur Brock viewed the war neurasthenic as dissociated from his social environment. Cure depended on 'a reintegration of the individual, a replacement of him in his *milieu*'.[97] Meanwhile, Millais Culpin included 'weak herd instinct', which he did not perceive as true psychoneurosis, in his classification of the psychoneuroses of peace and war. The shared characteristic of patients in this category was that 'their personal interests have overcome their patriotism'.[98] More harshly, John MacCurdy argued that the "shell-shocked" soldier's 'disinclination to return to the front' was 'essentially a selfish desire to avoid his responsibility as a citizen'. The patient had a conscious

[93] E. Prideaux, 'Suggestion and Suggestibility', *British Journal of Psychology*, 10:2 (March 1920), 237; Moran, *Anatomy of Courage*, pp. 150–3.
[94] Anon., 'Military Life and Physical Health', *BMJ*, 14 August 1915, 267. Anon., 'Insanity and the War', 553, asserted that rumours of neuroses among soldiers were most likely untrue as the majority of soldiers had 'so vivid a consciousness of the greatness and nobility of the principles for which they are contending that they are in a sense protected from the effects which sights and sounds of a terrifying nature might otherwise exercise over them'.
[95] Myers, 'Contributions to the Study of Shell Shock (IV)', 465. See also MacCurdy, *War Neuroses*, pp. 7, 28–9, 34, 86.
[96] E.W. Scripture, 'The Nature of Stuttering', *Practitioner*, 112:5 (May 1924), 325–6.
[97] Brock, 'Re-Education of the Adult', 26, 29–30.
[98] Culpin, *Psychoneuroses of Peace and War*, p. 32.

decision to make: he could either 'be a slacker or ... assume his share of the country's burden'.[99]

The view of "shell-shock" as selfish contrasted with explanations of the disorder as resulting from 'prolonged and stubborn resistance to the tendencies of individualism' which 'offended against the herd'.[100] David Eder sympathetically outlined this complex negotiation between individualistic and social tendencies in his account of an Australian sniper who developed amblyopia after a bullet hit the stock of his rifle while he was at his post. Although the soldier could have left his post, as the enemy had clearly located him, he decided to carry on. The 'egocentric instinct, self-preservation' asserted itself in unexplained eye-watering, forcing him to relinquish his position; at this point, the 'soldier's instinct' (which Eder here treated as synonymous with the gregarious instinct) came to the fore and the eye ceased to water. Eventually, the unconscious adopted 'a stronger attack' and the soldier developed blindness in his shooting eye. This disability allowed the man to retire with 'his safety guaranteed', and 'without loss of self-respect', and therefore represented the triumph of the 'egocentric instinct'. But Eder reminded readers that blindness, a disaster to a healthy young man, had proved this soldier's status as 'a first-class fighting man' who would not retreat until forced to do so. The unconscious solution of blindness was less a refuge than an alternative form of catastrophe.[101] There was no simple resolution to conflict between the instinct of self-preservation and the social values associated with the herd instinct – not for the men who suffered from "shell-shock", and not in the theories of doctors who tried to understand what led men to break down and what made them keep fighting.

The Herd, the Nation, and the Army

From the early days of the war, herd instinct was invoked to explain the strong urge towards national cohesion in wartime. W.H.B. Stoddart saw a 'latter-day exemplification of the herd instinct in the fact that the man who worries about the ultimate result of the war ceases to do so when he enlists in Kitchener's army'. The recruit who fulfilled his patriotic duty had 'the unconscious feeling of being within the fold'.[102] The classical scholar Gilbert Murray (1866–1957) more fully elucidated the role of herd instinct in war in his contribution to a lecture series on 'the

---

[99] MacCurdy, *War Neuroses*, p. 85.   [100] Chambers, 'Mental Wards', 156.
[101] Eder, *War-Shock*, pp. 68–9.
[102] Stoddart attributed this insight to Bernard Hart. Stoddart, 'Morison Lectures on the New Psychiatry. Lecture I', 584.

international crisis in its ethical and psychological aspects' held at the University of London in February and March 1915. Murray's discussion highlighted the ambiguous moral status of the gregarious instinct as source of both suggestibility and altruism, what this meant for individuals in wartime, and the dangers of the rule of instinct. In this lecture, Murray drew out the ethical problems raised by Trotter's analysis of the herd instinct, while remaining faithful to his conception of its nature, and articulated prevalent fears about the social effects of war.

Echoing popular opinion, Murray claimed that war had united the herd. In early 1914, 'our whole people seemed at strife with itself', but under external threat, internal dissidents such as militant suffragettes and trade union leaders agreed to sink their differences with the government.[103] However, the unity fostered by the herd instinct came at the cost of increased suggestibility. The crowd sanctioned normally suppressed desires and diminished the sense of individual responsibility, and therefore its rule led to an increase in socially reprehensible acts. As the herd instinct deadened individualistic emotions, people became more willing to subordinate their needs to the herd, as when soldiers with bleeding feet continued to march without remark or even awareness of pain.[104] Some might have emphasized the positive effects of individual submergence in the herd, but Murray viewed it with horror. He warned that 'if we yield to the stream of instinct and let scruples and doubts and inhibitions be swept away, we shall not really find life easier', as 'the powers to which we yield will only demand more and more'.[105] Under the apparent social cohesion of wartime lurked the anarchical tendencies of the crowd. In pursuit of the common goal, Britons had sunk not only their political differences but also their individuality, rationality, and responsibility. Any national unity originating in animal instinct rather than human intelligence constituted a seductive but potentially limitless descent from the standards of "civilized" social life.

The thoroughgoing pessimism of this vision, outlined by a future Liberal candidate for Parliament and chairman to the executive council of the League of Nations, provoked mixed reactions. Lord Bryce, head of the commission set up by Asquith to investigate war atrocities, approved of Murray's lecture, but McDougall criticized his emphasis on the negative aspects of the social instinct.[106] Nevertheless, others recognized the

---

[103] G. Murray, 'Herd Instinct and the War', in E.M. Sidgwick, G. Murray, A.C. Bradley, L.P. Jacks, G.F. Stout, and B. Bosanquet (eds.), *The International Crisis in Its Ethical and Psychological Aspects* (London: Oxford University Press, 1915), pp. 28–9.
[104] Murray, 'Herd Instinct and the War', pp. 25–6, 34–5.   [105] Ibid., p. 45.
[106] G. Murray, *Herd Instinct: For Good and Evil* (London: George Allen & Unwin, 1940), p. 3.

crowd latent in the nation. Osler mused on the 'contagion' of fear, 'a state in which the nerves were unstrung'. As evidence of how the herd instinct stripped reason from the crowd mind, Osler cited recent rumours of Russian troops passing through Britain, and the (unrelated) moral panic over a potential explosion of war babies. The nation 'needed steadying, more self-control, more cultivation of the will'. 'Nerves' must be replaced by 'nerve – that well-strung state so needful for our final victory'.[107] Later in the war, racial and xenophobic judgements tinged depictions of the crowd within the nation. A 1917 report on air raids praised the 'calm and grit' of most Londoners in the face of this German 'policy of frightfulness' but lamented the behaviour of 'certain elements of the alien population of the east end', who allegedly overran the public transport system in attempts to escape the city. The only solace was that 'if air raids and the measures taken for their repulse can produce such a state of nerves in these aliens, it is probable that raids over German towns would have a similar effect on their inhabitants'.[108]

The problem of how to achieve the right balance between individuality and social cohesion was often framed around national character. British commentators believed that Prussian militarism had produced 'a people strangely obedient to the voice of authority and unaccustomed to exercise individual judgement and personal initiative'. This kind of national con-sciousness was potentially a source of strength in wartime but also left Germans 'highly susceptible to the influence of mass-suggestion, and liable to the influx of waves of emotion overwhelming the reason'. In contrast, 'independence of thought and action' shielded Britons from the epidemics of emotion and irrationality associated with 'collective consciousness'.[109] In a similar vein, Trotter's 1916 publication on the herd instinct contrasted the bumbling development of the communal mind of the English people – 'the slow mingling and attrition of their ideas, and needs, and impulses' which created 'a store of moral power literally inexhaustible' – with the aggressive German form of herd instinct typified by the wolf pack. He insisted this was not mere analogy, but 'a real and gross identity'.[110] Freud's comment that Trotter's book did not 'entirely escape the antipathies that were set loose by the recent great war' was something of an understatement.[111]

[107] Anon., 'Nerve and Nerves: Address by Sir Wm. Osler, Bart.', *TMW*, 5 (July–December 1915), 492.
[108] Anon., 'The Air War', *BMJ*, 6 October 1917, 457. On investigations into the alleged behaviour of the Jewish population in air raids, see Kent, *Aftershocks*, p. 64.
[109] Anon., 'The Psychological Effect of War', *BMJ*, 13 March 1915, 476; Anon., 'Dr. G.L. Finlay on German "Nerves"', *TMW*, 4 (January–June 1915), 8.
[110] Trotter, *Instincts of the Herd*, pp. 191–2, 201, 204, 207.
[111] Freud, 'Group Psychology and the Analysis of the Ego', p. 118.

As both guardian of the nation and an organized crowd dependent on the subordination of the individual for its efficiency, the army became a locus for anxiety about the ambiguous effects of the herd mind. Military training inculcated automatic responses to ensure a unified and predictable response to the dangers of battle, but in order for discipline to be effective, soldiers must also internalize 'the voluntary spirit, the spirit of individual effort'.[112] Armstrong-Jones gave this predicament a nationalistic twist. He believed the war resulted from the German will to 'change the world without changing himself'. In the German military machine, cohesion was instilled 'by orders from without and not from within the troops themselves'. The 'collective will power' of the British army, on the other hand, was created 'from among themselves and from within', and the 'dissociated, uncertain, and disconnected "will powers"' of the mob reformed into a 'solid cohesive whole'. Yet even in the British army, units drilled to unity were often unprepared to meet unexpected events, 'for no over-drilled individual possesses the initiative or the originating capacity to construct new plans'. Armstrong-Jones maintained that the British army was 'composed of individuals who have not been dragooned into secondarily automatic machines' but he was not complacent about the nature of the 'collective mind'.[113]

Medical ambivalence about the relation between the individual and the group, whether regiment, army, state, or nation, deepened as the war continued. In March 1915, the *British Medical Journal* celebrated the impetus towards social cohesion since the outbreak of war. An editorial claimed that war had effected 'the sudden settlement of differences, the fusion of opposed bodies, the bending to a common purpose of antagonistic forces', and the direction of individual and national consciousness towards 'a single and plain duty'. Victory would depend on the ability of the British people to meet the demands of the state: the ability of fighting men 'to suffer and to go on suffering the terrific and nerve-shattering onslaught of modern gun-fire and still retain in their depleted ranks an effective and alert organisation', and the ability of civilians 'to suffer, proudly and gladly it may be, but to suffer and to go on suffering the increasing pinch of adversity and the loss of its bravest and best-loved sons'.[114] This kind of rhetoric remained powerful throughout the war, but as time went on, its force

---

[112] Recommendations of *RWOCESS*, pp. 208–9.
[113] Armstrong-Jones, 'Psychology of Fear', 356, 383; Armstrong-Jones, 'Mental States and the War. I', 238–9.
[114] Anon., 'Psychological Effect of War', 475.

depended more and more on the exclusion of those perceived to have let the side down. The "shell-shocked" soldier occupied an uncertain position in this economy of sacrifice: he had fought and suffered, but ultimately breakdown represented the triumph of individualistic tendencies over social needs.[115]

"Shell-shock" was always and inevitably a social problem. From the perspective of the governing elites, individual breakdown threatened the military success of the nation and burdened the state. After 1916, it became more common for doctors to put forward cost–benefit analyses of war neurosis. The broken soldier 'cost as much as a cartload of shells'; the 'money and energy' wasted on his training could have been expended more profitably on 'the manufacture of munitions'.[116] The success or failure of treatment meant 'the difference between a useless burden to the State and a useful civilian or even a useful soldier'.[117] If not treated, "shell-shocked" men would become 'a helpless drag upon themselves and an additional burden to the finances of the country'.[118] Medical pleas for the reform of military and civilian health services were presented as an economics of productive citizenry: true, it cost more on a daily basis to repair a car than to garage it, but the extra was gladly paid 'for the simple reasons that a motor car in its garage is of no use to us, and that the daily charge for housing the car would amount to a colossal figure if paid for many years'.[119] The application of principles of accountancy to the problems of war-damaged men feels wrong for all kinds of reasons, not least because emotional and economic structures are incommensurable. But more than this, dispassionate analyses of the economic costs of broken soldiers contradict the main lesson that "shell-shock" doctors claimed to have learnt from the war: that the human mind cannot be reduced to reason and consciousness but remains a seething mass of ineradicable instincts and emotions.

---

[115] On the ambiguous status of the war-wounded within the economy of sacrifice, see Gregory, *Last Great War*, p. 264.

[116] Mott, 'Chadwick Lecture', 40; Mott, 'Two Addresses on War Psycho-Neurosis. (I)', 128; G.H. Savage, 'Mental Disabilities for War Service', *JMS*, 62:259 (October 1916), 653.

[117] Adrian and Yealland, 'Treatment of Some Common War Neuroses', 867; Culpin, 'Practical Hints on Functional Disorders', 549; Tooth, 'Neurasthenia and Psychasthenia', 345; Grimbly, 'Neuroses and Psycho-Neuroses of the Sea', 253–4, 258.

[118] Veale, 'Some Cases of So-Called Functional Paresis', 614; Tombleson, 'An Account of Twenty Cases', 345–6.

[119] Smith and Pear, *Shell Shock and Its Lessons*, pp. 125–6; D.K. Henderson, 'War Psychoses: An Analysis of 202 Cases of Mental Disorder Occurring in Home Troops', *JMS*, 64:265 (April 1918), 177, 187.

Conclusion

In 1919, Wilfred Trotter added a postscript to *Instincts of the Herd in Peace and War*. In the first edition of the book, he had hymned the 'moral power, enthusiasm, courage, endurance, [and] enterprise' of the British people in response to war, and portrayed wartime unity as foreshadowing future national harmony.[120] This optimism had disappeared only a few months after the armistice. Trotter now grieved the resurgence of class divisions and class interests and the retreat of a state once again 'remote and quasi-hostile'. If possible, the nation was in a worse state than before the war. A people quickened by the joys of wartime social unity would not happily return to the 'tasteless social dietary of pre-war England', but no impetus to genuine cohesion now existed. He hinted at dark possibilities. The war had weakened conventional restraints on class hostility and accustomed the populace to change, violence, and irreverence for established traditions without permanently solving any of the social defects evident before its outbreak.[121] It was now apparent that the mirage of wartime social cohesion had only temporarily halted the steady crumbling of "civilization". Humans driven by instinct refused to use the intelligence which separated them from animals. The 'object lesson' of the war was not that the nation could triumph if it worked with one mind and one aim, but 'how easy it is for man, all undirected and unwarned as he is, to sink to the irresponsible destructiveness of the monkey'.[122]

Trotter was more pessimistic than most, but many social commentators shared the belief that war had revealed anew the "primitive" animal nature at the heart of human "civilization". For William Osler, war demonstrated that beneath 'a skin-deep civilisation were the same old elemental passions ready to burst forth'. The much-vaunted "progress" of the nineteenth century had not removed 'the savage instincts ground into the very fibre of [human] being'.[123] Harry Campbell concurred: all the concerted efforts to nurture children in the best possible way, or to alter the environment, had been in vain. No force in "civilization" or nature could 'change man's normal nature to its very depth' and 'eradicate all potentiality towards the primitive savage'. Education only covered 'with a thin veneer of moral polish the savage beneath', and 'the spots from which the veneer may be removed only appear the worse

---

[120] Trotter, *Instincts of the Herd*, pp. 142–3.
[121] Ibid., pp. 234–40. See also J. Lawrence, 'Forging a Peaceable Kingdom: War, Violence, and Fear of Brutalization in Post-First World War Britain', *Journal of Modern History*, 75:3 (September 2003), 566.
[122] Trotter, *Instincts of the Herd*, pp. 255–6.
[123] Osler, 'Address on Science and War', 796.

from contrast'.[124] The war was a harsh reminder that "civilization" was still in its own 'childhood', nothing more than 'a thin fringe like the layer of living polyps on the coral reef, capping the dead generations on which it rests'.[125] Unsurprisingly, psychoanalysts led this chorus, pointing out that 'the facts of the War itself accord with Freud's view of the human mind as containing beneath the surface a body of imperfectly controlled and explosive forces which in their nature conflict with the standards of civilisation'. War was an eruption of repressed impulses, a reaction against societal and ethical standards through 'reversion to a more primitive level of civilisation'.[126]

The dilemma revealed by war was the problem of instinct itself, the imperishable force which drove and constituted conflict at the individual, national, and international levels. In the gloomy post-war world, Mott assumed the mantle of seer and tried to imagine a future in which humanity could overcome the animal within. He concluded that it was impossible: no statute could abolish the 'predatory instinct of man', so war would continue as long as humanity itself survived.[127] On the cusp of another world war, Frederick Dillon reflected on his experiences at an NYDN centre in France two decades before. He believed it unlikely that neurosis could be avoided in a future war. 'Fear-inspiring conditions' would be 'similar but more intense' and would 'act on human beings with the same instincts, the same kinds of defence mechanisms, and similar neurotic proclivities'. The best to be hoped for was sensible management, not prevention.[128] Modern war had changed the methods of killing, but men remained the same: trapped in a 'primitive condition of existence' in trenches like caves, 'never knowing when some prehistoric beast, transformed in our civilised times into a shell or bullet, is going to make an end of them'.[129] "Shell-shock" forced the realization that the cerebral cortex and cumulative social achievements of two thousand years of "civilization" in the end supplied only the flimsiest cage for animal passions and emotions. This revelation indicted not only individuals but also war and "civilization" itself. The soldier might be restored to humanity, but humanity could not be saved from its state of perpetual embryonic crisis.

---

[124] H. Campbell, 'The Biological Aspects of Warfare', *Lancet*, 15 September 1917, 434; C.B. Moore, 'Some Psychological Aspects of War', *Pedagogical Seminary*, 23:3 (September 1916), 376–7.
[125] Osler, 'An Address on Science and War', 795.
[126] Jones, 'War Shock and Freud's Theory of the Neuroses', 25; Jones, 'War and Individual Psychology', 176–7.
[127] Mott, 'Neuroses and Psychoses in Relation to Conscription and Eugenics', 21–2.
[128] Dillon, 'Neuroses among Combatant Troops', 66.
[129] GHMSA: G/S6/14, unsigned, 'Physiology and the War' (undated, 1916–17), p. 11.

The broken soldier was an ominous reminder that only the thinnest and most fragile layer of neural tissue separated the human from the animal. "Shell-shock" was a great leveller. Whether perceived as the dominance of emotion, the recrudescence of instinct, or the loss of self-control, "shell-shock" always constituted a regression. Doctors adopted many different perspectives on war neurosis: they explored the physiology of emotion, psychobiology of instinct, and psychology of the unconscious in the attempt to understand "shell-shock". But all conceptualized the disorder as a struggle between the "higher" and "lower" in human nature and as damning evidence of animal origins. Even the noblest aspects of war, such as sacrifice of self-interest in a greater cause, could be explained as mere outgrowths of the herd instinct with its ugly underbelly of suggestibility and irrationality. The evolutionary framework of understanding aligned "shell-shock" with a much older complex of fears around human nature, "civilization", and the future development of both. These anxieties continued into the post-war era, deepened by the experience of four years of highly advanced and scientific bloodshed. War exposed the frailty not only of individual minds but also of the human condition. As "shell-shock" was dissected, concepts of the individual and the social inexorably bled into each other. The soldier represented and defended the nation; for many Britons, this meant "civilization" itself. On the body of the "shell-shocked" soldier, its pathologics were mapped out.

Conclusion
"Shell-Shock" and Post-War Medical Culture

Towards the end of the war, psychologist Charles Myers, the physician responsible for the first appearance of the word "shell-shock" in print, published a book on *Present-Day Applications of Psychology*. Disillusioned by his struggles with the military hierarchy, Myers had returned to civilian life and now threw his energies into showing that psychology could help with everyday problems, especially those of the industrial workplace. Myers, a former colleague of W.H.R. Rivers, spent some time outlining the role of repression in producing anxiety neurosis, as well as 'the modern method of treating hysterical and neurasthenic disorder' by persuasion and re-education developed by "analytic" doctors at Maghull and elsewhere. He described this theory and method as 'a totally new standpoint on the position of functional nervous disorders'. These illnesses, 'essentially of mental origin', demanded the attention of a 'new class of medical man, educated in ... psychological theories and practices'.[1] As an academic psychologist and trained physician, Myers had seen the value of both disciplines long before the war, but he presented his encounter with "shell-shock" as crucial to the realization that psychological methods must be applied to peacetime problems.

Myers echoed the sentiments of many of his professional brethren. As the war went on and doctors gained more experience in diagnosing and treating war neurosis, medical commentators frequently expressed their hopes that the lessons of "shell-shock" would be applied to the civilian sphere after the war. At a colloquium on medical education held shortly before the armistice, participants spoke of the urgent need for changes in medical approaches to nervous and mental disorders: doctors must be educated in "normal" as well as "abnormal" psychology; early diagnosis and treatment were essential; and the existing mental health system desperately required an overhaul, perhaps most of all in the provision

---

[1] Myers, *Present-Day Applications of Psychology*, pp. 43–4.

of outpatient clinics.[2] The experience of war had underscored the necessity of far-reaching changes to medical education and provision, and in the training course set up at Maghull Military Hospital, doctors even had a model for how to impart psychological knowledge to students within a relatively short space of time.[3] The desire for change was palpable, and the success of psychological approaches to "shell-shock" showed what could be achieved even under extreme pressure and constraints. As the war drew to its close, it seemed that "shell-shock" had provided the stimulus needed to transform British psychological medicine and that dramatic innovations in its theories, practices, and institutions were on the near horizon.

This transformation did happen, but not at the speed nor to the extent which seemed possible and desirable in 1918. In 1919, the Maudsley Hospital began to offer a course of instruction to prepare candidates for the diploma in psychological medicine, followed in 1921 by the Bethlem Hospital and the National Hospital for the Paralysed and Epileptic, Queen Square. In 1930, exactly the same institutions offered this instruction as in 1922.[4] In the 1920s, a handful of outpatient clinics and other facilities for the voluntary treatment of non-certifiable mental disorders opened, including the Maudsley Hospital, the Cassel Hospital, and the Tavistock Clinic. But the establishment of outpatient clinics on a grander scale did not follow until the Mental Treatment Act 1930 empowered local authorities to set up these facilities.[5] The same act of legislation finally fulfilled the aim of pre-war campaigns for the early treatment of mental disorders by making voluntary treatment in mental hospitals available to 'rate-aided persons' (the Act also discarded the terminology of 'lunatic asylums' and 'pauper lunatics').[6] A full twelve years after the end of the war, the major changes to the mental health system which

---

[2] Gulland, 'Teaching of Medicine', 23; Matthew, 'Teaching of Medicine'; J. Middlemass, 'Recent Advances in Medical Science: Mental Diseases', *EMJ*, 21 (July–December 1918), 118; Bramwell, 'Teaching of Neurology', 208.

[3] J. Mackenzie, 'Aim of Medical Education', 35–8; Hart, 'Psychology and the Medical Curriculum'; Robertson, 'The Teaching of Mental Diseases in Edinburgh', 229; Clarkson, 'The Teaching of Psychology to Medical Undergraduates', 240; Hart in 'Discussion: The Training of the Student of Medicine, XLII–XLVII', *EMJ*, 21 (July–December 1918), 248.

[4] Anon., 'Psychological Medicine', *BMJ*, 2 September 1922, 443–5; Anon., 'Psychological Medicine', *BMJ*, 6 September 1930, 389–91.

[5] By 1939 there were 187 psychiatric and psychological outpatient clinics in Britain. Shephard, *War of Nerves*, p. 161.

[6] J. Busfield, 'Restructuring Mental Health Services in Twentieth-Century Britain', in M. Gijswijt-Hofstra and R. Porter (eds.), *Cultures of Psychiatry and Mental Health Care in Postwar Britain and the Netherlands* (Amsterdam and Atlanta, GA: Rodopi, 1998), 13–15.

reformers had demanded for more than two decades were finally implemented. Administrative reform is almost always a drawn-out process. Nevertheless, this distance in time from the armistice makes it difficult to view the Act as a direct result of the "shell-shock" episode.

At issue here is the status of "shell-shock" within post-war psychological medicine and the long-term influence of the war on medical culture. Once again, this is an investigation of silence. In 1918, "shell-shock" was at the heart of demands for radical change to the mental health system. Yet after an initial flurry of books and articles in the early 1920s which pulled together or summarized doctors' conclusions on the war neuroses, "shell-shock" began to fade out of mainstream medical discourse.[7] After 1922, extended discussion of "shell-shock" slowly petered out of the published medical literature. This was the end of the first phase of the existence of "shell-shock", appropriately symbolized by the premature death of W.H.R. Rivers in June 1922 and the publication of the final report of the War Office Committee of Enquiry into "Shell-Shock" two months later.[8] Of course, the volume of debate on "shell-shock" could not be sustained in the aftermath of the war; still, there was far less discussion than might be expected. The experience of war was not entirely forgotten, but medical comments on "shell-shock" were scattered and often incidental. This is despite the flourishing of medical interest in psychology and psychoanalysis and the fact that "shell-shocked" soldiers did not disappear. In the immediate post-war period, a spate of criminal trials saw men claiming diminished responsibility through "shell-shock".[9] A decade afterwards, in March 1929, the government claimed it was still paying out 55,469 pensions for neurasthenia and "shell-shock".[10] As the government attempted to keep its pensions bill down, doctors had to assess and reassess war-related disabilities, and veterans' struggles were well publicized in charity appeals.[11] Yet *sustained*

---

[7] I owe this insight about the gradual waning of "shell-shock" from published medical literature in the early 1920s to Michael Roper's identification of a shift in psychoanalytical publications from discussion of the war neuroses to the analysis of children in the same period. M. Roper, 'From the Shell-Shocked Soldier to the Nervous Child: Psychoanalysis in the Aftermath of the First World War', *Psychoanalysis and History*, 18:1 (January 2016), 39–69.

[8] On the Report of the War Office Committee of Enquiry into "Shell-Shock", see Bogacz, 'War Neurosis and Cultural Change in England'.

[9] C. Emsley, 'Violent Crime in England in 1919: Post-War Anxieties and Press Narratives', *Continuity and Change*, 23:1 (2008), 173–95.

[10] The statistics for pensions awards in the post-war period are mired in confusion. For a full discussion, see E. Jones, I. Palmer and S. Wessely, 'War Pensions (1900–1945): Changing Models of Psychological Understanding', *British Journal of Psychiatry*, 180 (2002), 374–9; Jones and Wessely, *Shell Shock to PTSD*, pp. 150–6.

[11] On the post-war experiences of veterans, see Reid, *Broken Men*, pp. 71–162; Barham, *Forgotten Lunatics of the Great War*, especially pp. 181–98; P. Leese, 'Problems Returning

medical discussion of "shell-shock" or the problems of traumatized veterans was uncommon after the early 1920s.[12]

Doctors who had treated the disorder remained active in the medical world over the entire interwar period and often researched and wrote on topics with unstated but obvious connections to their wartime experiences – such as the cause of recent interest in psychotherapy, the uses of occupational therapy, or the diagnosis of traumatic neurasthenia.[13] Yet the war was either not discussed or passed over with the briefest of mentions. For example, when J.R. Lord considered 'the evolution of the "nerve" hospital in the progress of psychiatry' in 1929, he devoted much attention to the opening of outpatient clinics over the past decade but did not mention the war once.[14] Another strange absence is found in a 1935 address on psychotherapeutic clinics by Hugh Crichton-Miller, a doctor inspired by his treatment of "shell-shocked" soldiers to open in 1920 the Institute of Medical Psychology (later renamed the Tavistock Clinic), an outpatient clinic for patients with functional nervous disorders. In this address, Crichton-Miller did not once mention the war or war neurosis, although his account of the state of psychotherapy in Britain was liberally sprinkled with the names of "shell-shock" doctors, including Millais Culpin, William McDougall, W.H.R. Rivers, T.A. Ross (1875–1941), and Emanuel Miller (1892–1970).[15] This perfectly illustrates the prominence of "shell-shock" doctors in interwar medical discourse even as "shell-shock" became less visible in this forum.

This paradox has not been recognized, much less explained, but it is crucial to understanding the extent and nature of the influence of "shell-shock" on post-war psychological medicine. In the cultural sphere, it is widely accepted that "shell-shock" fundamentally affected how war was imagined even if it did not cancel out older heroic discourses. In contrast, historical interpretations of the effects of "shell-shock" on medical

Home: The British Psychological Casualties of the Great War', *Historical Journal*, 40:4 (December 1997), 1055–67; Leese, *Shell Shock*, pp. 141–58.

[12] For exceptions, see Somerville, 'War-Anxiety Neurotic of the Present Day'; H. Somerville, 'War Anxiety Neurotic of the Present Day: His "Dizzy Bouts" and Hallucinations', *British Journal of Medical Psychology*, 3:4 (1923), 309–19; A.F. Grimbly, 'A Problem in Diagnosis', *JMS*, 71:293 (April 1925), 278–83.

[13] E.F. Buzzard, 'Psycho-Therapeutics', *Lancet*, 17 February 1923, 330–2; Anon., 'Reports of Societies: "Occupation Cure" in Neurasthenia', *BMJ*, 3 February 1923, 190–1; M. Culpin, 'Some Cases of "Traumatic Neurasthenia"', *Lancet*, 1 August 1931, 233–7.

[14] J.R. Lord, 'The Evolution of the "Nerve" Hospital as a Factor in the Progress of Psychiatry', *JMS*, 75:309 (April 1929), 307–15.

[15] H. Crichton-Miller, 'Psychotherapeutic Clinics in Fact and Fancy', *BMJ*, 15 June 1935, 1205–8.

culture are divided.[16] As outlined in the introduction to this book, Martin Stone's influential interpretation portrayed the "shell-shock" episode as causing a transition to psychodynamic modes of understanding and treating mental illness, and as resulting in the creation of treatment sites outside the asylum.[17] Edgar Jones and Simon Wessely, on the other hand, argue that the long-term effects of "shell-shock" on civilian and military psychiatry were negligible, and 'much that had been achieved rapidly disappeared once the country had returned to peace'.[18] A halfway house between these opposed viewpoints is Mathew Thomson's contention that although the "shell-shock" episode was 'hugely important', it was still 'only a catalyst for what was taking place independently'.[19] The first interpretation assumes rather than firmly demonstrates the causal links between "shell-shock" and subsequent developments in psychological medicine, partly by depicting pre-1914 psychological medicine as utterly resistant to psychodynamic approaches. In the second and third interpretations, the effects of "shell-shock" are viewed as little more than an extension of processes in train before the outbreak of war.

None of these interpretations satisfactorily explains the coexistence of apparently contradictory factors in post-war medicine: genuine excitement at the end of the war about the possibilities of radical change in psychological medicine; the slow rate of reform; sea-changes in the type and quantity of commentary on psychology and psychoanalysis in the interwar period; the status of former "shell-shock" doctors as shapers of the culture of psychological medicine; and the diminished place of "shell-shock" within mainstream medical discourse. This conclusion suggests some of the ways in which the lessons of "shell-shock" were dispersed throughout medical culture even as discursive traces of the disorder faded. I argue that this waning of "shell-shock" was a by-product of two major successes: the triumph of wartime doctors in establishing that there was no fundamental difference between the neuroses of peace and war, and the achievement of psychologists in demonstrating the universal applicability of their research. Three important developments within

---

[16] Dawson, *Soldier Heroes*, p. 153; Hynes, *War Imagined*, pp. 214–15; J. Meyer, *Men of War: Masculinity and the First World War in Britain* (Basingstoke and New York: Palgrave Macmillan, 2009); Carden-Coyne, *Reconstructing the Body*, p. 313; M. Paris, *Warrior Nation: Images of War in British Popular Culture, 1850–2000* (London: Reaktion Books, 2000), pp. 112–85.

[17] Stone, 'Shellshock and the Psychologists'.

[18] Jones and Wessely, 'Impact of Total War', p. 147. See also Wessely, 'Twentieth-Century Theories on Combat Motivation', 273–4.

[19] Thomson, *Psychological Subjects*, p. 185.

post-war medical discourse, all of which can be related to wartime experiences of "shell-shock", together constituted a major shift: the extensive adoption of psychoanalytical language; the widespread employment of particular Freudian-derived concepts; and, perhaps most importantly, the scale of psychological debate after 1918. To describe this movement as an extension of pre-war trends does not adequately convey either the qualitative differences between pre- and post-war approaches to psychological matters or the massive quantitative increase in discussion of psychoanalysis and other "new" psychologies. At the same time, these changes were furthered by methods of assimilation familiar from the pre-war era, including eclecticism and the "translation" of radical concepts into the native idiom. This transformation might be best described as revolution via evolution.

"Shell-Shock" in the Civilian World

I have argued throughout this book that the war simultaneously provoked and contained interest in radical psychological ideas. The experience of treating "shell-shocked" soldiers inspired many doctors to explore new approaches to mind. Yet during the span of the war itself, the influence of "shell-shock" on existing frameworks and therapeutic practices was limited, both by the acknowledgement of war as an exceptional event, quite out of the everyday run of precipitating causes of neurosis, and by the constraints of military medicine, which demanded quick results from limited resources. The really far-reaching consequences of the "shell-shock" episode unfolded after the armistice, when doctors treating new cases of breakdown could no longer fall back on the get-out clause of the war to avoid following psychological theories to their logical conclusions, and when they had more freedom to explore and implement psychological approaches outside the system of military medicine. This happened despite the waning of "shell-shock" within published medical discourse and partially explains this disappearance. The flourishing of psychology within mainstream medical culture at the end of the war expressed the application of new psychological knowledges to civilian problems in directions not possible under wartime restrictions.

It is important to distinguish here between the effects of "shell-shock" on civilian psychological medicine and on military psychiatry. The claim that the experience of "shell-shock" had no real influence on military psychiatry in the interwar period is absolutely true. This lack of influence on post-war military medicine is at least partly a consequence of the status of "shell-shock" as a product of civilian medical expertise. As discussed in the introduction to this book, none of the doctors who contributed to published wartime medical debates on "shell-shock" were regular members of the RAMC. When the war ended, doctors who held temporary commissions returned to civilian practice. The expertise these doctors had accumulated in the field of military psychiatry was transferred to the civilian sphere. The structures of treatment also affected the type of knowledge of psychological disorders found in the military. After discharge or demobilization, men with war-related psychiatric disorders were treated outside military institutions. When the military authorities considered the problem of "shell-shock", they emphasized leadership, training, and morale not just because army culture encouraged a no-nonsense, non-medicalized approach to breakdown – though it certainly did – but because they could feasibly exert control over these practical measures. The army did not apply the lessons of "shell-shock" in the interwar period because the diagnosis had no firm roots in the institutions of military psychiatry. Given these limitations, it is even questionable whether military psychiatry was a separate field of medicine in the interwar years at all.

Of course, the shortcomings of interwar military psychiatry do not explain either the faded presence of "shell-shock" within civilian psychological medicine, or the explosion of interest in psychology within mainstream medical culture in this period. On the face of it, it might seem that war experience also exerted little influence on the professional lives of published "shell-shock" doctors. For the most part, doctors returned to their pre-war fields of specialism, and in many cases to exactly the same institutions and posts held before the war. The only inarguable exception to this rule is Millais Culpin, established as a surgeon before wartime experience of treating functional disorders led him towards medical psychology.[20] It is possible to make a case for the transformative effects of war on the careers of Joseph Prideaux (1884–1959) and W.H.R. Rivers, but the evidence is not wholly convincing in either instance. Joseph Prideaux graduated in 1908 and spent the next six years stationed in Fiji with the Colonial Service. He joined the RAMC in 1916 and his obituary records that work with "shell-shocked" men 'turned his interest to psychiatry', in which field he built an impressive career.[21] However, his career was not securely established before 1916, so we cannot know whether the war definitively altered his path. There is no doubt that personally, politically, and professionally, the war profoundly affected

---

[20] For Culpin's account of this "conversion", see M. Culpin, *The Nervous Patient* (London: H.K. Lewis, 1924), pp. 11–15.

[21] Anon., 'Obituary: Joseph Francis Engeldue Prideaux', *Lancet*, 28 November 1959, 978–9.

Rivers – but his diverse pre-war research interests had included psych-ology, and his post-war publications attempted to synthesize all his interests.

If we look at the post-war careers of those doctors too young to have firmly established themselves within particular specialisms before 1914, the influence of "shell-shock" is suddenly more apparent. Of the pub-lished "shell-shock" doctors who graduated between 1910 and 1918 and had not clearly taken up a distinct specialism before the war, at least seven later pursued careers in psychology, psychiatry, or neurology.[22] Most cut their teeth in special clinics set up by the Ministry of Pensions for the treatment of veterans suffering from "shell-shock" and allied disorders.[23] The post-war publications of these doctors also often explored subjects potentially connected to "shell-shock" (psychotherapy, psychoanalysis, functional nervous diseases) or problems prevalent among traumatized veterans in subsequent conflicts (insomnia, crime, alcoholism, and drug addiction).[24] In the squeezed post-war medical market, Ministry of Pensions clinics provided professional opportunities. Quite possibly, the psychological problems encountered in these clinics also shaped the future research interests of these young "shell-shock" doctors.[25]

The effects of war experience on doctors with established careers in psychology, psychoanalysis, or related fields is less clear-cut.[26] This group contained some of the most influential figures in interwar psych-ology and psychological medicine, including William Brown, Ernest

---

[22] Paul Bousfield, Alfred Carver, Philip Fenwick, Ronald Gray Gordon, Walter Reynell, Christopher Rixon, and Frederick Laughton Scott.

[23] Five of this subgroup are known to have worked in these clinics: Bousfield, Carver, Reynell, Rixon, and Scott.

[24] G.L. Scott, 'An Improved Method for Withdrawing Drugs of Addiction without Discomfort to the Patient', *Practitioner*, 118:1 (January 1927), 55–8; A. Carver, 'The Psychology of the Alcoholist', *British Journal of Medical Psychology*, 11:2 (1931), 117–24. For more information on these post-war publications, see Loughran, 'Shell-Shock in First World War Britain', pp. 240–89.

[25] This network of clinics was set up in late 1919. By October 1920, 29 clinics were in operation. In February 1921 it was estimated that 14,771 ex-servicemen were either attending boards for assessment or clinics for treatment. In addition to these clinics, the Ministry of Pensions also took over former military hospitals, and used these for the in-patient treatment of "shell-shocked" veterans. According to official statistics, the number of patients treated under the aegis of the Ministry of Pensions peaked in 1921 and declined steadily from the late 1920s onwards. E. Jones, 'Post-Combat Disorders: The Boer War to the Gulf', in H. Lee and E. Jones (eds.), *War and Health: Lessons from the Gulf War* (Chichester, West Sussex: John Wiley & Sons, 2007), p. 16.

[26] I have included in this group doctors drawn from academic psychology, psychoanalysis, and private nursing homes for nervous disorders: William Brown, Frederick Dillon, David Eder, David Forsyth, Ernest Jones, Charles Myers, W.H.R. Rivers, and Thomas Ross.

Jones, Charles Myers, and W.H.R. Rivers. All these doctors continued in the same fields after the war, but many altered the direction of their research while others adopted different explanatory mechanisms and treatments for psychological disorders. Until his death, W.H.R. Rivers' research probed instinct, the unconscious, and dreams, aspects of mind manifested in war neurosis which continued to fascinate him.[27] In several publications on suggestion, 'mental analysis', and psychotherapy, William Brown's investigations had a practical bent not always evident in his pre-war research.[28] Thomas Ross had shown keen interest in the common neuroses before the war, but afterwards concepts such as 'repression' and 'anxiety neurosis' entered his vocabulary, and he pursued more active and sophisticated forms of psychotherapy than the rest cure he had earlier endorsed (albeit with an emphasis on the "psychic" components of the treatment).[29] Finally, in the interwar period, Charles Myers almost single-handedly established the discipline of industrial psychology in Britain, starting with the foundation of the National Institute of Industrial Psychology in 1921.

This bare list of facts implies that the war decisively shaped these doctors' subsequent clinical practice and research interests. But after the early 1920s, few pushed the relation between "shell-shock" and their work in the civilian sphere, at least not until prompted to recall earlier experiences by the advent of another world war.[30] It is possible that some were ambivalent about the extent to which the war had influenced their opinions. In his preface to *The Group Mind* (1920), William McDougall explained that although the war 'is supposed by some to have revolutionised all our ideas of human nature and of national life', he had actually written substantial parts of the book before 1914. He asserted that the war had provided 'little reason to add to or to change what I had written'. However, his experiences during 1914–18 did prompt him finally to publish. After giving up 'five of the best years of my life ... to military

---

[27] Rivers, *Instinct and the Unconscious*; Rivers, *Conflict and Dream*.

[28] See for examples W. Brown, *Suggestion and Mental Analysis: An Outline of the Theory and Practice of Mind Cure* (London: University of London Press, 1922); W. Brown, 'Suggestion and Personality', *British Journal of Medical Psychology*, 5:1 (1925), 29–34; W. Brown, 'Theories of Suggestion', *BMJ*, 18 February 1928, 573–82.

[29] For example, compare Ross, 'Nature and Treatment of Neurasthenia'; Ross, 'Prevention of Relapse of Hysterical Manifestations'; T.A. Ross, 'Some Difficulties in Analytical Theory and Practice', *British Journal of Medical Psychology*, 10:1 (1930), 1–19.

[30] Many of the doctors in this subgroup of the cohort, including Ross, Brown, Myers and Dillon, published articles or books between 1939 and 1945 reflecting on their experiences of treating "shell-shock" in the First World War. For discussion of the contribution of doctors who had served during 1914–1918 to debates in the next war, see B. Shephard, '"Pitiless Psychology": The Role of Prevention in British Military Psychiatry in the Second World War', *History of Psychiatry*, 10 (1999), 494–6.

service and the practical problems of psycho-therapy', he realized that 'the years of a man's life are numbered', and that if he delayed publication until he was sure the book was absolutely ready, it might never come out.[31] McDougall simultaneously denied and acknowledged the influence of the war, possibly because of the difficulty of conceding its transformative effects without repudiating the valued achievements of the pre-war era. Many others doubtless felt similarly torn about the effects of the war on their professional lives.

Yet the submergence of "shell-shock" in the interwar publications of these psychologists did not result solely from ambivalent emotions as they tried to join up the threads of their pre-war, wartime, and post-war careers. Rather, this disappearance is to do with the nature of the lessons of "shell-shock". It was often claimed that "shell-shock" had shown that there was no essential difference between the neuroses of war and of peace. This led doctors to expect that wartime expertise in the diagnosis and treatment of functional disorders would be applied in the civilian sphere, not least in the service of damaged veterans.[32] In his inaugural address to the educational section of the British Psychological Society, Percy Nunn (1870–1944) claimed that psychologists had performed an 'invaluable service' to the nation 'in its hour of need'. During the war, psychologists had proved the worth of their discipline. In its aftermath, they must capitalize on the realization that 'there are great problems, of great moment to human efficiency and happiness, that cannot be solved except with the aid of psychological knowledge and psychological methods'.[33] Psychologists heeded this advice when they left explicit talk of "shell-shock" behind and threw themselves into the multifarious psychological problems of civilian life.

The post-war reconfiguration of the British Psychological Society (BPS) illustrates how the experience of "shell-shock" silently influenced

[31] W. McDougall, *The Group Mind: A Sketch of the Principles of Collective Psychology with Some Attempt to Apply Them to the Interpretation of National Life and Character* (Cambridge: Cambridge University Press, 1920), p. viii. For an example of this kind of rhetoric, see Parsons, *Mind and the Nation*, p. 140: 'To all such as survive the barriers have been broken down: new forces and old ones diversely applied, will be brought to bear upon the established institutions'.

[32] Anon., 'New Editions: M. Craig, Psychological Medicine, Third Edition', *EMJ*, 19 (July-December 1917), 338–9; Smith and Pear, *Shell Shock and Its Lessons*, pp. xiii-xv; Anon., 'Reviews: War Neuroses', *BMJ*, 26 April 1919, 520; Rivers, 'Psychology and Medicine', 190; J.M. Taylor, 'Common Motor Disorders, Disuse Cripplings, Neuroses, Post-Infective and Others', *TMW*, 14 (July-December 1920), 1016; Culpin, *Psychoneuroses of War and Peace*, unpaginated preface; J.G.P. Phillips, 'The Early Treatment of Mental Disorder: A Critical Survey of Out-Patient Clinics', *JMS*, 69:287 (October 1923), 474.

[33] T.B. Nunn, 'Psychology and Education', *British Journal of Psychology*, 10:2 (March 1920), 169.

the future development of psychology in Britain. In 1919, the constitution of the Society was altered to allow anyone with an interest in psychology to become a member. The previous rules had stipulated that members must be 'engaged in psychology'. This change in the regulations capitalized on post-war interest in psychology and led to an immediate increase in membership. At the same time, three special sections of the Society were set up to represent the fields of medicine, education, and industry. This development reflected the interests of key members of the Committee but was instituted to stave off the threat of autonomous institutions which dealt with these areas draining the Society's own membership.[34] However, the new sections can also be viewed as forums to investigate issues that "shell-shock" had forced to the forefront of the psychological agenda.

The great conundrum of "shell-shock" was not why some men broke down, but why so many did not under similar strains. To the extent that psychologists rejected heredity as sufficient explanation for this difference, they needed to formulate alternative explanations. The most prevalent response was that the conditions of early life shaped subsequent psychological reactions. The post-war development of child and educational psychology was one response to this realization. When psychologists tried to work out how to shape character and create psychological health, their research into child psychology formed an analogue to the military pursuit of more effective regimes of training to prevent psychological breakdown. This motivation is strikingly illustrated by the closing anecdote of a paper on 'the nervous child' by paediatrician Bernard Myers (1872–1957). Myers told how 'a certain British general' responded to the shock of witnessing at close quarters the death of a comrade in a shell explosion. The 'immediate shock' was so great that the general temporarily lost his nerve and 'felt an overwhelming desire to bolt for his life':

> However, it so happened that he had been brought up from early childhood to have complete control of himself. It then flashed through his mind that if he acted according to his first impulse, he would suffer severely from shell shock and be of no further use during the war. He therefore determined to remain, and, pulling himself together, quietly walked over to the spot where he and his brother officer had stood a few minutes previously. He stood at attention for five minutes, regained his nerve, and fought to the end of the war without suffering from shell-shock.

Myers concluded, 'It is this self-control and sense of duty we must endeavour to inculcate into every nervous child'.[35]

---

[34] Forrester, '1919: Psychology and Psychoanalysis, Cambridge and London', 45–7.
[35] B. Myers, 'The Nervous Child as Seen in Medical Practice', *BMJ*, 25 July 1925, 161–2.

The new sections of the BPS were founded to deal with practical problems, and their concerns bore little relation to the older traditions of either introspective or experimental psychology. The active support of Henry Head, William Brown, and Hugh Crichton-Miller for the British Institute of Philosophical Studies (founded 1925) suggests that former "shell-shock" doctors did appreciate the value of 'metaphysics' in attempts 'to distinguish between normal and abnormal conditions, physical or mental': but they saw this type of investigation as outside the newly drawn bounds of psychological medicine.[36] Instead, in different ways, the reformed sections of the BPS tackled a challenge familiar to military doctors: how to maintain the health and relative happiness of large numbers of people in order to pursue the goals of a particular organization with maximum efficiency. The origins of medical, educational, and industrial psychology can be traced back much further than the First World War.[37] Nevertheless, the development of these disciplines in Britain at this specific moment makes more sense if we think about the questions that "shell-shock" provoked.

As psychologists applied themselves to civilian psychology, the war faded into the background of their work. Of course, doctors did not need to explain the genesis of their ideas in every publication. But it is also possible that the exclusion of "shell-shock" was in part a conscious strategy designed to demonstrate the universal applicability of psychological insights. This interpretation is supported by different modes of presenting research problems to psychological audiences in the wartime and post-war era. In wartime publications on "shell-shock" for generalist medical journals, psychologists focused on practical problems of diagnosis and treatment. At meetings of the British Psychological Society, "shell-shock" doctors adopted a different tack, rarely presenting papers explicitly as contributions to debates on the war neuroses.[38] Instead, titles referred to universal attributes of mind or to general psychological questions, and doctors did not position their arguments as directly or solely based on work with "shell-shocked" men. However, the same concerns threaded through mainstream medical discourse on

[36] Dawson of Penn, T. Horder, T.W. Mitchell, W. Brown, and H. Crichton-Miller, 'Correspondence: British Institute of Philosophical Studies', *BMJ*, 9 April 1927, 699.

[37] Smith, *Between Mind and Nature*, pp. 70–136; Thomson, *Psychological Subjects*, pp. 109–206.

[38] From papers presented between 1915 and 1922, the exceptions are F.W. Mott, 'The Psychical Effects of Shell Shock' (20 November 1915); Millais Culpin, 'The Problem of the Neurasthenic Pensioner' (26 January 1921); and Gerald Fitzgerald and James Young, 'The Evolution of the War Neuroses' (14 December 1921). See 'Proceedings of the British Psychological Society', *British Journal of Psychology*, 8:2 (May 1916), 270; 11:3 (March 1921), 374; and 12:4 (April 1922), 394.

"shell-shock" and topics discussed at meetings of the Society. Between 1915 and 1922, published "shell-shock" doctors delivered papers on the physiology of emotion;[39] suggestion and hypnosis;[40] psychoanalysis;[41] "primitive" aspects of the mind, behaviour and culture;[42] and the nature and relation of instinct and the "unconscious".[43] The desire to position psychology as universally relevant, and to establish its value in solving the problems of everyday life and the "normal" mind, contributed to the diminished status of "shell-shock" in interwar psychological discourse. This absence is not a sign of the lack of influence of "shell-shock" on post-war psychological medicine. It is testament to the extent and depth of this influence.

'A Whole Climate of Opinion'[44]: Psychoanalysis and Post-War Medical Culture

In 1920, W.H.R. Rivers described the war as 'a vast crucible in which all our preconceived views concerning human nature have been tested'.[45] This view was common among psychologists who treated "shell-shocked" men. War demonstrated the driving force of the unconscious, especially the role of unconscious conflicts in nervous and mental

[39] J. Murray, 'The Involuntary Nervous System and the Involuntary Expression of Emotions', 13 May 1916; Alfred Carver, 'The Generation and Control of Emotion', 11 June 1919. See 'Proceedings of the British Psychological Society', *British Journal of Psychology*, 8:3 (September 1916), 394, and 10:1 (November 1919), 132.

[40] E. Prideaux, 'Suggestion and Suggestibility', 29 October 1919; discussion on 'The Revival of Emotional Memories and Its Therapeutic Value', featuring papers by W. Brown, C.S. Myers, and W. McDougall, 18 February 1920. 'Proceedings of the British Psychological Society', *British Journal of Psychology*, 10:2 (March 1920), 283, and 10:4 (July 1920), 352.

[41] W.H.R. Rivers, 'The Freudian Concept of the Censor', 25 January 1919; William Brown, 'Psycho-Analysis, Suggestion, and Education', 15 October 1919; Ernest Jones, 'Recent Advances in Psycho-Analysis', 21 January 1920. 'Proceedings of the British Psychological Society', *British Journal of Psychology*, 9:3 (May 1919), 376, and 10:2 (March 1920), 283.

[42] M.D. Eder, 'Destructiveness and Superstition', and W.H.R. Rivers, 'Dreams and Primitive Culture', both 26 January 1918. 'Proceedings of the British Psychological Society', *British Journal of Psychology*, 9:2 (October 1918), 260.

[43] Symposium on 'Why Is the "Unconscious" Unconscious?', including papers by Ernest Jones, W.H.R. Rivers, and Maurice Nicoll, 6 July 1918; symposium on 'Instinct and the Unconscious', featuring papers by W.H.R. Rivers, C.G. Jung, C.S. Myers, J. Drever, G. Wallas, and W. McDougall, 12 July 1919. 'Proceedings of the British Psychological Society', *British Journal of Psychology*, 9:3 (May 1919), 376, and 10:1 (November 1919), 132.

[44] W.H. Auden, 'In Memory of Sigmund Freud (d. Sept. 1939)': 'to us he is no more a person/ now but a whole climate of opinion/ under whom we conduct our different lives'.

[45] Rivers, *Instinct and the Unconscious*, p. 252.

disorders. At the end of the war, Thomas Pear believed that most doctors had realized the superiority of therapies tackling the unconscious origins of "shell-shock" and argued that as a result, methods based on the research of 'Freud, Jung, and others are now being widely used even by workers who do not necessarily agree with the theoretical views held by these writers'. In his view, the lasting influence of the war would be greater appreciation of the power of instinct, emotion, and 'non-rational beliefs to influence conduct'.[46] These reflections on how the war had influenced understandings of mind and behaviour anticipated the permeation of psychoanalytic ideas throughout British medical culture during the 1920s. In this period, words and concepts derived from Freud – repression, the unconscious, dream analysis – entered the everyday vocabulary of mainstream medical culture, although psychoanalytic methods did not become part of its standard practice. Alongside the infiltration of psychoanalytic ideas, a series of propositions about human nature, such as the primacy of instinct and emotion, became embedded in models of behaviour. In the British context, these propositions owed at least some of their success to their close fit with evolutionary frameworks of understanding, but they also coalesced with Freudian approaches to mind, and in the 1920s were more often expressed in the language of psychoanalysis.

The cultural appeal of psychoanalysis in British popular culture during the 1920s is well documented.[47] Graham Richards argues that this appeal was rooted in the 'unprecedented collective trauma' of the war but cannot be reduced to an offshoot of the effects of "shell-shock". The legacy of war stretched beyond specific diagnostic constructs, and instead embraced the totality of war experience: for soldiers and civilians, for the medically "shell-shocked", and for those quietly shaken. As individuals struggled to make sense of the catastrophe of war and its aftermath, they sought forms of psychological understanding which could explain and rectify 'the now glaring limitations and failures of "reason"'. The chaotic and rapid political, social, cultural, and technological changes of the 1920s – 'the General Strike and the airship, revolution and radium, Marxism, Modern Art, motor cars, movies, Marconi and Mussolini' – heightened the urgency of this mission. Psychoanalysis provided the vocabulary and concepts with which people

---

[46] Pear, 'War and Psychology', 88. See also Myers, 'Psychology and Industry'; McDougall, 'Presidential Address'.

[47] D. Rapp, 'The Reception of Freud by the British Press: General Interest and Literary Magazines, 1920–1925', *Journal of the History of the Behavioral Sciences*, 24 (1988), 191–201; Overy, *Morbid Age*, pp. 136–74.

made sense of human nature in this period of rapid transformation, when the world could only be seen as divided into the 'pre' and 'post' war.[48]

Richards' explanation of the appeal of psychoanalysis in the post-war period loosens the expectation of ironclad causal links to "shell-shock" and avoids the tendencies occasionally evident elsewhere in the historiography towards inflexible notions of what constitutes evidence of the success of psychoanalysis. There were some important differences between popular enthusiasm for psychoanalysis and medical responses to Freudianism, not least because most doctors viewed themselves as outside the psychoanalytic craze and sought to separate legitimate psychological inquiry from the taint of quackery and charlatanism. Nevertheless, Richards' account can be applied to medical culture too. In historical interpretations of the influence of "shell-shock", much hinges on perceptions of the extent of psychodynamic incursions into psychological medicine before 1914. For Stone, pre-war movements in this direction were negligible, and so post-war engagement with psychoanalysis demonstrates the transformative effects of the "shell-shock" episode.[49] For Jones and Wessely, the development of modified psychoanalytic approaches before the war is evidence that "shell-shock" had little real effect on attitudes towards Freud.[50] Evidence of post-war hostility towards psychoanalysis is also invoked to support claims that the apparent wartime successes of psychodynamic psychology were superficial and short-lived.[51] But as shown in earlier discussions of wartime attitudes towards psychoanalysis, there is no real contradiction between increased support for a particular position and the simultaneous existence of widespread antagonism towards it. In some circumstances, clearer articulation of a position provokes more distinct critiques.

It does not always make sense to focus arguments around "for" and "against", or continuity and change. The prosaic and undeniable truth is that there was some support for psychoanalysis before the war, and some hostility towards it afterwards. The importance of both pre-war support and post-war antagonism should not be underestimated. Before 1914, doctors "translated" the key terms of Freudian theory into the native idiom. Wartime doctors furthered these specific approaches in their explorations of "shell-shock", and both during and after the war, these "translations" enabled increasing numbers of non-"analytic" doctors to

---

[48] Richards, 'Britain on the Couch', 187, 199–200, 221.
[49] Stone, 'Shellshock and the Psychologists', especially pp. 242–4, 265–6.
[50] Jones and Wessely, 'Impact of Total War', pp. 136–7.
[51] Bourke, *Dismembering the Male*, p. 121; Jones and Wessely, 'Impact of Total War', p. 137.

accept many aspects of psychoanalysis. But in turn, the gradual normalization of psychoanalysis in mainstream medical culture provoked venomous repudiations of Freudianism, and this also had far-reaching effects. After 1918, hostility towards psychoanalysis contributed to the inward turn of the British psychoanalytic movement, as manifested in new restrictions on membership of the British Psychoanalytical Society and in its adoption of an orthodox Freudianism far apart from the eclecticism of mainstream medical psychologies.[52] Neither championship of Freud before the war nor rejection of psychoanalysis in its aftermath represents the full spectrum of medical opinion. Neither trend proves that wartime events did not shape the subsequent relation of psychoanalysis to psychological medicine in Britain. In retrospect, it might look very much as though Britain was on the cusp of a psychological revolution in 1914: there was an active campaign for the early treatment of mental disorders; new psychiatric outpatient facilities and psychological clinics had been established;[53] new associational forums for the pursuit of psychological research had been founded;[54] proponents of the 'new psychology' had formulated and published important modifications of Freudian theory.[55] But this perspective all depends on that crucial formulation, 'in retrospect'. If we assume that subsequent changes would have occurred regardless of the war, we are guilty of determinism.

Of course, some of the approaches developed within pre-war psychological medicine anticipated and no doubt facilitated wartime lines of research. In July 1914, the British Psychological Society held a combined meeting with the Aristotelian Society and the Mind Association on 'the role of repression in forgetting'.[56] After the meeting, participants might

---

[52] Richards, 'Britain on the Couch', 204, 216; Raitt, 'Early British Psychoanalysis', 63, 79–81; E.R. Valentine, '"A Brilliant and Many-Sided Personality": Jessie Margaret Murray, Founder of the Medico-Psychological Clinic', *Journal of the History of the Behavioral Sciences*, 45:2 (2009), 158–9.

[53] On the campaign for early treatment and the provision of outpatient facilities see the introduction to this volume, and Raitt, 'Early British Psychoanalysis', which charts the foundation and history of the Medico-Psychological Clinic from its opening in 1913.

[54] The British Psychological Society (1904); the Section of Psychiatry of the Royal Society of Medicine (1912); a special subsection for Psychology within the Physiology Section of the British Association for the Advancement of Science (1913); the London Psycho-Analytical Society (1913).

[55] The most important publications were Stoddart, *Mind and Its Disorders* (first edition 1908, second edition 1912), and Hart, *Psychology of Insanity*.

[56] 'Proceedings of the British Psychological Society', *British Journal of Psychology*, 7:2 (September 1914), 264. In January 1915 Ernest Jones presented a paper to the Society on 'Some Points Concerning the Theory of Repression in its Relation to Memory': 'Proceedings of the British Psychological Society', *British Journal of Psychology*, 7:4 (March 1915), 492.

have relaxed by reading a few chapters of David Eder's newly published English translation of Freud's *Über den Traum*. But these were all very recent developments. Psychodynamic approaches had not established roots within British psychological medicine. We do not know what would have happened in the absence of war. But we do know that after 1918, the hum of medical interest in Freud, which had steadily escalated before the outbreak of war, built to a crescendo. Adoption of "pure" psychoanalysis remained a minority pursuit, and it was not the only form of psychology to flourish. It coexisted and often merged with other forms of psychology as 'a practical tool within regimes of self-improvement'. As in the "analytic" therapies discussed in Chapter 5, this practical psychology often assimilated and furthered traditional concepts of character and self-help.[57] Nevertheless, the diffusion of psychoanalytic vocabulary and concepts is one of the most conspicuous differences between medical discourse in 1914 and in 1918. This change in the tone, tempo, and volume of engagement with psychoanalytic approaches represents a definitive shift in British medicine's relationship to Freud. By the early 1920s, psychoanalytic modes of thought had taken firm hold within psychological medicine.

Revolution via Evolution: "Translation", Eclecticism, and the Assimilation of Psychoanalysis

If the post-war incursion of psychoanalytic ideas into mainstream psychological medicine does not always seem very novel, this is at least partly because wittingly or unwittingly, doctors often underplayed the radicalism of these approaches. I have argued that British doctors "translated" new psychological theories into the native idiom, and that this process involved the selective appropriation and combination of different elements of "psychic" and psychological therapies. This argument goes some way towards resolving different interpretations of the state of psychological knowledge and practice in Britain before 1914. Although doctors had started to branch out in "psychological" directions, engagement with psychological ideas took eclectic forms and was often presented in deliberately anti-theoretical terms, or as little more than the extension of much older methods. In this manner, radical ideas were tamed and normalized, while new psychological vocabularies and concepts entered the mainstream of British psychological medicine by stealth and gradually expanded its framework of understanding. This was a process of

[57] Thomson, *Psychological Subjects*, pp. 17–53. Quotation p. 19.

evolution, but the explosion of interest in psychodynamic approaches after the war represents such a step change in attitudes that it starts to look, even just for that moment, very much like a revolution.

Not everyone endorsed newer psychological forms. In July 1922, the psychotherapist Robert Macdonald Ladell wrote a fairly innocuous letter to the *British Medical Journal* suggesting that instruction in psychotherapy and basic psychoanalysis should form part of the medical curriculum. This sparked a chain of correspondence lasting until May 1923, and eventually numbering thirty-nine letters from twenty-two correspondents, and provoked an editorial and a statement (rapidly overturned) that the correspondence could not continue. The grounds of debate shifted quite quickly from the desirability of teaching students psychoanalysis to the truth of key psychoanalytic concepts, the potential harm it did to patients, the relation between mind and matter (and physiology and psychology), and the ideal model of a psychiatric clinic.[58]

This long and complicated correspondence demonstrates several points about the nature of opposition to psychoanalysis in the interwar period. First, even aggressive repudiations demonstrate the extent to which psychoanalysis was a live issue dominating the agendas of psychological medicine. Second, the correspondence rocked to-and-fro between defenders and critics of psychoanalysis; it perfectly illustrates how articulation of a distinct position generated detailed deconstructions of that stance. Third, there were different levels of acceptance and criticism of psychoanalysis. Correspondents approved or rejected different parts of Freud's theories. For many contemporaries, engagement with psychoanalysis was not a simple matter of "for" or "against". Qualified assimilation extended beyond this correspondence and can be seen (for example) in Hugh Crichton-Miller's criticism of the 'exceedingly elaborate closed system' of psychoanalysis, even while he relied on some of its key concepts to understand the 'repression of infantile experience' in many "functional" nervous cases.[59] Fourth, debate on psychoanalysis inevitably drew comparisons to other techniques and schools of thought, such as suggestion, Couéism, and Christian Science. Eclecticism was still

---

[58] See correspondence under the headings 'The Teaching of Psychotherapy', 'Psycho-Analysis', 'The Teaching of Psychology and Psycho-Therapy to Medical Students', 'Psychiatric Clinics', and 'Physiology and Psychology', *BMJ*, 29 July 1922–5 May 1923, and the editorial by Anon., 'Psycho-Analysis', *BMJ*, 6 January 1923. A similar debate kicked off in 1924, despite the editor's warning that 'we cannot open our columns to the discussion of Freudian doctrines generally', and closed only when he refused to print any more letters. See correspondence under the heading 'Freudian Doctrine', *BMJ*, 20 December 1924–7 February 1925.

[59] KCHMSA: KHU/C1/M10, H. Crichton-Miller, 'Psychotherapy in General Practice' (21 November 1928).

the order of the day. It is clear that many drew no hard and fast lines between different methods. Finally, while it makes sense that supporters of psychoanalysis used its insights to diagnose the causes of resistance among its critics, we also see critics of psychoanalysis employing its methods to underscore the errors of its proponents. For example, Horatio Bryan Donkin (1845–1927) recommended reading Freud's discussion of 'the psychology of errors' in order to understand 'the mental trend and dialectical method of the psycho-analyst'.[60] Such comments were intended to be humorous but reveal the extent to which psychoanalysis had infiltrated medical culture by the early 1920s.

The tendency of critics of psychoanalysis to pseudo-diagnose its supporters as suffering from unresolved complexes and perversions demonstrates one of the crooked paths by which psychoanalytic languages and concepts gradually became part of the mainstream of medical thought. In most cases, the processes of assimilation followed the same forms outlined in my earlier discussions of how pre-war psychological medicine engaged with the "psychological". Selective appropriation was common. Many saw some value in psychoanalytic therapies but objected to the theoretical edifice of psychoanalysis.[61] Quite often, the defence of psychoanalytic therapies rested on denigration of Freud's supporters, who were (wrongly) held responsible for the distortion of a system more or less unobjectionable in its original form. Xenophobia is evident in the approach of an anonymous contributor to *The Medical World* who blamed Freud's German supporters for emphasizing sex, thereby degrading psychoanalysis 'into a bestial mystery more fitted for discussion by a conclave of satyrs than by mixed gatherings of decent men and women' while reminding readers that Freud was Austrian, not German.[62] Insistence that the concepts and methods of psychoanalysis were not really novel ('they are old ideas expressed with new terms taken from chemistry, physics, physiology, and other sciences') doubtless did much to normalize psychoanalytic ideas, even if it did not further understanding.[63] A variant of this approach combined older and newer languages of psychological explanation, as in one description of stammering

---

[60] H.B. Donkin, 'Correspondence: Psycho-Analysis', *BMJ*, 16 December 1922, 1191.

[61] Read, 'Unconscious', 298; T. Beaton, 'The Psychogenic Factor in the Causation of Mental Disorder', *JMS*, 70:288 (January 1924), 64–5.

[62] Anon., 'Psycho-Analysis', *TMW*, 14 (July–December 1920).

[63] Naccarati, 'Hormones and Emotions', 1835; L.A. Weatherly, 'Correspondence', *TMW*, 14 (July–December 1920); Anon., 'Open Confession', *TMW*, 17 (January–June 1923), 456; Anon., 'Reports of Societies: Psychotherapy', 326; M.J. Nolan, 'Some Considerations on the Present-Day Knowledge of Psychiatry, and Its Application to Those Under Care in Public Institutions for the Insane', *JMS*, 70:291 (October 1924), 513.

as 'a neurosis, caused by repression and conflict within the mind, by an inhibition of the will weakening the controlling forces, generally from the influence of an "external agent"'.[64] Such formulations familiarized and rendered knowable complex psychoanalytic ideas.

However, the most important mode of transmission of psychoanalytic approaches was their incorporation into eclectic therapeutic regimes. This method of assimilation carried over from pre-war medical culture into treatments devised for "shell-shock", and continued right through the interwar period. Millais Culpin, a more theoretically adept doctor than most, explained in his post-war book on 'the psychoneuroses of war and peace' that his preference for particular therapeutic methods did not stop him using any technique that worked. His blunt assertion that the object was 'not so much to find a theoretical explanation as to seek a means of cure' fitted into the self-consciously empiricist tradition of British medicine.[65] In the 1920s and after, British doctors continued to insist that individual cases had to be assessed on their own merits: hypnosis, persuasion, and psychoanalysis were all 'valuable when they are applied in the right way and to the right type of case'.[66] Psychotherapists elevated eclecticism to the highest of therapeutic virtues. In 1935, Hugh Crichton-Miller identified seven 'sects' among the psychotherapists. His own sympathies lay with 'the eclectics', defined as 'those who try to incorporate in their technique and theory such elements as appear to be most valuable and compatible'. Crichton-Miller conjured the ghost of "shell-shock" when he described these doctors as working in the tradition of 'tolerant eclecticism' espoused by W.H.R. Rivers.[67] The evolution of psychological modes of understanding proceeded in higgledy-piggledy fashion, and as it did so, secured a quiet revolution.

The uptake of psychoanalytic ideas in the mainstream depended on large numbers of practitioners agreeing that it was possible to take a "modern" approach to diagnosis and treatment of neurosis without being 'compelled to accept the entire Freudian gospel'.[68] The psychoanalytic movement did not accept this principle and became increasingly insulated and self-enclosed over the interwar period.[69] This divergence

[64] M.H. Wigglesworth, 'Stammering', *TMW*, 17 (January–June 1923), 494.
[65] Culpin, *Psychoneuroses of War and Peace*, p. 123. See also T.S. Good, 'The Use of Analysis in Diagnosis', *JMS*, 68:282 (July 1922), 229; I. Skottowe, 'The Utility of the Psychiatric Out-Patient Clinic', *JMS*, 77:317 (April 1931), 316–17.
[66] Anon., 'Psycho-Analysis', *TMW*, 14, 26 August 1921; KCHMSA: KHU/C1/M9, S.A.K. Wilson, 'The Treatment of Functional Nervous Disease' (29 November 1922).
[67] Crichton-Miller, 'Psychotherapeutic Clinics in Fact and Fancy', 1207.
[68] T.H. Gandy, 'Correspondence', *TMW*, 14 (January–June 1921), 1261.
[69] Richards, 'Britain on the Couch', 217; Forrester, '1919: Psychology and Psychoanalysis, Cambridge and London', 50–1.

between orthodox psychoanalytic practitioners and eclectic psychotherapists has obscured the extent of medical consensus on some of the basic principles of psychoanalytic theory by the end of the 1920s. As early as 1923, Sir George Newman (1870–1948), first Chief Medical Officer to the Ministry of Health, and hardly a radical, outlined a model for teaching psychological medicine as part of the ordinary medical curriculum which included instruction in 'the concept of the Unconscious Mind', and how it could be studied via 'tricks of conduct, lapses of attention, dreams', as well as 'mental factors' such as 'mental trauma, prolonged mental stress, the repression and operation of "complexes," and subconscious states'.[70] Some of the correspondents to the *British Medical Journal* might have been distressed to hear it, but by this date most medical students were probably already familiar with these concepts.

This chapter opened with Charles Myers' statement of belief in the need to train a new breed of medical psychologist fully equipped to understand the mental tribulations of harassed modern citizens. Myers recommended forms of "analytic" thought which drew on psychoanalytic ideas and concepts and which had already filtered down to the next generation of doctors by the early 1920s. The records of the associational life of medical schools demonstrate casual familiarity with psychoanalysis in this period. The *King's College Hospital Gazette* regularly referenced psychoanalysis throughout the 1920s. Some of this commentary was sober and evangelical, as in an extended account of psychoanalysis as the only method able to convert 'a discontented and nervous invalid into a happy man or woman with the initiative and courage to grasp life's opportunities, to enjoy its pleasures and its battles, and cheerfully to endure its misfortunes'.[71] Much more of the coverage was humorous, as in this exuberant rhyme: 'There was a young lady called Psyche,/ Who was heard to ejaculate "Pcryche!"/ For when riding her Pbych/ She ran over a Ptych,/ And fell on some rails that were Pspyche'.[72]

The jokes were often terrible, but comedic takes pinpoint a moment in the history of psychoanalysis when the theory was familiar enough for the joke to make sense but still new enough to seem intrinsically funny. In another example, in 1922, the *Gazette* reported on the activities of a new student organization, the Neuropathological and Psycho-Pathological Society (NAPS). The first two papers the society heard were from

[70] Newman, *Recent Advances in Medical Education*, pp. 138–41.
[71] R.C. McWatters, 'Common Misconceptions Concerning Freud's Psycho-Analysis', *King's College Hospital Gazette*, 1 (1921–2), 43.
[72] Anon., untitled poem, *King's College Hospital Gazette*, 10 (1931), 45; J.M. 'Psycho-Analysis', *King's College Hospital Gazette*, 1 (1921–2), 58.

William Aldren Turner and David Forsyth, both "shell-shock" doctors, and it was reported that both meetings were well attended and 'thoroughly enjoyed'. A wag later wrote in to ask whether the society was called NAPS 'because it deals with dreams'.[73] Yes, another bad joke, but also proof of familiarity with psychoanalysis and a tantalising hint of how "shell-shock" made this possible. These comedians, the post-"shell-shock" generation of doctors, eventually took these ideas for granted and carried them into the new era, into their own relations with patient and with future generations of medical students.

Concluding Reflections

On the tenth anniversary of the outbreak of war, an editorial in the *British Medical Journal* reflected on its legacy. Nowadays, the war might

seldom be discussed in its more personal or intimate details, but it is still an active factor in the lives of most of us ... This is inevitable. The great war was less a war than a cataclysm, and one whose social and economic effects must be felt not merely by the present generation but by many generations to come.[74]

Most of the time, we do not know exactly how the war affected individuals or historical events. We know that there was a before and an after, and the best we can do is try to draw causal links between these two states. The war is not in itself sufficient explanation for any post-war event, but it is the necessary precondition for all the "afters". When the war broke out, British psychological medicine was in a state of flux, still wedded to the somatic paradigm, but poised on the brink of new forms of understanding. For the most part, doctors who treated "shell-shocked" men were not experts in mind, nerves, or brain. Under the immense pressures of wartime, faced with the outbreak of nervous and mental disorder on an unanticipated scale, they fell back on existing knowledges gleaned from medical education and general medical culture. They formulated theories of "shell-shock" within the dominant frameworks of pre-war psychological medicine, but the evolutionary paradigm proved able to accommodate surprisingly diverse approaches. Within its confines, doctors experimented with different psychological, physiological, and neurological explanations for "shell-shock". At the war's end, these experiments took flight. Doctors who had treated "shell-shock" went off into different niches of civilian medicine. Although "shell-shock" faded

---

[73] Anon., 'Cabbages and "King's"', *King's College Hospital Gazette*, 2 (1922–3), 104 (see also 212).

[74] Anon., 'Ten Years', *BMJ*, 2 August 1924, 202.

somewhat within medical discourse, its legacies can be read between the lines, not least in the explosion of interest in psychoanalysis in the interwar period.

If it is not always easy to make sense of the legacies of "shell-shock", this is partly because contemporaries emerged out of the shadow of war blinking, bewildered, and unsure how to find their bearings in the rubble of the old world. On 14 November 1918, the neurologist Henry Head addressed the neurological section of the Royal Society of Medicine. He invoked "shell-shock" in the attempt to convey shared disbelief that the 'long nightmare' of war had finally ended: 'As with many of its victims, who came under our care, the horror has been so oppressive that the dream still haunts our first waking hours'.[75] Identification with the "shell-shocked" soldier illustrates the prevalent sense of disorientation at the end of the war. Adrian Gregory has argued that depictions of Britain in the 1920s as 'a traumatised society, with a shattered sense of itself' should be understood as 'constructions to cover up a much more complex social reality of winners and losers, continuities and changes'.[76] Portrayals of Britain as a "shell-shocked" nation undoubtedly served such purposes, but they also testified to genuine, powerful, and widespread feelings of grief, tiredness, and uncertainty about the future which were as much a part of social reality as class antagonism, wrangling over pensions, or unemployment. These were people living self-consciously in a period of "after", not knowing what would come next. This sense of dislocation lingered for months, if not years. In the understated words of one appeal for help for veterans, 'Everyone is tired, and no one knows what will happen next, and a reaction has set in after the war'.[77] The language of "shell-shock" powerfully encapsulated the mood of the era.

To echo Charles Myers, this book is a contribution to the study of "shell-shock". It is not a definitive statement. I have tried to explain how doctors made sense of "shell-shock", to reconstruct their mental worlds, and in doing so, to understand the shifting shapes and contexts of psychological knowledge in the early twentieth century. As I draw towards the end of this project, I am surprised at how much I have left unsaid and how much I still do not know. Above all, it is difficult to know where to end. Any frame is a 'simulacrum of meaning, order and design' designed to draw the eye away from the mess beyond its edges.[78] There

---

[75] Head, 'Some Principles of Neurology', 344.   [76] Gregory, *Last Great War*, p. 257.
[77] S.K. Vesey, 'Future Care of Shell Shock Cases', *TMW*, 14 (January–June 1920), 79.
[78] M. Drabble, *The Pattern in the Carpet: A Personal History with Jigsaws* (London: Atlantic Books, 2010), p. 388.

are some forms of chaos out of which it is not possible to make order. The doctors I have written about attempted to contain the protean symptoms of soldiers within diagnostic boundaries, but "shell-shock" still twitched and jerked and refused to remain confined to the pages of medical journals. The potential histories of "shell-shock" branch out in hundreds of directions: for every sufferer, witness, or attempt to understand how this could possibly happen, there is another history to be written. These untold stories haunt this ending, awaiting their own historians.

Bibliography

ABBREVIATIONS

ANP	*Archives of Neurology and Psychiatry*
BMJ	*British Medical Journal*
EMJ	*Edinburgh Medical Journal*
JMS	*Journal of Mental Science*
KCHR	*King's College Hospital Reports*
PRSM	*Proceedings of the Royal Society of Medicine*
SBHR	*St Bartholomew's Hospital Reports*
TMW	*The Medical World*

PRIMARY SOURCES

MANUSCRIPT SOURCES

Guy's Hospital Medical School Archives (GHMSA)
G/S6. Guy's Hospital Physiological Society Papers.
G/S7. Guy's Hospital Pupil's Physical Society Papers.
G/PUB/6/1. Guy's Hospital Examination Papers 1889–1890.
G/PUB1/1/1. *Guy's Hospital Reports*, 50 (1893).
G/PUB 1/1/1/2. *Guy's Hospital Neurological Studies*, 67 (1913).

King's College Hospital and Medical School Archive (KCHMSA)
KHU/C1. Minutes of the Meetings of the King's College Hospital Medical Society.
KH/SYL1/1. *The Medical School of King's College Hospital 1910–1911.*
KH/SYL1/2. *King's College Hospital Medical School 1911–1912 Abridged Syllabus.*

St Bartholomew's Hospital Archive (SBHA)
MS 20. St Bartholomew's School Calendars.

OFFICIAL PUBLICATIONS

Report of the War Office Committee of Enquiry into "Shell-Shock" (London: Imperial War Museum, 2004) [1922].

234

Macpherson, W.G., Herringham, W.P., Elliott, T.R., and Balfour, A. (eds.), *History of the Great War Based on Official Documents. Medical Services: Diseases of the War*, 2 vols. (London: HMSO, 1923).
Mitchell, T.J., and Smith, G.M., *History of the Great War Based on Official Documents. Medical Services: Casualties and Medical Statistics of the Great War* (London: HMSO, 1931).
Newman, G., *Recent Advances in Medical Education in England: A Memorandum Addressed to the Minister of Health* (London: HMSO, 1923).

JOURNALS

'Discussion on Functional Cases', Laryngological Section, *PRSM*, 8:2 (1914–15), 117–20.
'Discussion: The Psychology of Traumatic Amblyopia Following Explosion of Shells', Neurological Section, *PRSM*, 8:2 (1914–15), 65–8.
'Special Discussion on Shell Shock without Visible Signs of Injury', Sections of Psychiatry and Neurology (Combined Meeting), *PRSM*, 9:3 (1915–16), i–xliv.
'Discussion: The Repression of War Experience', Section of Psychiatry, *PRSM*, 11:3 (1917–18), 18–20.
'Discussion: War Neuroses', Section of Laryngology, *PRSM*, 11 (Parts 1 and 2) (1917–18), 185–200.
'Discussion: Functional Gastric Disturbance in the Soldier', *JMS*, 63:260 (January 1917), 144–8.
'Discussion: Observations on the Rolandic Area in a Series of Cases of Insanity', *JMS*, 64:267 (October 1918), 363–5.
'Discussion: War Psychoses and Psychoneuroses', *JMS*, 64:265 (April 1918), 234–8.
'Discussion: The Teaching of Medicine', *EMJ*, 21 (July–December 1918), 30–42.
'Discussion: The Training of the Student of Medicine, XLII–XLVII', *EMJ*, 21 (July–December 1918), 244–8.
'Discussion on the Nervous Child', *BMJ*, 24 November 1923, 63–71.
Anon., 'The Medical Society', *KCHR*, 5 (1897–8), 237.
'Medico-Psychological Association of Great Britain and Ireland: General Meeting', *JMS*, 46:194 (July 1900), 601–2.
'A New Journal', *JMS*, 49:206 (July 1903), 523–4.
'Medical Societies: Edinburgh Medico-Chirurgical Society', *Lancet*, 1 January 1910, 27–8.
'Medical Societies: Liverpool Medical Institution', *Lancet*, 9 April 1910, 1001–2.
'Freud's Theory of Hysteria and Other Psychoneuroses', *Lancet*, 21 May 1910, 1424–5.
'Emotion as a Factor in the Development of Neuropathic and Psychopathic Symptoms', *Lancet*, 20 August 1910, 572–3.
'Modern Views of Hysteria', *Lancet*, 8 April 1911, 951–2.
'The British Medical Association Seventy-Ninth Annual Meeting in Birmingham: Section of Neurology and Psychological Medicine', *Lancet*, 12 August 1911, 450–1.

'Review: La Neurasthénie Rurale by Dr Raymond Belbèze', *Lancet*,
    30 September 1911, 351.
'Medical Societies: Nottingham Medico-Chirurgical Society', *Lancet*,
    11 November 1911, 1338.
'The Increase of Nervous Instability', *Lancet*, 2 December 1911, 1572.
'Review: The Conquest of Nerves by J.W. Courtney', *Lancet*, 27 July 1912,
    239–40.
'Sheffield Medico-Chirurgical Society: Some Recent Conceptions of Hysteria',
    Lancet, 12 April 1913, 1024–5.
'Freud's Theory of Dreams', *Lancet*, 10 May 1913, 1327.
'Medical Societies: Medical Society of London', *Lancet*, 22 and 29 November
    1913, 1469–72, 1542–4.
'The Science and Philosophy of Instinct', *Nature*, 92 (September
    1913–February 1914), 627.
'Treatment by Hypnotism and Suggestion', *EMJ*, 12 (January–June 1914), 277.
'Review: Modern Problems in Psychiatry', *EMJ*, 12 (January–June 1914),
    277–8.
'Mental and Nervous Shock among the Wounded', *BMJ*, 7 November 1914,
    802–3.
'French Wounded from Some Early Actions', *BMJ*, 14 November 1914,
    853–4.
'Dr. G.L. Finlay on German "Nerves"', *TMW*, 4 (January–June 1915), 8.
'The War and Nervous Breakdown', *Lancet*, 23 January 1915, 189–90.
'The Psychological Effect of War', *BMJ*, 13 March 1915, 475–6.
'Shell Explosions and the Special Senses', *Lancet*, 27 March 1915, 663–4.
'The Mental Treatment Bill', *BMJ*, 1 May 1915, 771–2.
'Medical Notes in Parliament: Early Treatment of Mental Disorder', *BMJ*,
    1 May 1915, 777.
'Nerve and Nerves: Address by Sir Wm. Osler, Bart.', *TMW*, 5
    (July–December 1915), 492.
'Medical Notes in Parliament: The Naval and Military War Pensions Bill',
    BMJ, 17 July 1915, 106–7.
'The Commotional Syndrome in War', *BMJ*, 31 July 1915, 185–6.
'The Neurology of War', *BMJ*, 14 August 1915, 264.
'The Pathology of Shell Concussion', *BMJ*, 14 August 1915, 264–5.
'Military Life and Physical Health', *BMJ*, 14 August 1915, 267.
'Insanity and the War', *Lancet*, 4 September 1915, 553–4.
'Reviews: Sane Psycho-Therapy', *BMJ*, 23 October 1915, 605.
'Special Hospitals for Officers: Lord Knutsford's Appeal', *Lancet*,
    20 November 1915, 1155–7.
'Lord Knutsford's Special Hospitals for Officers', *Lancet*, 27 November 1915,
    1201–2.
'Review: *The New Psychiatry* by W.H.B. Stoddart', *EMJ*, 16 (January–June
    1916), 152.
'A Discussion on Shell Shock', *Lancet*, 5 February 1916, 306.
'High Explosives and the Central Nervous System', *Nature*, 97 (March 1916),
    112–14.

'Medical Societies: Brighton and Sussex Medico-Chirurgical Society', *Lancet*, 20 May 1916, 1042.
'The War: Nervous and Mental Shock', *BMJ*, 10 June 1916, 830–2.
'The Disabled Soldier in France', *BMJ*, 7 October 1916, 499.
'The Maudsley Hospital', *BMJ*, 13 January 1917, 51.
'Scotland', *BMJ*, 24 February 1917, 277–8.
'The Management of Neurasthenia and Allied Disorders in the Army', *TMW*, 8 (January–June 1917), 642–3.
'Shell Shock, Gas Poisoning, and War Neuroses', *BMJ*, 19 May 1917, 656.
'Neurasthenia in Soldiers', *Lancet*, 23 June 1917, 962–3.
'Cure of Shell-Shock', *Times*, 14 June 1917.
'Reports of Societies: Shell Shock', *BMJ*, 21 July 1917, 81.
'The Mind of the Soldier', *BMJ*, 11 August 1917, 188–9.
'The Effect of the War Upon Psychiatry in England', *Lancet*, 1 September 1917, 352–3.
'The Air War', *BMJ*, 6 October 1917, 457–8.
'Review: G. Elliot Smith and T.H. Pear, Shell-Shock and Its Lessons', *EMJ*, 19 (July–December 1917), 272–3.
'New Editions: M. Craig, Psychological Medicine, Third Edition', *EMJ*, 19 (July–December 1917), 338–9.
'The Psychical Factor in Therapeutics', *BMJ*, 22 December 1917, 836–7.
'Army Horses: Animal Sufferers from Shell Shock', *Times*, 28 December 1917.
'Shell Shock in Cows', *Lancet*, 2 February 1918, 187–8.
'Reports of Societies: War Neuroses', *BMJ*, 23 March 1918, 345–6.
'Medical Societies: Royal Society of Medicine', *Lancet*, 23 March 1918, 437–9.
'Hysterical Disorders of Warfare', *BMJ*, 10 August 1918, 134.
'Review: Hysterical Disorders of Warfare', *Lancet*, 24 August 1918, 242.
'The Interdependence of the Sympathetic and Central Nervous Systems', *BMJ*, 26 October 1918, 471.
'Reviews: The Treatment of Hysteria', *BMJ*, 9 November 1918, 515–16.
'The Treatment of War Psycho-Neuroses', *BMJ*, 7 December 1918, 634.
'Reviews: Charles Myers, Present-Day Applications of Psychology with Special Reference to Industry, Education and Nervous Breakdown', *British Journal of Psychology*, 9:2 (October 1918), 259.
'Functional Anosmia', *BMJ*, 25 January 1919, 110.
'Notes and News: The Medico-Psychological Association of Great Britain and Ireland', *JMS*, 55:229 (April 1919), 391–3.
'Reviews: "War Shock"', *BMJ*, 5 April 1919, 413–14.
'Reviews: War Neuroses', *BMJ*, 26 April 1919, 520.
'British Medical Association Special Clinical Meeting, Section of Medicine: War Neuroses', *Lancet*, 26 April 1919, 709–11.
'Review: H. Crichton-Miller (ed.), *Functional Nerve Disease*', *British Journal of Psychology*, 10:4 (July 1920), 350–1.
'Psycho-Analysis', *TMW*, 14 (July–December 1920), 1195.
'Notes and News: The Late Dr. C.A. Mercier', *JMS*, 67:145 (January 1921), 146.
'A Psychiatrist's Review', *BMJ*, 12 March 1921, 394.

'Section of Obstetrics and Gynaecology', *BMJ*, 29 October 1921, 699–705.
'Psycho-Analysis', *TMW*, 14 (July–December 1921), 2055.
'Keep Smiling', *TMW*, 15 (July–December 1921), 341.
'Psychological Medicine', *BMJ*, 2 September 1922, 443–5.
'Ninetieth Annual Meeting of the British Medical Association: Section of Medicine: Discussion of Exophthalmic Goitre', *BMJ*, 11 November 1922, 908–14.
'Reports of Societies: Psychotherapy', *BMJ*, 24 February 1923, 327.
'Endocrines and Psychoneuroses', *BMJ*, 24 March 1923, 514.
'Open Confession', *TMW*, 17 (January–June 1923), 456–7.
'Reports of Societies: "Occupation Cure" in Neurasthenia', *BMJ*, 3 February 1923, 190–1.
'Cabbages and "King's"', *King's College Hospital Gazette*, 2 (1922–3), 103–6.
'Review: The English Review', *King's College Hospital Gazette*, 3:1 (February 1924), 366.
'Ten Years', *BMJ*, 2 August 1924, 202.
'Some Methods of Treatment Exercised by the Ancient Australian Medicine Men', *King's College Hospital Gazette*, 3 (October 1924), 508–11.
'Obituary: Sir Frederick Mott', *Lancet*, 19 June 1926, 1228–30.
'Obituary: Thomas Claye Shaw', *BMJ*, 22 January 1927, 169.
'Mental Disorder in Relation to Eugenics', *BMJ*, 26 February 1927, 386.
'Traumatic Neurasthenia and the "Litigation Neurosis"', *BMJ*, 17 December 1927, 1145.
'Psychological Medicine', *BMJ*, 6 September 1930, 389–91.
'Obituary: Lewis Ralph Yealland', *Lancet*, 13 March 1954, 577–8.
'Obituary: Joseph Francis Engeldue Prideaux', *Lancet*, 28 November 1959, 978–9.
Abrahams, A., 'A Case of Hysterical Paraplegia', *Lancet*, 24 July 1915, 178–9.
'The Medical Officer in Charge of a Division', *Journal of the RAMC*, 33:1 (July 1919), 79–94.
Adrian, E.D., and Yealland, L.R., 'The Treatment of Some Common War Neuroses', *Lancet*, 9 June 1917, 867–72.
Alcock, J.A.M., 'Review: W.A. White, Foundations of Psychiatry', Medical Section, *British Journal of Psychology*, 2:4 (1922), 339–41.
Allbutt, T.C., 'President's Address on the Universities in Medical Research and Practice', *BMJ*, 3 July 1920, 1–8.
[Armstrong-]Jones, R., 'Para-Myo-Clonus Multiples and Insanity', *SBHR*, 46 (1910), 19–30.
'An Address on Temperaments: Is There a Neurotic One?' *Lancet*, 1 July 1911, 1–6.
Armstrong-Jones, R., 'Correspondence: Psycho-Analysis', *BMJ*, 13 January 1917, 64–5.
'Dreams and Their Interpretation', *Practitioner*, 98:3 (March 1917), 201–19.
'Psychological Medicine', *Nature*, 99 (March–August 1917), 301–2.
'The Psychology of Fear and the Effects of Panic Fear in War Time', *JMS*, 63:262 (July 1917), 346–89.
'Mental States and the War – The Psychological Effects of Fear. I', *Journal of State Medicine*, 25:8 (August 1917), 238–49.

'Mental States and the War – The Psychological Effects of Fear. II', *Journal of State Medicine*, 25:10 (October 1917), 289–99.

'The Psychopathy of the Barbed Wire', *Nature*, 100 (September 1917–February 1918), 1–3.

'Mental and Nervous States in Connection with the War and Their Mechanism', *Practitioner*, 103:5 (November 1919), 321–34.

'In Memoriam, Thomas Claye Shaw', *SBHR*, 60 (1927), 1–6.

Ash, E.L., 'The Combined Psycho-Electrical Treatment of Neurasthenia and Allied Neuroses', *Practitioner*, 91:1 (July 1913), 123–31.

Bainbridge, F.A., 'Some Neuroses of Children', *SBHR*, 37 (1901), 343–53.

Balfour, B., 'Botany in Medical Education', *EMJ*, 20 (January–June 1918), 114–17.

Ballard, E.F., 'A Case of Aggravated Hysteroid Movements', *JMS*, 56:233 (April 1910), 317–20.

'The Psychoneurotic Temperament and Its Reactions to Military Service', *JMS*, 64:267 (October 1918), 365–77.

Bastian, H.C., 'On Different Kinds of Aphasia, with Special Reference to Their Classification and Ultimate Pathology', *BMJ*, 5 November 1887, 985–90.

Beaton, T., 'The Psychogenic Factor in the Causation of Mental Disorder', *JMS*, 70:288 (January 1924), 58–68.

Berry, J.A., 'A Plea for a National Laboratory for the Study of Mental Abnormality', *BMJ*, 14 January 1928, 46–7.

Bird, C., 'From Home to the Charge: A Psychological Study of the Soldier', *American Journal of Psychology*, 28:3 (July 1917), 315–48.

Birley, J.L., 'Goulstonian Lectures on the Principles of Medical Science as Applied to Military Aviation', *Lancet*, 29 May 1920, 1147–51.

Bond, C.H., 'The Position of Psychological Medicine in Medical and Allied Services', *JMS*, 67:279 (October 1921), 404–49.

Bousfield, P., 'The Relation of Blood-Pressure to the Psycho-Neuroses', *Practitioner*, 101:5 (November 1918), 266–70.

Bramwell, E., 'Recent Advances in Medical Science: Neurology', *EMJ*, 14 (January–June 1915), 477–9.

'Recent Advances in Medical Science: Neurology', *EMJ*, 15 (July–December 1915), 434–8.

'The Teaching of Neurology', *EMJ*, 21 (July–December 1918), 209–12.

Brock, A.J., '"Ergotherapy" in Neurasthenia', *EMJ*, 6 (January–June 1911), 430–4.

'Habit as a Pathological Factor', *EMJ*, 13 (July–December 1914), 129–46.

'The Re-Education of the Adult. 1: The Neurasthenic in War and Peace', *Sociological Review*, 10:1 (Summer 1918), 25–40.

Brown, W., 'Freud's Theory of Dreams', *Lancet*, 19 and 26 April 1913, 1114–18, 1182–4.

'The Treatment of Cases of Shell Shock in an Advanced Neurological Centre', *Lancet*, 17 August 1918, 197–200.

'War Neurosis: A Comparison of Early Cases Seen in the Field with Those Seen at the Base', *Lancet*, 17 May 1919, 833–6.

'Hypnosis, Suggestion, and Dissociation', *BMJ*, 14 June 1919, 734–6.

'Suggestion and Personality', *British Journal of Medical Psychology*, 5:1 (1925), 29–34.

'Theories of Suggestion', *BMJ*, 18 February 1928, 573–82.

Brown, W.L., 'The Croonian Lectures on the Role of the Sympathetic Nervous System in Disease. I', *Lancet*, 17 May 1919, 826–33.

'The Croonian Lectures on the Role of the Sympathetic Nervous System in Disease. IV', *Lancet*, 7 June 1919, 965–70.

'A Presidential Address on Hunter, Gaskell, and the Evolution of the Nervous System', *Lancet*, 20 March 1920, 641–8.

'A British Medical Association Lecture on Minor Endocrine Disturbances and Their Metabolic and Psychical Effects', *BMJ*, 8 December 1923, 1073–7.

Burton-Fanning, F.W., 'Neurasthenia in Soldiers of the Home Forces', *Lancet*, 16 June 1917, 907–11.

Bury, J.S., 'Remarks on the Pathology of the War Neuroses', *Lancet*, 27 July 1918, 97–9.

'The Physical Element in the Psycho-Neuroses', *Lancet*, 10 July 1920, 66–8.

Buzzard, E.F., 'Warfare on the Brain', *Lancet*, 30 December 1916, 1095–9.

'Psycho-Therapeutics', *Lancet*, 17 February 1923, 330–2.

Calwell, W., 'An Address on Elementary Psychology in General Hospital Teaching', *BMJ*, 21 May 1921, 736–8.

Campbell, H., 'The Feelings', *JMS*, 46:193 (April 1900), 219–42.

'War Neuroses', *Practitioner*, 96:5 (May 1916), 501–9.

'The Biological Aspects of Warfare', *Lancet*, 15 September 1917, 433–5.

Carmalt-Jones, D.W., 'War-Neurasthenia, Acute and Chronic', *Brain*, 42:3 (October 1919), 171–213.

Carver, A., 'Some Observations Bearing Upon the Commotional Factor in the Aetiology of Shell Shock', *Lancet*, 2 August 1919, 193–6.

'The Generation and Control of Emotion', *British Journal of Psychology*, 10:1 (November 1919), 51–65.

'Forgetting: Psychological Repression', *BMJ*, 10 January 1920, 46–7.

'The Search for a Kingdom', Medical Section, *British Journal of Psychology*, 2:4 (1922), 273–91.

'Primary Identification and Mysticism', *British Journal of Medical Psychology*, 4:2 (1924), 102–14.

'The Psychology of the Alcoholist', *British Journal of Medical Psychology*, 11:2 (1931), 117–24.

Carver, A., and Dinsley, A., 'Some Biological Effects due to High Explosives', Section of Neurology, *PRSM*, 12 (Parts 1 and 2) (1918–19), 36–51.

Chambers, W.D., 'Mental Wards with the British Expeditionary Force: A Review of Ten Months' Experience', *JMS*, 65:270 (July 1919), 152–80.

Clarke, E., 'Neurasthenia and Eyestrain', *Practitioner*, 86:1 (January 1911), 24–8.

Clarke, J.M., 'Some Neuroses of the War', *Bristol Medico-Chirurgical Journal*, 34:130 (July 1916), 49–72.

Clarkson, R.D., 'The Teaching of Psychology to Medical Undergraduates', *EMJ*, 21 (July–December 1918), 240–4.

Clouston, T.S., 'The Possibility of Providing Suitable Means of Treatment for
    Incipient and Transient Mental Diseases in Our Great General Hospitals',
    JMS, 48:203 (October 1902), 697–709.
'The Position of Psychiatry and the Role of General Hospitals in Its
    Improvement', *JMS*, 61:252 (January 1915), 1–17.
Cobb, I.G., 'Neurasthenia – Its Causes and Treatment', *Practitioner*, 95
    (July–December 1915), 224–44.
Collie, J., 'Neurasthenia: What It Costs the State', *Journal of the RAMC*, 26:4
    (April 1916), 525–44.
'The Management of Neurasthenia and Allied Disorders Contracted in the
    Army', *Journal of State Medicine*, 26:1 (January 1918), 2–17.
Cooper, P.R., 'Correspondence: Treatment of "Shell Shock"', *BMJ*, 12 August
    1916, 242.
Core, D.E., 'Some Mechanisms at Work in the Evolution of Hysteria', *Lancet*,
    9 March 1918, 365–70.
'Correspondence: Hypnosis in Hysteria', *Lancet*, 5 October 1918, 471.
'Some Clinical Aspects of Certain Emotions', *British Journal of Medical
    Psychology*, 5:4 (1925), 310–28.
Crawfurd, R., 'Graves' Disease: An Emotional Disorder', *KCHR*, 3 (1895–96),
    44–56.
Crichton-Browne, J., 'The First Maudsley Lecture', *JMS*, 66:274 (July 1920),
    199–225.
Crichton-Miller, H., 'Rest-Cures in Theory and Practice', *Practitioner*, 89
    (July–December 1912), 834–45.
'The Psychic and Endocrine Factors of Functional Disorders, *BMJ*,
    23 September 1922, 551–4.
'Psychotherapeutic Clinics in Fact and Fancy', *BMJ*, 15 June 1935, 1205–8.
Culpin, M., 'Practical Hints on Functional Disorders', *BMJ*, 21 October 1916,
    548–9.
'The Early Stage of Hysteria', *BMJ*, 13 April 1918, 225–6.
'Correspondence: The Discussion on War Neuroses', *BMJ*, 19 April 1919,
    501.
'Dreams and Their Value in Treatment', *Practitioner*, 102:3 (March 1919),
    156–62.
'Some Cases of "Traumatic Neurasthenia"', *Lancet*, 1 August 1931, 233–7.
Davy, H., 'An Address on Some War Diseases', *BMJ*, 27 December 1919,
    837–40.
Dawson of Penn, Horder, T., Mitchell, T.W., Brown, W., and Crichton-Miller, H.,
    'Correspondence: British Institute of Philosophical Studies', *BMJ*, 9 April
    1927, 699.
Devine, H., 'Reviews: Psycho-Analysis', *BMJ*, 29 March 1924, 578–9.
Dickinson, D.E., 'The Training of Medical Students for General Practice:
    Recollections and Reflections', *EMJ*, 21 (July–December 1918), 361–5.
Dillon, F., 'The Analysis of a Composite Neurosis', *Lancet*, 11 January 1919, 57–60.
'The Methods of Psychotherapy', *JMS*, 71:292 (January 1925), 48–59.
'Neuroses among Combatant Troops in the Great War', *BMJ*, 8 July 1939, 63–6.
Donkin, H.B., 'Correspondence: Psycho-Analysis', *BMJ*, 16 December 1922, 1191.

Drummond, D., 'Correspondence: War Psycho-Neurosis', *Lancet*, 2 March 1918, 349.

Eager, R., 'An Investigation as to the Therapeutic Value of Thyroid Feeding in Mental Diseases', *JMS*, 58:242 (July 1912), 424–47.

'War Psychoses Occurring in Cases with a Definite History of Shell Shock', *BMJ*, 13 April 1918, 422–5.

'A Record of Admissions to the Mental Section of the Lord Derby War Hospital, Warrington, from June 17th, 1916, to June 16th, 1917', *JMS*, 64:266 (July 1918), 272–96.

'The Early Treatment of Mental Disorders', *Lancet*, 27 September 1919, 558–63.

'Head Injuries in Relation to the Psychoses and Psycho-Neuroses', *JMS*, 66:273 (April 1920), 111–31.

Eder, M.D., 'An Address on the Psycho-Pathology of the War Neuroses', *Lancet*, 12 August 1916, 264–8.

Elliott, T.R., 'Transient Paraplegia from Shell Explosions', *BMJ*, 12 December 1914, 1005–6.

Evans, J.J., 'Organic Lesions from Shell Concussion', *BMJ*, 11 December 1915, 848.

Ewart, J.C., 'The Connection of Zoology with Medicine', *EMJ*, 20 (January–June 1918), 117–21.

Farquharson, A., 'The Oxford Conference on the Correlation of the Social Sciences', *Sociological Review*, 15:1 (January 1923), 48–52.

Fearnsides, E.G., 'Essentials of Treatment of Soldiers and Discharged Soldiers Suffering from Functional Nervous Disorders', Neurological Section, *PRSM* 11 (1917–18), 42–8.

Feiling, A., 'Loss of Personality from "Shell Shock"', *Lancet*, 10 July 1915, 63–6.

Fenwick, P.C.C., 'Entero-Spasm Following Shell Shock', *Practitioner*, 98:4 (April 1917), 391.

Ferrier, D., 'Neurasthenia and Drugs', *Practitioner*, 86:1 (January 1911), 11–15.

Fitzgerald, G.H., 'Some Aspects of the War Neurosis', Medical Section, *British Journal of Psychology*, 2:2 (January 1922), 109–20.

Fleming, R.A., 'Neurasthenia and Gastralgia', *Practitioner*, 86:1 (January 1911), 29–37.

Forster, F.C., 'The Management of Neurasthenia, Psychasthenia, Shell-Shock, and Allied Conditions', *Practitioner*, 100:1 (January 1918), 85–90.

Forsyth, D., 'Functional Nerve Disease and the Shock of Battle: A Study of the So-Called Traumatic Neuroses Arising in Connexion with the War', *Lancet*, 25 December 1915, 1399–403.

Fothergill, C.F., 'The Treatment of Neurasthenia', *Practitioner*, 92 (January–June 1914), 723–5.

Fowler, J.S., 'Recent Literature: Critical Summaries and Abstracts. Medicine: Modern Theories of Hysteria – Babinski, Janet, and Freud', *EMJ*, 6 (January–June 1911), 443–8.

France, J.I., 'Nervous and Mental Symptoms of Heart Disease', *TMW*, 4 (January–June 1915), 355–7.

Fraser, J.S., 'War Injuries of the Ear: A Résumé of Recent Literature', *EMJ*, 18 (January–June 1917), 107–19.

'The "Nasal" Neuroses, Regarded as Sensitisations of the Respiratory Tract: A Résumé of Recent Literature', *EMJ*, 19 (July–December 1917), 91–107.

Gandy, T.H., 'Correspondence', *TMW*, 14 (January–June 1921), 1261.

Gardner, H.W., 'A Case of Periodic Paralysis', *Brain*, 35:3 (February 1913), 243–53.

Garton, W., 'Shell Shock and Its Treatment by Cerebro-Spinal Galvanism', *BMJ*, 28 October 1916, 584–6.

Glynn, T.R., 'Abstract of the Bradshaw Lecture on Hysteria in Some of Its Aspects', *Lancet*, 8 November 1913, 1303.

Golla, F., 'The Organic Basis of the Hysterical Syndrome', Section of Psychiatry, *PRSM*, 16 (1923), 1–11.

Good, T.S., 'The Use of Analysis in Diagnosis', *JMS*, 68:282 (July 1922), 229–36.

Goodwin, J., 'An Address on the Army Medical Service as a Career', *Lancet*, 11 October 1919, 631–3.

Gordon, H.L., 'Eye-Colour and the Abnormal Palate in Neuroses and Psychoses', *Lancet*, 5 July 1919, 9–10.

Gordon, R.G., 'War Neuroses', *Practitioner*, 103:5 (November 1919), 358–65.

Grant, J.W.G., 'The Traumatic Neuroses – Some Points in Their Aetiology, Diagnosis, and Medico-Legal Aspects', *Practitioner*, 93 (1914), 26–43.

Green, E., 'Blood Pressure and Surface Temperature in 110 Cases of Shell Shock', *Lancet*, 22 September 1917, 456–7.

Grimbly, A.F., 'The Cure of Spinal Concussion in Warfare by Suggestion', *Practitioner*, 100:3 (March 1918), 292.

'Neuroses and Psycho-Neuroses of the Sea', *Practitioner*, 102:5 (May 1919), 243–58.

'A Problem in Diagnosis', *JMS*, 71:293 (April 1925), 278–83.

Gulland, G.L., 'The Teaching of Medicine', *EMJ*, 21 (July–December 1918), 19–23.

Hale-White, W., 'An Address on Some Applications of Experience Gained by the War to the Problems of Civil Medical Practice', *BMJ*, 23 August 1919, 227–30.

Hall, A.J., 'How Far Is Trauma a Possible Factor in the Production of Disease', *Practitioner*, 88:6 (June 1912), 831–44.

Harris, W., 'The Value of Sleep', *Practitioner*, 122:1 (January 1929), 19–20.

Hart, B., 'The Psychology of Freud and His School', *JMS*, 56:234 (July 1910), 431–52.

'Freud's Conception of Hysteria', *Brain*, 33:3 (January 1911), 339–66.

'Psychology and the Medical Curriculum', *EMJ*, 21 (July–December 1918), 213–24.

'Review: T.W. Mitchell, Problems in Psychopathology', *British Journal of Medical Psychology*, 8:2 (1928), 161–2.

Harwood, T.E., 'A Preliminary Note on the Nature and Treatment of Concussion', *BMJ*, 15 April 1916, 551.

'Three Cases Illustrating the Functional Consequences of Head-Injuries', *Lancet*, 2 September 1916, 431.

Head, H., 'Some Principles of Neurology', *Brain*, 41:3–4 (November 1918), 344–54.
'Observations on the Elements of the Psycho-Neuroses', *BMJ*, 20 March 1920, 389–92.

Head, H., and Fearnsides, E.G., 'The Clinical Effects of Syphilis of the Nervous System in the Light of the Wassermann Reaction and Treatment with Neosalvarsan', *Brain*, 37:1 (September 1914), 1–140.

Henderson, D.K., 'War Psychoses: An Analysis of 202 Cases of Mental Disorder Occurring in Home Troops', *JMS*, 64:265 (April 1918), 165–89.

Herringham, W.P., 'Cases of Mental Disturbance after Operations', *SBHR*, 21 (1885), 165–7.

Hertz [Hurst], A., 'Paresis and Involuntary Movements Following Concussion Caused by a High Explosive Shell', Neurological Section, *PRSM*, 8:2 (1914–15), 83–4.

Hewat, A.F., 'Clinical Cases from Medical Division, Royal Victoria Hospital, Netley', *EMJ*, 18 (January–June 1917), 210–15.

Hill, L., 'Correspondence: Death from High Explosives without Wounds', *BMJ*, 19 May 1917, 665.

Holmes, G., 'The Sexual Element in the Neurasthenia of Men', *Practitioner*, 86:1 (January 1911), 50–60.

Holmes, G., and Lister, W.T., 'Disturbances of Vision from Cerebral Lesions, with Special Reference to the Cortical Representation of the Macula', *Brain*, 39:1–2 (June 1916), 34–73.

Hotchkis, R.D., 'Renfrew District Asylum as a War Hospital for Mental Invalids: Some Contrasts in Administration. With an Analysis of Cases Admitted during the First Year', *JMS*, 63:261 (April 1917), 238–49.

Hunter, P.D., 'Neurasthenia and Emotion', *Practitioner* 103:5 (November 1919), 343–57.

Hurst, A.F., 'Observations on the Etiology and Treatment of War Neuroses', *BMJ*, 29 September 1917, 409–14.
'Cinematograph Demonstration of War Neuroses', Section of Neurology, *PRSM*, 11:2 (1917–18), 39–42.
'The Bent Back of Soldiers', *BMJ*, 7 December 1918, 621–3.
'Nerves and the Men (the Mental Factor in the Disabled Soldier)', *Reveille*, 2 (November 1918), 260–8.
'Hysteria in the Light of the Experience of War', *ANP*, 2:5 (November 1919), 562–72.
'The War Neuroses and the Neuroses of Civil Life', *Guy's Hospital Reports*, 70 (1922), 125–55.

Hurst, A.F., and Peters, E.A., 'A Report on the Pathology, Diagnosis, and Treatment of Absolute Hysterical Deafness in Soldiers', *Lancet*, 6 October 1917, 517–19.

Hurst, A.F., and Symns, J.L.M., 'The Rapid Cure of Hysterical Symptoms in Soldiers', *Lancet*, 3 August 1918, 139–41.

Jacob, E., 'Remarks on Functional Aphemia', *BMJ*, 13 September 1890, 622–3.

James, A., 'Trauma as a Factor in Disease. II', *EMJ*, 8 (January–June 1912), 312–23.

James, W., 'What Is an Emotion?', *Mind*, 9 (1884), 188–205.

Jeffrey, G.R., 'Some Points of Interest in Connection with the Psychoneuroses of War', *JMS*, 66:273 (April 1920), 131–42.

J.M., 'Psycho-Analysis', *King's College Hospital Gazette*, 1 (1921–2), 58.

Johnson, W., 'Hysterical Tremor', *BMJ*, 7 December 1918, 627–8.
'Symptoms of Hyperthyroidism Observed in Exhausted Soldiers', *BMJ*, 22 March 1919, 335–7.

Jones, E., 'War and Individual Psychology', *Sociological Review*, 8:3 (July 1915), 167–80.
'Correspondence: Functional Nervous Disease', *Lancet*, 11 March 1916, 588–9.
'War Shock and Freud's Theory of the Neuroses', Section of Psychiatry, *PRSM*, 11:3 (April 1918), 21–36.
'Why Is the "Unconscious" Unconscious? II', *British Journal of Psychology*, 9:2 (October 1918), 247–56.
'The Psychopathology of Anxiety', *British Journal of Medical Psychology*, 9:1 (1929), 17–25.

Keay, J., 'The Presidential Address on the War and the Burden of Insanity', *JMS*, 64:267 (October 1918), 323–44.

Knowles, T.E., 'An Address on Some of the Causes of Our C3 Population', *BMJ*, 17 December 1921, 1020–3.

Ladell, R.M., 'Correspondence: A French View of Freudism', *BMJ*, 3 October 1925, 769.

Leslie, R.M., 'Medical Report for the Year 1901', *KCHR*, 8 (1901), 81–187.

Littlejohn, H., and Pirie, J.H.H., 'Medical Jurisprudence: Mental Disturbances Following Traumatism', *EMJ*, 7 (July–December 1911), 88–9.

Lord, J.R., 'The Evolution of the "Nerve" Hospital as a Factor in the Progress of Psychiatry', *JMS*, 75:309 (April 1929), 307–15.
'Psychology the Science of Mind', *JMS*, 73:314 (July 1930), 543–5.
'Review: Psychopathology; A Survey of Modern Approaches', *JMS*, 77:316 (January 1931), 207–8.

Loveday, T., 'The Role of Repression in Forgetting (IV)', *British Journal of Psychology*, 7:2 (September 1914), 161–5.

M.E.R., 'Dr. Trotter on the Herd Instinct', *Sociological Review*, 9:1 (Autumn 1916), 60.

M.N., 'Dr. Weatherly's Offensive', *TMW*, 11 (July–December 1918), 202.

McDougall, W., 'Presidential Address: The Present Position in Clinical Psychiatry', *JMS*, 65:270 (July 1919), 141–52.
'Instinct and the Unconscious. VI', *British Journal of Psychology*, 10:1 (November 1919), 35–42.

McDowall, C., 'Functional Gastric Disturbance in the Soldier', *JMS*, 63:260 (January 1917), 76–88.
'Mutism in the Soldier and Its Treatment', *JMS*, 64:264 (January 1918), 54–64.
'The Genesis of Delusions: Clinical Notes', *JMS*, 65:270 (July 1919), 187–94.

McWatters, R.C., 'Common Misconceptions Concerning Freud's Psycho-Analysis', *King's College Hospital Gazette*, 1 (1921–2), 39–43.

246   Bibliography

Mackenzie, J., 'The Aim of Medical Education', *EMJ*, 20 (January–June 1918), 31–48.
Macnaughton-Jones, H., 'The Sexual Element in the Neurasthenia of Women', *Practitioner*, 86:1 (January 1911), 61–75.
  'The Relation of Puberty and the Menopause to Neurasthenia', *Lancet*, 29 March 1913, 879–81.
Marett, R.R., 'The Primitive Medicine-Man', Section of the History of Medicine, *PRSM*, 11 (Parts 1 and 2) (1917–18), 48–9.
Matthew, E., 'The Teaching of Medicine', *EMJ*, 21 (July–December 1918), 24–30.
Mercier, C.A., 'Correspondence: Psycho-Analysis', *BMJ*, 13 January 1917, 65.
Middlemass, J., 'Recent Advances in Medical Science: Mental Diseases', *EMJ*, 21 (July–December 1918), 118–22.
Middlemiss, J.E., 'Notes on a Case of Hysteria', *JMS*, 56:234 (July 1910), 502–6.
  'Correspondence: The Treatment of War Psycho-Neuroses', *BMJ*, 21 December 1918, 700.
Miles, A., and Fowler, J.S., 'Editorial Notes: Annus 1915', *EMJ*, 16 (January–June 1916), 1–4.
Milligan, E.T.C., 'A Method of Treatment of "Shell Shock"', *BMJ*, 15 July 1916, 73–4.
Milligan, W., 'A Note on Treatment of "Functional Aphonia" in Soldiers from the Front', Laryngological Section, *PRSM*, 9:2 (1915–16), 83–5.
  'Correspondence: Treatment of "Shell Shock"', *BMJ*, 12 August 1916, 242–3.
Milligan, W., and Westmacott, F.H., 'Warfare Injuries and Neuroses: Introductory Paper', Laryngological Section, *PRSM*, 8:2 (1914–15), 109–14.
Moore, C.B., 'Some Psychological Aspects of War', *Pedagogical Seminary*, 23:3 (September 1916), 367–86.
Mott, F.W., 'Preface', *Archives of Neurology*, 3 (1907), iii–vii.
  'On Alcohol and Insanity', *BMJ*, 28 September 1907, 797–803.
  'Heredity and Insanity', *Eugenics Review*, 2:4 (January 1911), 257–81.
  'Neurasthenia and Some Associated Conditions', *Practitioner*, 86:1 (January 1911), 1–10.
  'Sanity and Insanity', *Journal of the Royal Sanitary Institute*, 33 (1912–13), 228–51.
  'A Study of the Neuropathic Inheritance', *American Journal of Insanity*, 69 (1912–13), 907–38.
  'Is Insanity on the Increase?' *Sociological Review*, 6:1 (January 1913), 1–29.
  'The Application of Physiology and Pathology to the Study of the Mind in Health and Disease', *Section of Psychiatry*, PRSM, 8:3 (1914–15), 1–16.
  'The Study of Character by the Dramatists and Novelists', *JMS*, 61:254 (July 1915), 339–44.
  'The Psychic Mechanism of the Voice in Relation to the Emotions', *BMJ*, 11 December 1915, 845–7.
  'Opening Paper and Concluding Response: Special Discussion on Shell Shock without Visible Signs of Injury', Sections of Psychiatry and Neurology, *PRSM*, 9:3 (1915–16), i–xxiv, xli–xliv.

'The Lettsomian Lectures on the Effects of High Explosives Upon the Central Nervous System. I', *Lancet*, 12 February 1916, 331–8.

'The Lettsomian Lectures on the Effects of High Explosives Upon the Central Nervous System. II', *Lancet*, 26 February 1916, 441–9.

'The Lettsomian Lectures on the Effects of High Explosives Upon the Central Nervous System. III', *Lancet*, 11 March 1916, 545–53.

'Punctiform Haemorrhages of the Brain in Gas Poisoning', *BMJ*, 19 May 1917, 637–41.

'The Chadwick Lecture on Mental Hygiene and Shell Shock during and after the War', *BMJ*, 14 July 1917, 39–42.

'The Microscopic Examination of the Brains of Two Men Dead of Commotio Cerebri (Shell Shock) without Visible Injury', *Journal of the RAMC*, 29:6 (December 1917), 662–78.

'Two Addresses on War Psycho-Neurosis. (I) Neurasthenia: The Disorders and Disabilities of Fear', *Lancet*, 26 January 1918, 127–9.

'Two Addresses on War Psycho-Neurosis. (II): The Psychology of Soldiers' Dreams', *Lancet*, 2 February 1918, 169–72.

'War Psychoses and Psychoneuroses', *JMS*, 64:265 (April 1918), 230–4.

'The Neurological Aspects of Shock', *Lancet*, 12 March 1921, 519–22.

'The Psychopathology of Puberty and Adolescence', *JMS*, 67:278 (July 1921), 279–381.

'The Second Maudsley Lecture', *JMS*, 67:278 (July 1921), 319–39.

'Body and Mind: The Origin of Dualism', *Lancet*, 7 January 1922, 1–5.

'The Neuroses and Psychoses in Relation to Conscription and Eugenics', *Eugenics Review*, 14:1 (April 1922), 13–22.

'Mental Hygiene in Relation to Insanity and Its Treatment', *Lancet*, 14 October 1922, 793–5.

'A British Medical Association Lecture on Psychology and Medicine', *BMJ*, 10 March 1923, 403–8.

'Heredity in Relation to Mental Disease and Mental Deficiency', *BMJ*, 19 June 1926, 1023–6.

Muirhead, I.B., '"Shock" Psychology', *TMW*, 9 (July–December 1917), 309–10.

'The Mental Factor', *TMW*, 11 (July–December 1918), 170–2.

Myers, B., 'The Nervous Child as Seen in Medical Practice', *BMJ*, 25 July 1925, 158–62.

Myers, C.S., 'A Contribution to the Study of Shell Shock: Being an Account of Three Cases of Loss of Memory, Vision, Smell, and Taste, Admitted into the Duchess of Westminster's War Hospital, Le Touquet', *Lancet*, 13 February 1915, 316–20.

'Contributions to the Study of Shell Shock (II): Being an Account of Certain Cases Treated by Hypnosis', *Lancet*, 8 January 1916, 65–9.

'Contributions to the Study of Shell Shock (III): Being an Account of Certain Disorders of Cutaneous Sensibility', *Lancet*, 18 March 1916, 608–13.

'Contributions to the Study of Shell Shock (IV): Being an Account of Certain Disorders of Speech, with Special Reference to Their Causation and Their Relation to Malingering', *Lancet*, 9 September 1916, 461–7.

'Correspondence: The Justifiability of Therapeutic Lying', *Lancet*, 27 December 1919, 1213–14.

'A Final Contribution to the Study of Shell Shock: Being a Consideration of Unsettled Points Needing Investigation', *Lancet*, 11 January 1919, 51–4.

'Treatment of a Case of Narcolepsy', *Lancet*, 28 February 1920, 491–3.

'Psychology and Industry', *British Journal of Psychology*, 10:2 (March 1920), 177–82.

Naccarati, S., 'Hormones and Emotions', *TMW*, 14 (January–June 1921), 1831–6.

Nicoll, M., 'The Conception of Regression in Psychological Medicine', *Lancet*, 8 June 1918, 797–8.

Nolan, M., 'Some Considerations on the Present-Day Knowledge of Psychiatry, and Its Application to Those under Care in Public Institutions for the Insane', *JMS*, 70:291 (October 1924), 507–19.

Nunn, T.B., 'Psychology and Education', *British Journal of Psychology*, 10:2 (March 1920), 169–76.

Oldfield, C., 'Some Pelvic Disorders in Relation to Neurasthenia', *Practitioner*, 91:3 (September 1913), 335–43.

Ormerod, J.A., 'Two Theories of Hysteria', *Brain*, 33:3 (January 1911), 269–87.

'The Lumleian Lectures on Some Modern Theories Concerning Hysteria. I', *Lancet*, 25 April 1914, 1163–9.

'The Lumleian Lectures on Some Modern Theories Concerning Hysteria. II', *Lancet*, 2 May 1914, 1233–9.

Ormond, A.W., 'The Treatment of "Concussion Blindness"', *Journal of the RAMC*, 26:1 (January 1916), 43–9.

Orr, D., and Rows, R.G., 'The Interdependence of the Sympathetic and Central Nervous Systems', *Brain*, 41:1 (June 1918), 1–22.

Osler, W., 'An Address on Science and War', *Lancet*, 9 October 1915, 795–801.

Paget, J., 'Clinical Lectures on the Nervous Mimicry of Organic Diseases. Lecture I', *Lancet*, 11 October 1873, 511–13.

Palmer, F.S., 'Traumatic Neuroses and Psychoses', *Practitioner*, 86 (1911), 808–20.

Parsons, J.H., 'The Psychology of Traumatic Amblyopia Following Explosion of Shells', Neurological Section, *PRSM*, 8:2 (1914–15), 55–65.

Pear, T.H., 'The War and Psychology', *Nature*, 102:2253 (3 October 1918), 88–9.

Pearn, O.P.N., 'Psychoses in the Expeditionary Forces', *JMS*, 65:269 (April 1919), 101–8.

Pegler, L.H., 'Case of (?) Nervous or Functional Aphonia', Laryngological Section, *PRSM*, 9:2 (1915–16), 118–20.

Pemberton, H.S., 'The Psychology of Traumatic Amblyopia Following the Explosion of Shells', *Lancet*, 8 May 1915, 967.

Phillips, J.G.P., 'The Early Treatment of Mental Disorder: A Critical Survey of Out-Patient Clinics', *JMS*, 69:287 (October 1923), 471–82.

Potter, C., 'Case of Gunshot Wound of the Neck with Laryngeal Symptoms for Diagnosis and Opinions as to Treatment', Laryngological Section, *PRSM*, 8:2 (1914–15), 116.

'Case of Aphonia in a Soldier', Laryngological Section, *PRSM*, 9:2 (1915–16), 90–2.

Prideaux, E., 'Stammering in the War Psycho-Neuroses', *Lancet*, 8 February 1919, 217–18.

'Suggestion and Suggestibility', *British Journal of Psychology*, 10:2 (March 1920), 228–41.

Raw, N., 'Fear and Worry', *JMS*, 75:311 (October 1929), 573–83.

Read, C., 'The Unconscious', *British Journal of Psychology*, 9:3 (May 1919), 281–98.

Read, C.S., 'A Survey of War Neuro-Psychiatry', *Mental Hygiene*, 2:3 (July 1918), 359–87.

Reynell, W.R., 'Hysterical Vomiting in Soldiers', *Lancet*, 4 January 1919, 18–20.

Rippon, T.S., 'The Wear and Tear of Flying', *TMW*, 12 (July–December 1919), 326–7.

Ritchie, J., 'Neurasthenia', *EMJ*, 12 (January–June 1914), 113–20.

Rivers, W.H.R., 'The Fitzpatrick Lectures on Medicine, Magic, and Religion. II', *Lancet*, 15 January 1916, 117–23.

'Sociology and Psychology', *Sociological Review*, 9:1 (Autumn 1916), 1–13.

'Freud's Psychology of the Unconscious', *Lancet*, 16 June 1917, 912–14.

'A Case of Claustrophobia', *Lancet*, 18 August 1917, 237–40.

'An Address on the Repression of War Experience', *Lancet*, 2 February 1918, 173–7.

'War-Neurosis and Military Training', *Mental Hygiene*, 2:4 (October 1918), 513–33.

'Why Is the "Unconscious" Unconscious? II', *British Journal of Psychology*, 9:2 (October 1918), 236–46.

'Psychology and Medicine', *British Journal of Psychology*, 10:2 (March 1920), 183–93.

Riviere, C., 'Neurasthenia in Children', *Practitioner*, 86:1 (January 1911), 38–49.

Rixon, C.H.L., 'The Hysterical Perpetuation of Symptoms', *Lancet*, 15 March 1919, 417–19.

Robertson, G.M., 'The Employment of Female Nurses in the Male Wards of Mental Hospitals in Scotland', *EMJ*, 16 (January–June 1916), 193–203.

'The Teaching of Mental Diseases in Edinburgh', *EMJ*, 21 (July–December 1918), 225–31.

Robinson, Prof., 'The Place of Anatomy in the Medical Curriculum', *EMJ*, 20 (January–June 1919), 185–7.

Rolleston, H.D., 'Treatment by Hypnotic Suggestion', *SBHR*, 25 (1889), 115–26.

'In Memoriam Joseph Arderne Ormerod', *SBHR*, 59 (1926), 1–8.

Ross, T.A., 'The Nature and Treatment of Neurasthenia', *EMJ*, 12 (January–June 1914), 296–315.

'The Prevention of Relapse of Hysterical Manifestations', *Lancet*, 19 October 1918, 516–17.

'Certain Inter-Relations between Peace and War Neuroses', Section of Neurology, *PRSM*, 12 (Parts 1 and 2) (1918–19), 13–20.

'Some Difficulties in Analytical Theory and Practice', *British Journal of Medical Psychology*, 10:1 (1930), 1–19.

Rows, R.G., 'The Development of Psychiatric Science as a Branch of Public Health', *JMS*, 58:240 (January 1912), 25–39.

'Mental Conditions Following Strain and Nerve Shock', *BMJ*, 25 March 1916, 441–3.

Russell, J.S.R., 'The Treatment of Neurasthenia', *Lancet*, 22 November 1913, 1453–6.

Savage, G.H., 'Suicide as a Symptom of Mental and Nervous Disorder', *Guy's Hospital Reports*, 35 (1894), 7–41.
'An Address on Mental Disorders', *Lancet*, 26 October 1912, 1134–7.
'Mental Disabilities for War Service', *JMS*, 62:259 (October 1916), 653–79.
'Mental War Cripples', *Practitioner*, 100:1 (January 1918), 1–7.

Schäfer, E., 'Presidential Address on the Nature, Origin, and Maintenance of Life,' *Lancet*, 7 September 1912, 675–85.

Scott, G.L., 'Ten Consecutive Cases Treated by Hypnotism', *Guy's Hospital Neurological Studies*, 67 (1913), 114–19.
'Hysterical "Paralysis" of Long Standing', *Practitioner*, 101:2 (August 1918), 97–9.
'The Anxiety State – An Aspect of Treatment', *Practitioner*, 102:4 (April 1919), 222–4.
'An Improved Method for Withdrawing Drugs of Addiction without Discomfort to the Patient', *Practitioner*, 118:1 (January 1927), 55–8.

Scripture, E.W., 'The Nature of Stuttering', *Practitioner*, 112:5 (May 1924), 318–26.

Shaw, T.C., 'On Degradation of Type in the Insane', *SBHR*, 20 (1884), 169–80.
'On the Forecast of Destructive Impulses in the Insane', *SBHR*, 21 (1885), 1–21.
'Suicide and Sanity', *Lancet*, 20 April 1907, 1067–9.
'A Contribution to the Analysis of the Mental Process in Criminal Acts', *Lancet*, 9 November 1907, 1306–9.
'A Lecture on the Special Psychology of Women', *Lancet*, 2 May 1908, 1263–7.
'Considerations on the Occult', *BMJ*, 18 June 1910, 1472–7.
'A Lecture on the Mental Processes in Sanity and Insanity', *Lancet*, 27 January 1912, 211–15.

Skottowe, I., 'The Utility of the Psychiatric Out-Patient Clinic', *JMS*, 77:317 (April 1931), 311–20.

Smith, G.E., 'Shock and the Soldier. I', *Lancet*, 15 April 1916, 813–17.
'Shock and the Soldier. II', *Lancet*, 22 April 1916, 853–7.
'Correspondence: Functional Nervous Disease', *Lancet*, 6 May 1916, 971.
'Correspondence: "The Psychoneuroses of War"', *BMJ*, 22 September 1917, 402.

Smith, G.E., and Pear, T.H., 'Letters to the Editor: Shell Shock and Its Lessons', *Nature*, 100 (September 1917–February 1918), 64–6.

Smurthwaite, H., 'War Neuroses', Section of Laryngology, *PRSM*, 11 (Parts 1 and 2) (June 1918), 182–5.

Somerville, H., 'The War-Anxiety Neurotic of the Present Day: A Clinical Sketch', *JMS*, 69:285 (April 1923), 170–80.
'The War Anxiety Neurotic of the Present Day: His "Dizzy Bouts" and Hallucinations', *British Journal of Medical Psychology*, 3:4 (1923), 309–19.

Stewart, J.P., 'The Treatment of War Neuroses', *ANP*, 1:1 (January 1919), 14–24.

Stoddart, W.H.B., 'The New Psychiatry. Lecture I', *EMJ*, 14 (January–June 1915), 244–60.

'The New Psychiatry. Lecture II', *EMJ*, 14 (January–June 1915), 339–59.

'The New Psychiatry. Lecture III', *EMJ*, 14 (January–June 1915), 443–61.

'The Morison Lectures on the New Psychiatry. Lecture I', *Lancet*, 20 March 1915, 583–90.

'The Morison Lectures on the New Psychiatry. Lecture II', *Lancet*, 27 March 1915, 639–43.

Stopford, J.S.B., 'So-Called Functional Symptoms in Organic Nerve Injuries', *Lancet*, 8 June 1918, 795–6.

Suttie, I.D., 'Correspondence: Psycho-Analysis', *BMJ*, 23 December 1922, 1243–4.

Symns, J.L.M., 'Hysteria as Seen at a Base Hospital', *Practitioner*, 101:2 (August 1918), 90–6.

Taylor, J.M., 'Common Motor Disorders, Disuse Cripplings, Neuroses, Post-Infective and Others', *TMW*, 14 (July–December 1920), 1015–17.

Temple, R.C., 'Administrative Value of Anthropology', *Nature*, 92 (September 1913–February 1914), 207–13.

Thom, D.A., 'War Neuroses: Experiences of 1914–1918', *Journal of Laboratory and Clinical Medicine*, 28:1 (1942–3), 499–508.

Thomas, J.L., 'Correspondence: Death from High Explosives without Wounds', *BMJ*, 5 May 1917, 599.

Thomson, D.G., 'The Teaching of Psychiatry', *JMS*, 54:226 (July 1908), 550–9.

'Correspondence: Psycho-Analysis', *BMJ*, 6 January 1917, 32–3.

Thomson, H.C., 'Mental Therapeutics in Neurasthenia', *Practitioner*, 86:1 (January 1911), 76–83.

'Traumatic Neurasthenia', *JMS*, 59:247 (October 1913), 582–96.

Thorburn, W., 'Presidential Address: The Traumatic Neuroses', Neurological Section, *PRSM*, 7:2 (1913–14), 1–14.

Thursfield, H., 'Review of Children's Diseases', *Practitioner*, 87:1 (July 1911), 117–22.

Tippet, J.A., 'Correspondence: Psycho-Analysis', *BMJ*, 23 December 1922, 1244.

Tombleson, J.B., 'An Account of Twenty Cases Treated by Hypnotic Suggestion', *Journal of the RAMC*, 29:3 (September 1917), 340–6.

Tooth, H.H., 'Neurasthenia and Psychasthenia', *Journal of the RAMC*, 28:3 (March 1917), 328–45.

Tredgold, A.F., 'Neurasthenia and Insanity', *Practitioner*, 86:1 (January 1911), 84–95.

Trotter, R.H., 'Neurasthenic and Hysterical Cases in General Military Hospitals', *Lancet*, 23 November 1918, 703–4.

Trotter, W., 'Herd Instinct and Its Bearing on the Psychology of Civilised Man', *Sociological Review*, 1:3 (July 1908), 227–48.

'Sociological Application of the Psychology of the Herd Instinct', *Sociological Review*, 2:1 (January 1909), 36–54.

Turner, W.A., 'Remarks on Cases of Nervous and Mental Shock Observed at the Base Hospitals in France', *BMJ*, 15 May 1915, 833–5.

'Arrangements for the Care of Cases of Nervous and Mental Shock Coming from Overseas', *Lancet*, 27 May 1916, 1073–5.

'The Bradshaw Lecture on Neuroses and Psychoses of War', *Lancet*, 9 November 1918, 613–17.

Van Ness Dearborn, G., 'Kinesthesia and the Intelligent Will', *American Journal of Psychology*, 24:2 (April 1913), 204–55.

Veale, R.A., 'Some Cases of So-Called Functional Paresis Arising out of the War and Their Treatment', *Journal of the RAMC*, 29:5 (November 1917), 607–14.

Vesey, S.K., 'Future Care of Shell Shock Cases', *TMW*, 14 (January–June 1920), 79–81.

Ward, G., 'A Few Consecutive Cases from General Practice', *King's College Hospital Gazette*, 4 (1925), 161–5.

Waterson, D., 'The Teaching of Anatomy', *EMJ*, 20 (January–June 1918), 180–5.

Weatherly, L.A., 'The War and Neurasthenia, Psychasthenia and Mild Mental Disorders. I', *TMW*, 11 (July–December 1918), 217.

'The War and Neurasthenia, Psychasthenia and Mild Mental Disorders. II', *TMW*, 11 (July–December 1918), 265–6.

'Correspondence', *TMW*, 14 (July–December 1920), 1235–7.

Weber, F.P., 'The Association of Hysteria with Malingering: The Phylogenetic Aspect of Hysteria as Pathological Exaggeration (or Disorder) of Tertiary (Nervous) Sex Characters', *Lancet*, 2 December 1911, 1542–3.

West, S., 'Five Cases of Functional Nervous Disorder', *SBHR*, 21 (1885), 59–64.

White, E.W., 'Psychological Medicine in Relation to the Medical Practitioner', *KCHR*, 1 (1893–4), 49–54.

'Observations on Shell Shock and Neurasthenia in the Hospitals in the Western Command', *BMJ*, 13 April 1918, 421–2.

Wigglesworth, M.H., 'Stammering', *TMW*, 17 (January–June 1923), 494–5.

Williamson, R.T., 'Remarks on the Treatment of Neurasthenia and Psychasthenia Following Shell Shock', *BMJ*, 1 December 1917, 713–15.

Willmore, W.S., 'Correspondence: The Teaching of Psychotherapy', *BMJ*, 26 August 1922, 401.

Wilson, J.G., 'The Effects of High Explosives on the Ear', *BMJ*, 17 March 1917, 353–5.

'Further Report on the Effects of High Explosives on the Ear', *BMJ*, 5 May 1917, 578–9.

Wilson, S.A.K., 'Some Modern French Conceptions of Hysteria', *Brain*, 33:3 (January 1911), 293–338.

Wiltshire, H., 'A Contribution to the Etiology of Shell Shock', *Lancet*, 17 June 1916, 1207–12.

Wolfsohn, J.M., 'The Predisposing Factors of War Psycho-Neuroses', *Lancet*, 2 February 1918, 177–80.

Yealland, L.R., 'Hysterical Fits: With Some Reference to Their Treatment', *Lancet*, 15 September 1923, 551–5.

Young, J., 'Two Cases of War Neurosis', Medical Section, *British Journal of Psychology*, 2:3 (April 1922), 230–6.

BOOKS

Anon., 'The Mental Factor in Modern War: Shell Shock and Nervous Injuries', in *The Times History of the War* (London: The Times, 1916), pp. 313–48.

Allbutt, T.C., 'Neurasthenia', in T.C. Allbutt (ed.), *A System of Medicine*, 8 vols. (London and New York: Macmillan, 1898), vol. 8, pp. 134–66.

Arndt, R., 'Neurasthenia', in D.H. Tuke (ed.), *A Dictionary of Psychological Medicine*, 2 vols. (London: J. & A. Churchill, 1892), vol. 2., pp. 840–50.

Babinski, J., and Froment, J., *Hysteria or Pithiatism and Reflex Nervous Disorders in the Neurology of War* (London: University of London Press, 1918).

Bain, A., *The Emotions and the Will* (London: John W. Parker and Son, 1859).

Ballard, E.F., *An Epitome of Mental Disorders: A Practical Guide to Aetiology, Diagnosis, and Treatment for Practitioners, Asylum and R.A.M.C. Medical Officers* (London: J. & A. Churchill, 1917).

Bastian, H.C., *Various Forms of Hysterical or Functional Paralysis* (London: H.K. Lewis, 1893).

Bernheim, H., 'Suggestion and Hypnotism', in D.H. Tuke (ed.), *A Dictionary of Psychological Medicine*, 2 vols. (London: J. & A. Churchill, 1892), vol. 2, pp. 1213–17.

Bousfield, P., *"An Outline of Psychotherapy": A Lecture Delivered before the Deputy Commissioner of Medical Service* (London: Balliere, Tindall and Cox, 1919).

Brown, W., *Suggestion and Mental Analysis: An Outline of the Theory and Practice of Mind Cure* (London: University of London Press, 1922).

Buttar, E., 'Physiology of the Brain and Nervous System', in G. Rhodes (ed.), *The Mind at Work: A Handbook of Applied Psychology* (London: Thomas Murby, 1914), pp. 28–43.

Buzzard, T., 'Simulation of Hysteria by Organic Disease of the Nervous System', in D.H. Tuke (ed.), *A Dictionary of Psychological Medicine*, 2 vols. (London: J. & A. Churchill, 1892), vol. 1, pp. 1161–3.

Cannon, W.B., *Bodily Changes in Pain, Hunger, Fear and Rage: An Account of Recent Researches into the Function of Emotional Excitement* (New York and London: D. Appleton, 1920).

Clarke, J.M., *Hysteria and Neurasthenia* (London and New York: John Lane, 1905).

Cole, R.H., *Mental Diseases: A Text-Book of Psychiatry for Medical Students and Practitioners* (London: University of London Press, 1913).

Mental Diseases: A Text-Book of Psychiatry for Medical Students and Practitioners, 2nd edn (London: University of London Press, 1919).

Colvin, S.S., 'Education', in W.A. White and S.E. Jelliffe (eds.), *The Modern Treatment of Nervous and Mental Diseases, by American and British Authors* (London: Henry Kimpton, 1913), pp. 56–99.

Conklin, E.S., *Principles of Abnormal Psychology* (London: George Allen & Unwin, 1928).

Coupland, W.C., 'Philosophy of Mind', in D.H. Tuke (ed.), *A Dictionary of Psychological Medicine*, 2 vols. (London: J. & A. Churchill, 1892), vol. 1, pp. 27–49.

Craig, M., *Psychological Medicine: A Manual on Mental Diseases for Practitioners and Students*, 3rd edn (London: J. & A. Churchill, 1917).

Culpin, M., *Psychoneuroses of Peace and War* (Cambridge: Cambridge University Press, 1920).

The Nervous Patient (London: H.K. Lewis, 1924).

Darwin, C., *The Descent of Man, and Selection in Relation to Sex*, 2nd edn (London: Penguin, 2004) [1879].

The Expression of the Emotions in Man and Animals, 2nd edn (London: Fontana Press, 1999) [1889].

Eder, M.D., *War-Shock: The Psycho-Neuroses in War Psychology and Treatment* (London: William Heinemann, 1917).

Ellis, H., *Man and Woman: A Study of Human Secondary Sexual Characters*, 5th edn (New York and Melbourne: Walter Scott Publishing, 1914).

Foley, E.J., 'Consciousness and Sensation', in G. Rhodes (ed.), *The Mind at Work: A Handbook of Applied Psychology* (London: Thomas Murby, 1914), pp. 58–66.

'Modes of Consciousness', in G. Rhodes (ed.), *The Mind at Work: A Handbook of Applied Psychology* (London: Thomas Murby, 1914), pp. 67–101.

'Cognition and Ideation', in G. Rhodes (ed.), *The Mind at Work: A Handbook of Applied Psychology* (London: Thomas Murby, 1914), pp. 154–87.

Freud, S., 'Thoughts for the Times on War and Death' [1915], in *The Standard Edition of the Complete Works of Sigmund Freud* [*SE*], translated from the German under the General Editorship of James Strachey in collaboration with Anna Freud, assisted by Alix Strachey and Alison Tyson, vol. 14, pp. 275–300.

'Group Psychology and the Analysis of the Ego' [1921], in *The Standard Edition of the Complete Works of Sigmund Freud* [*SE*], translated from the German under the General Editorship of James Strachey in collaboration with Anna Freud, assisted by Alix Strachey and Alison Tyson, vol. 18, pp. 69–143.

Harris, W., *Nerve Injuries and Shock* (London: Oxford University Press, 1915).

Hart, B., *The Psychology of Insanity* (Cambridge: Cambridge University Press, 1912).

Psychopathology: Its Development and Its Place in Medicine (London: Cambridge University Press, 1927).

Henderson, D.K., and Gillespie, R.D., *A Text-Book of Psychiatry for Students and Practitioners*, 3rd edn (London: Humphrey Milford/Oxford University Press, 1932).

Herringham, W.P., *A Physician in France* (London: Edward Arnold, 1919).

Hobhouse, L.T., *Mind in Evolution* (London: Macmillan, 1901).

Hurst, A.F., *Medical Diseases of the War* (London: Edward Arnold, 1917).

Medical Diseases of the War, 2nd edn (London: Edward Arnold, 1918).

Medical Diseases of War, 4th edn (London: Edward Arnold, 1944).

Janet, P., *Mental State of Hystericals: A Study of Mental Stigmata and Mental Accidents*, trans. C. Corson (New York: G.P. Putnam's Sons, 1901).

Jones, E., *Free Associations: Memories of a Psycho-Analyst* (London: Hogarth Press, 1959).

Kernahan, J.C., *The Experiences of a Recruiting Officer* (London: Hodder and Stoughton, 1915).

Kipling, R., *Something of Myself: For My Friends Known and Unknown* (London: Penguin, 1988) [1937].

Lépine, J., *Mental Disorders of War* (London and Paris: University of London Press/Masson et Cie, 1919).

Léri, A., *Shell Shock: Commotional and Emotional Aspects* (London: University of London Press, 1919).

Lord, J.R. (ed.), *Contributions to Psychiatry, Neurology and Sociology Dedicated to the Late Sir Frederick Mott, K.B.E.* (London: H.K. Lewis, 1929).

McDougall, W., *An Introduction to Social Psychology* (Bristol and Tokyo: Thoemmes Press and Maruzen, 1998) [1908].

Psychology: The Study of Behaviour (London: Williams and Norgate, 1914).

The Group Mind: A Sketch of the Principles of Collective Psychology with Some Attempt to Apply Them to the Interpretation of National Life and Character (Cambridge: Cambridge University Press, 1920).

Outline of Abnormal Psychology (New York: Charles Scribner's Sons, 1926).

MacCurdy, J.T., *War Neuroses* (Cambridge: Cambridge University Press, 1918).

Marr, H.C., *Psychoses of the War, Including Neurasthenia and Shell Shock* (London: Henry Frowde and Hodder & Stoughton, 1919).

Maudsley, H., *Body and Mind: An Inquiry into Their Connection and Mutual Influence, Specially in Reference to Mental Disorders* (New York: D. Appleton, 1871).

Body and Will (London: Kegan Paul, Trench, 1883).

Mitchell, P.C., 'Evolution', *Encyclopaedia Britannica*, 11th edn, 29 vols. (Cambridge: Cambridge University Press, 1910), vol. 10, pp. 22–37.

Moran, Lord, *The Anatomy of Courage* (London: Sphere Books, 1968) [1945].

Morgan, C.L., 'Instinct', *Encyclopaedia Britannica*, 11th edn, 29 vols. (Cambridge: Cambridge University Press, 1910), vol. 14, pp. 648–50.

Mott, F.W., *Syphilis of the Nervous System* (London: Henry Frowde and Hodder and Stoughton, 1910).

Nature and Nurture in Mental Development (London: John Murray, 1914).

War Neuroses and Shell Shock (London: Hodder and Stoughton, 1919).

'Alcohol and Its Relations to Problems in Mental Disorders', in E.H. Starling, *The Action of Alcohol on Man* (London: Longmans, Green, 1923), pp. 183–212.

Murray, G., 'Herd Instinct and the War', in E.M. Sidgwick, G. Murray, A.C. Bradley, L.P. Jacks, G.F. Stout, and B. Bosanquet (eds.), *The International Crisis in Its Ethical and Psychological Aspects* (London: Oxford University Press, 1915), pp. 22–45.

Herd Instinct: For Good and Evil (London: George Allen & Unwin, 1940).

Myers, C.S., *Present-Day Applications of Psychology with Special Reference to Industry, Education and Nervous Breakdown* (London: Methuen, 1918).

Shell Shock in France 1914–1918: Based on a War Diary (Cambridge: Cambridge University Press, 1940).

Nagel, J.D., *Nervous and Mental Diseases: A Manual for Students and Practitioners* (London: Hodder and Stoughton, 1905).

Ormerod, J.A., 'Hysteria', in T.C. Allbutt (ed.), *A System of Medicine*, 8 vols. (London and New York: Macmillan, 1898), vol. 8, pp. 88–127.

Page, H.W., 'Shock from Fright', in D.H. Tuke (ed.), *A Dictionary of Psychological Medicine*, 2 vols. (London: J. & A. Churchill, 1892), vol. 2, pp. 1157–60.

Parsons, J.H., *Mind and the Nation* (London: Bale, Sons and Danielsson, 1918).

Playfair, W.S., 'Neuroses, Functional, the Systematic Treatment of (So-Called Weir Mitchell Treatment)', in D.H. Tuke (ed.), *A Dictionary of Psychological Medicine*, 2 vols. (London: J. & A. Churchill, 1892), vol. 2, pp. 850–7.

Potts, C.S., *Nervous and Mental Diseases for Students and Practitioners*, 2nd edn (London: Henry Kimpton, 1908).

Pye-Smith, P.H., *Syllabus of a Course of Lectures on Physiology Delivered at Guy's Hospital* (London: J. & A. Churchill, 1885).

Rhodes, G., 'Introduction', in G. Rhodes (ed.), *The Mind at Work: A Handbook of Applied Psychology* (London: Thomas Murby, 1914), pp. 1–13.

'Mechanism of the Will', in G. Rhodes (ed.), *The Mind at Work: A Handbook of Applied Psychology* (London: Thomas Murby, 1914), pp. 88–93.

Ribot, T., 'Will, Disorders of', in D.H. Tuke Hack Tuke (ed.), *A Dictionary of Psychological Medicine*, 2 vols. (London: J. & A. Churchill, 1892), vol. 2, pp. 1366–8.

The Psychology of the Emotions, 2nd edn (New York and Melbourne: Walter Scott Publishing, 1911).

Rivers, W.H.R., 'Preface', in J.T. MacCurdy, *War Neuroses* (Cambridge: Cambridge University Press, 1918), pp. v–ix.

Instinct and the Unconscious: A Contribution to a Biological Theory of the Psycho-Neuroses (Cambridge: Cambridge University Press, 1920).

Conflict and Dream (London: Kegan Paul, Trench, Trubner, 1923).

Rixon, C.H.L, and Matthew, D., *Anxiety Hysteria: Modern Views on Some Neuroses* (London: H.K. Lewis, 1920).

Romanes, G., 'Instinct', in D.H. Tuke (ed.), *A Dictionary of Psychological Medicine*, 2 vols. (London: J. & A. Churchill, 1892), vol. 2, pp. 704–6.

Ross, T.A., 'Shell Shock', in H. Joules (ed.), *The Doctor's View of War* (London: George Allen and Unwin, 1938), pp. 48–55.

'Anxiety Neuroses of War', in A.F. Hurst, *Medical Diseases of War* (London: Edward Arnold, 1944), pp. 149–72.

Roussy, G., and Lhermitte, J., *The Psychoneuroses of War* (London and Paris: University of London Press/Masson et Cie, 1918).

Savill, T.D., *Lectures on Hysteria and Allied Vaso-Motor Conditions* (London: Henry J. Glaister, 1909).

Shand, A.F., *The Foundations of Character: Being a Study of the Tendencies of the Emotions and Sentiments* (London: Macmillan, 1914).

Shaw, T.C., *Ex Cathedra: Essays on Insanity* (London: Adlard and Son, 1904).

Smith, G.E., 'Preface', in W.H.R. Rivers, *Conflict and Dream* (London: Kegan Paul, Trench, Trubner, 1923), pp. v–ix.

Smith, G.E., and Pear, T.H., *Shell Shock and Its Lessons*, 2nd edn (Manchester: Manchester University Press, 1918).

Southard, E.E., *Shell-Shock and Other Neuropsychiatric Problems, Presented in Five Hundred and Eighty-Nine Case Histories from the War Literature, 1914–1918* (Boston, MA: W.M. Leonard, 1919).

Stewart, J.P., *The Diagnosis of Nervous Diseases* (London: Edward Arnold, 1906).

Stoddart, W.H.B., *Mind and Its Disorders: A Text-Book for Students and Practitioners* (London: H.K. Lewis, 1908).

Mind and Its Disorders: A Text-Book for Students and Practitioners, 2nd edn (London: H.K. Lewis, 1912).

The New Psychiatry (London: Baillière, Tindall and Cox, 1916).

Sully, J., 'Introduction', in B. Perez, *The First Three Years of Childhood* (London: Swan Sönnenschein, 1889), pp. iii–xxiv.

Trotter, W., *Instincts of the Herd in Peace and War* (London: Ernest Benn, 1919).
Tuke, D.H. (ed.), *A Dictionary of Psychological Medicine*, 2 vols. (London: J. & A. Churchill, 1892).
Wittkower, E., and Spillane, J.P., 'A Survey of the Literature of Neuroses in War', in E. Miller (ed.), *The Neuroses in War* (London: Macmillan, 1940), pp. 1–32.
White, W.A., and Jelliffe, S.E. (eds.), *The Modern Treatment of Nervous and Mental Diseases, by American and British Authors* (London: Henry Kimpton, 1913).
Wright, A., *The Unexpurgated Case against Woman Suffrage* (New York: Paul Hoeber, 1913).
Wyllie, J., *The Disorders of Speech* (Edinburgh: Oliver and Boyd, 1894).
Yealland, L.R., *Hysterical Disorders of Warfare* (London: Macmillan, 1918).

SECONDARY SOURCES

JOURNALS

Atenstaedt, R.L., 'The Organisation of the RAMC During the Great War', *Journal of the RAMC*, 152 (2006), 81–5.
Bogacz, T., 'War Neurosis and Cultural Change in England, 1914–22: The Work of the War Office Committee of Enquiry into "Shell-Shock"', *Journal of Contemporary History*, 24 (1989), 227–56.
Cantor, D., 'Between Galen, Geddes, and the Gael: Arthur Brock, Modernity, and Medical Humanism in Early-Twentieth-Century Scotland', *Journal of the History of Medicine and Allied Sciences*, 60:1 (2005), 1–41.
Collins, M., 'The Fall of the English Gentleman: The National Character in Decline, c. 1918–1970', *Historical Research*, 75:187 (February 2000), 90–111.
Collins, T., 'Return to Manhood: The Cult of Masculinity and the British Union of Fascists', *International Journal of the History of Sport*, 16:4 (2000), 145–62.
Doan, L., 'A Challenge to Change? New Perspectives on Women and the Great War', *Women's History Review*, 15:2 (April 2006), 337–43.
Emsley, C., 'Violent Crime in England in 1919: Post-War Anxieties and Press Narratives', *Continuity and Change*, 23:1 (2008), 173–95.
Feudtner, C., '"Minds the Dead Have Ravished": Shell Shock, History, and the Ecology of Disease Systems', *History of Science*, 31 (1993), 377–420.
Forrester, J., '1919: Psychology and Psychoanalysis, Cambridge and London – Myers, Jones and MacCurdy', *Psychoanalysis and History*, 10:1 (2008), 37–94.
Francis, M., 'Attending to Ghosts: Some Reflections on the Disavowals of British Great War Historiography', *Twentieth Century British History*, 25:3 (2014), 347–67.
Gagen, W.J., 'Remastering the Body, Renegotiating Gender: Physical Disability and Masculinity during the First World War, the Case of J.B. Middlebrook', *European Review of History*, 14:4 (2007), 525–41.
Greisman, H.C., 'Herd Instinct and the Foundations of Biosociology', *Journal of the History of the Behavioral Sciences*, 15 (1979), 357–69.
Harrison, M., 'The Medicalization of War – The Militarization of Medicine', *Social History of Medicine*, 9:2 (1996), 267–76.
Higgonet, M., 'Authenticity and Art in Trauma Narratives of WWI', *Modernism/Modernity*, 9:1 (2002), 91–107.

Holdorff, B., and Dening, T., 'The Fight for "Traumatic Neurosis", 1889–1916: Hermann Oppenheim and His Opponents in Berlin', *History of Psychiatry*, 22:4 (2011), 465–76.

Humphries, M., 'War's Long Shadow: Masculinity, Medicine, and the Gendered Politics of Trauma, 1914–1939', *Canadian Historical Review*, 91:3 (September 2010), 503–31.

Humphries, M., and Kurchinski, K., 'Rest, Relax and Get Well: A Re-Conceptualisation of Great War Shell Shock Treatment', *War & Society* [University of New South Wales], 27:2 (2008), 89–110.

Ismail, S., 'A "Creative Tension": The Royal Army Medical Corps and the Interplay of Psychological and Physiological in the Rise of a Psychoanalytic Synthesis, 1915–22', *Psychoanalysis and History*, 7:2 (2005), 171–203.

Jacyna, L.S., 'Somatic Theories of Mind and the Interests of Medicine in Britain, 1850–1879', *Medical History*, 26 (1982), 233–58.

Jones, E., 'The Psychology of Killing: The Combat Experience of British Soldiers during the First World War', *Journal of Contemporary History*, 41:2 (2006), 229–46.

'Shell Shock at Maghull and the Maudsley: Models of Psychological Medicine in the UK', *Journal of the History of Medicine and Allied Sciences*, 65:3 (2010), 368–95.

'War Neuroses and Arthur Hurst: A Pioneering Medical Film about the Treatment of Psychiatric Battle Casualties', *Journal of the History of Medicine and Allied Sciences*, 67:3 (2012), 345–73.

Jones, E., Fear, N.T., and Wessely, S., 'Shell Shock and Mild Traumatic Brain Injury: A Historical Review', *American Journal of Psychiatry*, 164 (2007), 1641–5.

Jones, E., Palmer, I., and Wessely, S., 'War Pensions (1900–1945): Changing Models of Psychological Understanding', *British Journal of Psychiatry*, 180 (2002), 374–9.

Kaufmann, D., 'Science as Cultural Practice: Psychiatry in the First World War and Weimar Germany', *Journal of Contemporary History*, 34 (1999), 125–44.

Koven, S., 'Remembering and Dismemberment: Crippled Children, Wounded Soldiers and the Great War in Britain', *American Historical Review*, 99:4 (October 1994), 1167–202.

Lawrence, C., 'Incommunicable Knowledge: Science, Technology and the Clinical Art in Britain, 1850–1914', *Journal of Contemporary History*, 20 (1985), 503–20.

Lawrence, J., 'Forging a Peaceable Kingdom: War, Violence, and Fear of Brutalization in Post-First World War Britain', *Journal of Modern History*, 75:3 (September 2003), 557–89.

Leese, P., 'Problems Returning Home: The British Psychological Casualties of the Great War', *Historical Journal*, 40:4 (December 1997), 1055–67.

Lerner, P., 'Hysterical Cures: Hypnosis, Gender and Performance in World War I and Weimar Germany', *History Workshop Journal*, 45 (1998), 79–101.

Leys, R., 'Traumatic Cures: Shell Shock, Janet, and the Question of Memory', *Critical Inquiry*, 20 (Summer 1994), 623–62.

Linden, S.C., and Jones, E., '"Shell Shock" Revisited: An Examination of the Case Records of the National Hospital in London', *Medical History*, 58:4 (2014), 519–45.

Link-Heer, U., '"Male Hysteria": A Discourse Analysis', *Cultural Critique*, 15 (1990), 191–220.

Loughran, T., 'Hysteria and Neurasthenia in Pre-1914 British Medical Discourse and in Histories of Shell-Shock', *History of Psychiatry*, 19:1 (March 2008), 25–46.

'Shell-Shock and Psychological Medicine in First World War Britain', *Social History of Medicine*, 22:1 (2009), 79–95.

'Shell Shock, Trauma, and the First World War: The Making of a Diagnosis and Its Histories', *Journal of the History of Medicine and Allied Sciences*, 67:1 (January 2012), 94–119.

'A Crisis of Masculinity? Re-Writing the History of Shell-Shock and Gender in First World War Britain', *History Compass*, 11:9 (2013), 727–38.

May, C., 'Lord Moran's Memoir: Shell-Shock and the Pathology of Fear', *Journal of the Royal Society of Medicine*, 91 (1998), 95–100.

Mayou, R., 'The History of General Hospital Psychiatry', *British Journal of Psychiatry*, 155 (1989), 764–76.

Meyer, J., 'Separating the Men from the Boys: Masculinity and Maturity in Understandings of Shell Shock in Britain', *Twentieth Century British History*, 20:1 (2009), 1–22.

Micale, M., 'Hysteria and Its Historiography: The Future Perspective', *History of Psychiatry*, 1 (1990), 33–124.

'Charcot and the Idea of Hysteria in the Male: Gender, Mental Science, and Medical Diagnosis in Late Nineteenth-Century France', *Medical History*, 34 (1990), 363–411.

'On the "Disappearance" of Hysteria: A Study in the Clinical Deconstruction of a Diagnosis', *Isis*, 84 (1993), 496–526.

Nye, R., 'Degeneration, Neurasthenia and the Culture of Sport in *Belle Époque* France', *Journal of Contemporary History*, 17 (1982), 51–68.

Otis, L., 'Organic Memory and Psychoanalysis', *History of Psychiatry*, 4 (1993), 349–72.

Porter, D., '"Enemies of the Race": Biologism, Environmentalism, and Public Health in Edwardian England', *Victorian Studies*, 34 (1991), 159–78.

Raitt, S., 'Early British Psychoanalysis and the Medico-Psychological Clinic', *History Workshop Journal*, 58 (Autumn 2004), 63–85.

Rapp, D., 'The Reception of Freud by the British Press: General Interest and Literary Magazines, 1920–1925', *Journal of the History of the Behavioral Sciences*, 24 (1988), 191–201.

Ray, L.J., 'Models of Madness in Victorian Asylum Practice', *Archives Européenes de Sociologie*, 22 (1981), 229–64.

Richards, G., 'Britain on the Couch: The Popularization of Psychoanalysis in Britain 1918–1940', *Science in Context*, 13:2 (June 2000), 183–230.

Roper, M., 'Between Manliness and Masculinity: The "War Generation" and the Psychology of Fear in Britain, 1914–1950', *Journal of British Studies*, 44:2 (April 2005), 343–62.

'Nostalgia as an Emotional Experience in the Great War', *Historical Journal*, 54:2 (2011), 421–51.

'From the Shell-Shocked Soldier to the Nervous Child: Psychoanalysis in the Aftermath of the First World War', *Psychoanalysis and History*, 18:1 (January 2016), 39–69.

Roudebush, M., 'A Patient Fights Back: Neurology in the Court of Public Opinion in France during the First World War', *Journal of Contemporary History*, 35:1 (2000), 29–38.

Schmiedebach, H-P., 'Post-Traumatic Neurosis in Nineteenth-Century Germany: A Disease in Political, Juridical and Professional Context', *History of Psychiatry*, 10 (1999), 27–57.

Shephard, B., '"Pitiless Psychology": The Role of Prevention in British Military Psychiatry in the Second World War', *History of Psychiatry*, 10 (1999), 491–524.

Sicherman, B., 'The Uses of a Diagnosis: Doctors, Patients, and Neurasthenia', *Journal of the History of Medicine and Allied Sciences*, 32 (1977), 33–54.

Smith, R, 'Does the History of Psychology Have a Subject?', *History of the Human Sciences*, 1:2 (1988), 147–77.

Soffer, R., 'New Elitism: Social Psychology in Prewar England', *Journal of British Studies*, 8:2 (May 1969), 111–40.

Thomson, M., '"The Solution to His Own Enigma": Connecting the Life of Montague David Eder (1865–1936), Socialist, Psychoanalyst, Zionist and Modern Saint', *Medical History*, 55 (2011), 61–84.

Tosh, J., 'Masculinities in an Industrializing Society: Britain, 1800–1914', *Journal of British Studies*, 44 (2005), 330–42.

Valentine, E.R., '"A Brilliant and Many-Sided Personality": Jessie Margaret Murray, Founder of the Medico-Psychological Clinic', *Journal of the History of the Behavioral Sciences*, 45:2 (2009), 145–61.

Walk, A., 'Medico-Psychologists, Maudsley and the Maudsley', *British Journal of Psychiatry*, 128 (1976), 19–30.

Weisz, G., 'Reconstructing Paris Medicine', *Bulletin of the History of Medicine*, 75:1 (2001), 105–19.

Wessely, S., 'Twentieth-Century Theories on Combat Motivation and Breakdown', *Journal of Contemporary History*, 41:2 (2006), 269–86.

Winter, J., 'Shell-Shock and the Cultural History of the Great War', *Journal of Contemporary History*, 35:1 (2000), 7–11.

Young, A., 'W.H.R. Rivers and the War Neuroses', *Journal of the History of the Behavioral Sciences*, 35:4 (1999), 359–78.

BOOKS

Allderidge, P., 'The Foundation of the Maudsley Hospital', in G.E. Berrios and H. Freeman (eds.), *150 Years of British Psychiatry, 1841–1991* (London: Gaskell, 1991), pp. 79–88.

Anning, S.T., and Walls, W.K.J., *A History of the Leeds School of Medicine: One and a Half Centuries, 1831–1981* (Leeds: Leeds University Press, 1982).

Barham, P., *Forgotten Lunatics of the Great War* (New Haven, CT, and London: Yale University Press, 2004).

Barrett, M., *Casualty Figures: How Five Men Survived the First World War* (London: Verso, 2007).

Bet-El, I., 'Men and Soldiers: British Conscripts, Concepts of Masculinity, and the Great War', in B. Melman (ed.), *Borderlines: Genders and Identities in War and Peace, 1870–1930* (London: Routledge, 1998), pp. 73–95.

Conscripts: Lost Legions of the Great War (Stroud: Sutton, 1999).

Binneveld, H., *From Shell Shock to Combat Stress: A Comparative History of Military Psychiatry* (Amsterdam: Amsterdam University Press, 1997).

Bourke, J., *Dismembering the Male: Men's Bodies, Britain and the Great War* (London: Reaktion Books, 1999).

Bourne, J., 'The British Working Man in Arms', in H. Cecil and P.H. Liddle (eds.), *Facing Armageddon: The First World War Experienced* (London: Leo Cooper, 1996), pp. 336–52.

Braybon, G., 'Winners or Losers: Women's Symbolic Role in the War Story', in G. Braybon (ed.), *Evidence, History, and the Great War: Historians and the Impact of 1914–18* (Oxford: Berghahn Books, 2003), pp. 86–112.

Busfield, J., 'Restructuring Mental Health Services in Twentieth-Century Britain', in M. Gijswijt-Hofstra and R. Porter (eds.), *Cultures of Psychiatry and Mental Health Care in Postwar Britain and the Netherlands* (Amsterdam and Atlanta, GA: Rodopi, 1998), pp. 9–28.

Cantor, D., 'The Diseased Body', in R. Cooter and J. Pickstone (eds.), *Companion to Medicine in the Twentieth Century* (London and New York: Routledge, 2003), pp. 347–66.

Carden-Coyne, A., *Reconstructing the Body: Classicism, Modernism, and the First World War* (Oxford: Oxford University Press, 2009).

Clark, M.J., 'The Rejection of Psychological Approaches to Mental Disorder in Late Nineteenth-Century British Psychiatry', in A. Scull (ed.), *Madhouses, Mad-Doctors and Madmen: The Social History of Psychiatry in the Victorian Era* (Philadelphia, PA: University of Pennsylvania Press, 1981), pp. 271–312.

Collini, S., *Public Moralists: Political Thought and Intellectual Life in Britain, 1850–1930* (Oxford: Clarendon Press, 1991).

Cooter, R., 'Malingering in Modernity: Psychological Scripts and Adversarial Encounters during the First World War', in R. Cooter, M. Harrison, and S. Sturdy (eds.), *War, Medicine and Modernity* (Stroud: Sutton, 1999), pp. 125–48.

Corrigan, G., *Mud, Blood and Poppycock: Britain and the Great War* (London: Cassell Military Paperbacks, 2004).

Crammer, J.L., 'Training and Education in British Psychiatry 1770–1970', in H. Freeman and G.E. Berrios (eds.), *150 Years of British Psychiatry. Volume 2: The Aftermath* (London: Athlone, 1996), pp. 209–42.

Crook, P., *Darwinism, War and History: The Debate over the Biology of War from the Origin of Species to the First World War* (Cambridge and New York: Cambridge University Press, 1994).

Crouthamel, J., *The Great War and German Memory: Society, Politics and Psychological Trauma, 1914–1945* (Exeter: University of Exeter Press, 2009).

Cunningham, A., 'Transforming Plague: The Laboratory and the Identity of Infectious Disease', in A. Cunningham and P. Williams (eds.), *The Laboratory Revolution in Medicine* (Cambridge: Cambridge University Press, 1992), pp. 209–44.

Danto, E.A., *Freud's Free Clinics: Psychoanalysis and Social Justice, 1918–1938* (New York and Chichester, West Sussex: Columbia University Press, 2005).

Das, S., *Touch and Intimacy in First World War Literature* (Cambridge and New York: Cambridge University Press, 2005).

Daston, L.J., 'The Theory of Will versus the Science of Mind', in W.R. Woodward and M.G. Ash (eds.), *The Problematic Science: Psychology in Nineteenth-Century Thought* (New York: Praeger, 1982), pp. 88–115.

Davidoff, L., *Worlds between: Historical Perspectives on Gender and Class* (Cambridge: Polity, 1995).

Dawson, G., *Soldier Heroes: British Adventure, Empire and the Imagining of Masculinities* (London and New York: Routledge, 1994).

Digby, A., *The Evolution of British General Practice 1850–1948* (Oxford: Oxford University Press, 1999).

Dixon, T., *The Invention of Altruism: Making Moral Meanings in Modern Britain* (Oxford and New York: Oxford University Press, 2008).

Drabble, M., *The Pattern in the Carpet: A Personal History with Jigsaws* (London: Atlantic Books, 2010).

Drinka, G.F., *The Birth of Neurosis: Myth, Malady and the Victorians* (New York: Simon and Schuster, 1984).

Eksteins, M., *Rites of Spring: The Great War and the Birth of the Modern Age* (London: Papermac, 2000).

Figlio, K., 'How Does Illness Mediate Social Relations? Workmen's Compensation and Medico-Legal Practices, 1890–1940', in P. Wright and A. Treacher (eds.), *The Problem of Medical Knowledge: Examining the Social Construction of Medicine* (Edinburgh: Edinburgh University Press, 1982), pp. 174–224.

Forrest, D., *Hypnotism: A History* (London: Penguin, 1999).

Forrester, J., 'The English Freud: W.H.R. Rivers, Dreaming, and the Making of the Early Twentieth-Century Human Sciences', in S. Alexander and B. Taylor (eds.), *History and Psyche: Culture, Psychoanalysis, and the Past* (Basingstoke and New York: Palgrave Macmillan, 2012), pp. 71–104.

Fussell, P., *The Great War and Modern Memory* (London, Oxford, and New York: Oxford University Press, 1975).

Gijswijt-Hofstra, M., 'Introduction: Cultures of Neurasthenia from Beard to the First World War', in M. Gijswijt-Hofstra and R. Porter (eds.), *Cultures of Neurasthenia from Beard to the First World War* (Amsterdam and New York: Rodophi, 2001), pp. 1–30.

Glover, E., 'Eder as Psycho-Analyst', in J.B. Hobman (ed.), *David Eder: Memoirs of a Modern Pioneer* (London: Victor Gollancz, 1945), pp. 89–116.

Goebel, S., *The Great War and Medieval Memory: War, Remembrance and Medievalism in Britain and Germany* (Cambridge and New York: Cambridge University Press, 2006).

Grayzel, S., *Women's Identities at War: Gender, Motherhood, and Politics in Britain and France during the First World War* (Chapel Hill, NC and London: University of North Carolina Press, 1999).

Gregory, A., *The Last Great War: British Society and the First World War* (Cambridge and New York: Cambridge University Press, 2008).

Gullace, N., *"The Blood of Our Sons": Men, Women, and the Renegotiation of British Citizenship during the Great War* (New York and Basingstoke: Palgrave Macmillan, 2002).

Hacking, I., 'Making Up People', in T.C. Heller *et al.* (eds.), *Reconstructing Individualism: Autonomy, Individuality and the Self in Western Thought* (Stanford, CA: Stanford University Press, 1986), pp. 222–36.

'The Looping Effects of Human Kinds', in D. Sperber, D. Premack, and A.J. Premack (eds.), *Causal Cognition: A Multidisciplinary Approach* (Oxford: Clarendon Press, 1994), pp. 351–94.

'Memory Sciences, Memory Politics', in P. Antze and M. Lambek (eds.), *Tense Past: Cultural Essays in Trauma and Memory* (New York and London: Routledge, 1996), pp. 67–88.

Hallett, C., *Containing Trauma: Nursing Work in the First World War* (Manchester: Manchester University Press, 2009).

Harrington, R., 'The Railway Accident: Trains, Trauma, and Technological Crises in Nineteenth-Century Britain', in M. Micale and P. Lerner (eds.), *Traumatic Pasts: History, Psychiatry, and Trauma in the Modern Age, 1870–1930* (Cambridge: Cambridge University Press, 2001), pp. 31–56.

Harris, R., *Murders and Madness: Medicine, Law, and Society in the Fin de Siècle* (Oxford: Clarendon, 1989).

Heathorn, S., 'Representations of War and Martial Heroes in English Elementary School Reading and Rituals, 1885–1914', in J. Marten (ed.), *Children and War: A Historical Anthology* (New York and London: New York University Press, 2002), pp. 103–15.

Horne, J., 'Masculinity in Politics and War in the Age of Nation-States and World Wars, 1850–1950', in S. Dudlink, K. Hagemann, and J. Tosh (eds.), *Masculinities in Politics and War: Gendering Modern History* (Manchester and New York: Manchester University Press, 2004), pp. 22–40.

Hunting, P., *The History of the Royal Society of Medicine* (London: Royal Society of Medicine Press, 2002).

Hynes, S., *A War Imagined: The First World War and English Culture* (New York: Atheneum, 1991).

Jones, E., 'Post-Combat Disorders: The Boer War to the Gulf', in H. Lee and E. Jones (eds.), *War and Health: Lessons from the Gulf War* (Chicester, West Sussex: John Wiley & Sons, 2007), pp. 5–40.

Jones, E., and Wessely, S., 'The Impact of Total War on the Practice of British Psychiatry', in R. Chickering and S. Förster (eds.), *The Shadows of Total War: Europe, East Asia, and the United States, 1919–1939* (Cambridge: Cambridge University Press, 2003), pp. 129–48.

Shell Shock to PTSD: Military Psychiatry from 1900 to the Gulf War (Hove, East Sussex and New York: Psychology Press, 2005).

Jones, G.S., *Outcast London: A Study in the Relationship between Classes in Victorian Society* (Harmondsworth: Penguin, 1984).

Kaarsholm, P., 'Kipling and Masculinity', in R. Samuel (ed.), *Patriotism: The Making and Unmaking of British National Identity. Volume 3: National Fictions* (London: Routledge, 1989), pp. 215–26.

Kent, S.K., *Making Peace: The Reconstruction of Gender in Interwar Britain* (Princeton, NJ: Princeton University Press, 1993).

Aftershocks: Politics and Trauma in Britain, 1918–1931 (Basingstoke: Palgrave Macmillan, 2009).

King, H., 'Once Upon a Text: Hysteria from Hippocrates', in S. Gilman *et al.*
(eds.), *Hysteria Beyond Freud* (Berkeley, Los Angeles, and London:
University of California Press), pp. 3–89.

Köhne, J.B., 'Visualising "War Hysterics": Strategies of Feminization and
Re-Masculinization in Scientific Cinematography, 1916–1918', in
C. Hämmerle, O. Überegger, and B. Bader Zaar (eds.), *Gender and the First
World War* (Basingstoke and New York: Palgrave Macmillan, 2014),
pp. 72–88.

Koureas, G., *Memory, Masculinity and National Identity in British Visual
Culture, 1914–1930: A Study of 'Unconquerable Manhood'* (Aldershot:
Ashgate, 2007).

Leed, E., *No Man's Land: Combat and Identity in World War One* (Cambridge:
Cambridge University Press, 1979).

Leese, P., '"Why Are They Not Cured?" British Shellshock Treatment during the
Great War', in M. Micale and P. Lerner (eds.), *Traumatic Pasts: History,
Psychiatry and Trauma in the Modern Age, 1870–1930* (Cambridge:
Cambridge University Press, 2001), pp. 205–21.

Shell Shock: Traumatic Neurosis and the British Soldiers of the First World War
(Basingstoke: Palgrave, 2002).

Lerner, P., 'From Traumatic Neurosis to Male Hysteria: The Decline and Fall of
Hermann Oppenheim, 1889–1919', in M. Micale and P. Lerner (eds.),
*Traumatic Pasts: History, Psychiatry, and Trauma in the Modern Age,
1870–1930* (Cambridge: Cambridge University Press, 2001), pp. 140–71.

*Hysterical Men: War, Psychiatry and the Politics of Trauma in Germany,
1890–1930* (Ithaca, NY and London: Cornell University Press, 2003).

Light, A., *Forever England: Femininity, Literature and Conservatism between the
Wars* (London and New York: Routledge, 1991).

Lutz, T., 'Neurasthenia and Fatigue Syndromes: Social Section', in G.E. Berrios
and R. Porter (eds.), *A History of Clinical Psychiatry: The Origin and History of
Psychiatric Disorders* (London: Athlone, 1995), pp. 533–44.

'Varieties of Medical Experience: Doctors and Patients, Psyche and Soma in
America', in M. Gijswijt-Hofstra and R. Porter (eds.), *Cultures of
Neurasthenia: From Beard to the First World War* (Amsterdam and New York:
Rodophi, 2001), pp. 51–76.

McLaren, A., *Impotence: A Cultural History* (Chicago, IL and London: University
of Chicago, 2007).

Marland, H., '"Uterine Mischief": W.S. Playfair and His Neurasthenic Patients',
in M. Gijswijt-Hofstra and R. Porter (eds.), *Cultures of Neurasthenia: From
Beard to the First World War* (Amsterdam and New York: Rodophi, 2001),
pp. 117–39.

Marwick, A., *The Deluge: British Society and the First World War* (Basingtoke:
Macmillan, 1965).

*War and Social Change in the Twentieth Century: A Comparative Study of Britain,
France, Germany, Russia, and the United States* (Basingstoke: Palgrave
Macmillan, 1974).

Meyer, J., *Men of War: Masculinity and the First World War in Britain* (Basingstoke
and New York: Palgrave Macmillan, 2009).

Micale, M., 'Hysteria Male/Hysteria Female: Reflections on Comparative Gender Construction in Nineteenth-Century France and Britain', in M. Benjamin (ed.), *Science and Sensibility: Gender and Scientific Enquiry, 1780–1945* (Oxford: Basil Blackwell, 1991), pp. 200–39.

Approaching Hysteria: Disease and Its Interpretations (Princeton, NJ: Princeton University Press, 1995).

'Jean-Martin Charcot and *les névroses traumatiques*: From Medicine to Culture in French Trauma Theory of the Late Nineteenth Century', in M. Micale and P. Lerner (eds.), *Traumatic Pasts: History, Psychiatry, and Trauma in the Modern Age, 1870–1930* (Cambridge: Cambridge University Press, 2001), pp. 115–39.

Hysterical Men: The Hidden History of Male Nervous Illness (Cambridge, MA, and London: Harvard University Press, 2008).

Micale, M., and Lerner, P., 'Trauma, Psychiatry, and History: A Conceptual and Historiographical Introduction', in M. Micale and P. Lerner (eds.), *Traumatic Pasts: History, Psychiatry, and Trauma in the Modern Age, 1870–1930* (Cambridge: Cambridge University Press, 2001), pp. 1–27.

Micale, M., and Lerner, P. (eds.), *Traumatic Pasts: History, Psychiatry and Trauma in the Modern Age, 1870–1930* (Cambridge: Cambridge University Press, 2001).

Mosse, G., *The Image of Man: The Creation of Modern Masculinity* (New York and Oxford: Oxford University Press, 1996).

Neve, M., 'Public Views of Neurasthenia: Britain, 1880–1930', in M. Gijswit-Hofstra and R. Porter (eds.), *Cultures of Neurasthenia: From Beard to the First World War* (Amsterdam and New York: Rodophi, 2001), pp. 141–60.

Oppenheim, J., *"Shattered Nerves": Doctors, Patients, and Depression in Victorian England* (Oxford and New York: Oxford University Press, 1991).

Otis, L., *Organic Memory: History and the Body in the Late Nineteenth and Early Twentieth Centuries* (Lincoln, NE and London: University of Nebraska Press, 1994).

Overy, R., *The Morbid Age: Britain and the Crisis of Civilization, 1919–1939* (London: Penguin Books, 2010).

Paris, M., *Warrior Nation: Images of War in British Popular Culture, 1850–2000* (London: Reaktion Books, 2000).

Pick, D., *Faces of Degeneration: A European Disorder, c. 1848–c. 1918* (Cambridge: Cambridge University Press, 1989).

War Machine: The Rationalisation of Slaughter in the Modern Age (New Haven, CT, and London: Yale University Press, 1993).

Svengali's Web: The Alien Enchanter in Modern Culture (New Haven, CT, and London: Yale University Press, 2000).

'Maladies of the Will: Freedom, Fetters and the Fear of Freud', in R. Bivins and J.V. Pickstone (eds.), *Medicine, Madness and Social History: Essays in Honour of Roy Porter* (Basingstoke: Palgrave Macmillan, 2007), pp. 197–209.

Pines, M., 'The Development of the Psychodynamic Movement', in G.E. Berrios and H. Freeman (eds.), *150 Years of British Psychiatry, 1841–1991* (London: Gaskell, 1991), pp. 206–31.

Porter, R., 'Nervousness, Eighteenth and Nineteenth Century Style: From Luxury to Labour', in M. Gijswijt-Hofstra and R. Porter (eds.), *Cultures of Neurasthenia: From Beard to the First World War* (Amsterdam and New York: Rodophi, 2001), pp. 31–49.

Poynter, D.J., '"Regeneration" Revisited: W.H.R. Rivers and Shell Shock during the Great War', in M. Hughes and M. Seligmann (eds.), *Leadership in Conflict 1914–1918* (Barnsley, South Yorkshire: Leo Cooper, 2000), pp. 227–43.

Read, D., *The Age of Urban Democracy: England 1868–1914*, rev. edn (Essex: Longman, 1994).

Reader, W.J., *At Duty's Call: A Study in Obsolete Patriotism* (Manchester and New York: Manchester University Press, 1988).

Reed, J., *Victorian Will* (Athens, OH: Ohio University Press, 1989).

Reid, F., *Broken Men: Shell Shock, Treatment and Recovery in Britain 1914–1930* (London and New York: Continuum, 2010).

Robb, G., *British Culture and the First World War* (Basingstoke and New York: Palgrave, 2002).

Romani, R., *National Character and Public Spirit in Britain and France, 1750–1914* (Cambridge: Cambridge University Press, 2002).

Roper, M., *The Secret Battle: Emotional Survival in the Great War* (Manchester and New York: Manchester University Press, 2009).

Rose, N., *The Psychological Complex: Psychology, Politics and Society in England 1869–1939* (London: Routledge & Kegan Paul, 1985).

Roudebush, M., 'A Battle of Nerves: Hysteria and Its Treatments in France during World War I', in M. Micale and P. Lerner (eds.), *Traumatic Pasts: History, Psychiatry, and Trauma in the Modern Age, 1870–1930* (Cambridge: Cambridge University Press, 2001), pp. 253–79.

Rousseau, G.S., *Nervous Acts: Essays on Literature, Culture and Sensibility* (Basingstoke: Palgrave Macmillan, 2004).

Rutherford, J., *Forever England: Reflections on Race, Masculinity and Empire* (London: Lawrence and Wishart, 1997).

Schivelbusch, W., *The Railway Journey: The Industrialization of Time and Space in the 19th Century* (Leamington Spa, Hamburg, and New York: Berg, 1986).

Scull, A., *The Most Solitary of Afflictions: Madness and Society in Britain, 1700–1900* (New Haven, CT, and London: Yale University Press, 1993).

Searle, G., *Eugenics and Politics in Britain, 1900–1914* (Leyden: Noordhoff, 1976).

Sengoopta, C., '"A Mob of Incoherent Symptoms"? Neurasthenia in British Medical Discourse, 1860–1920', in M. Gijswijt-Hofstra and R. Porter (eds.), *Cultures of Neurasthenia: From Beard to the First World War* (Amsterdam and New York: Rodophi, 2001), pp. 97–116.

Shamdasani, S., 'Claire, Lise, Jean, Nadia, and Gisèle: Preliminary Notes Towards a Characterisation of Pierre Janet's Psychasthenia', in M. Gijswijt-Hofstra and R. Porter (eds.), *Cultures of Neurasthenia: From Beard to the First World War* (Amsterdam and New York: Rodophi, 2001), pp. 363–85.

Sheffield, G., 'Office-Man Relations, Discipline and Morale in the British Army of the Great War', in H. Cecil and P.H. Liddle (eds.), *Facing Armageddon: The First World War Experienced* (London: Leo Cooper, 1996), pp. 413–24.

Leadership in the Trenches: Officer-Man Relations, Morale and Discipline in the British Army in the Era of the First World War (Basingstoke and New York: Macmillan Press, 2000).

Shephard, B., '"The Early Treatment of Mental Disorders": R.G. Rows and Maghull 1914–1918', in H. Freeman and G.E. Berrios (eds.), *150 Years of British Psychiatry. Volume 2: The Aftermath* (London: Athlone, 1996), pp. 434–64.

'Shell-Shock', in H. Freeman (ed.), *A Century of Psychiatry*, 2 vols. (London: Mosby-Wolfe Medical Communications, 1999), vol. 2, pp. 33–40.

A War of Nerves: Soldiers and Psychiatrists, 1914–1994 (London: Pimlico, 2002).

Shepherd, M., 'Psychiatric Journals and the Evolution of Psychological Knowledge', in W.F. Bynum, S. Lock, and R. Porter (eds.), *Medical Journals and Medical Knowledge: Historical Essays* (London and New York: Routledge, 1992), pp. 188–206.

Showalter, E., *The Female Malady: Women, Madness and English Culture, 1830–1980* (London: Virago, 1987).

'Rivers and Sassoon: The Inscription of Male Gender Anxieties', in M. Higgonet *et al.* (eds.), *Behind the Lines: Gender and the Two World Wars* (New Haven, CT and London: Yale University Press, 1987), pp. 61–9.

'Hysteria, Feminism and Gender', in S. Gilman *et al.* (eds.), *Hysteria Beyond Freud* (Berkeley, Los Angeles, and London: University of California Press, 1993), pp. 286–344.

Hystories: Hysterical Epidemics and Modern Culture (London and Basingstoke: Picador, 1997).

Smith, R., *The Fontana History of the Human Sciences* (London: Fontana Press, 1997).

Free Will and the Human Sciences in Britain, 1870–1910 (London and Brookfield, VT: Pickering and Chatto, 2013).

Between Mind and Nature: A History of Psychology (London: Reaktion Books, 2013).

Stone, M., 'Shellshock and the Psychologists', in W.F. Bynum, R. Porter, and M. Shepherd (eds.), *The Anatomy of Madness: Essays in the History of Psychiatry. Volume 1: People and Ideas* (London and New York: Tavistock, 1985), pp. 242–71.

Strachan, H., 'Liberalism and Conscription, 1789–1919', in H. Strachan (ed.), *The British Army: Manpower and Society into the Twenty-First Century* (London: Frank Cass, 2000), pp. 3–15.

Stryker, L., 'Mental Cases: British Shellshock and the Politics of Interpretation', in G. Braybon (ed.), *Evidence, History and the Great War: Historians and the Impact of 1914–18* (New York and Oxford: Berghahn Books, 2003), pp. 154–71.

Sulloway, F.G., *Freud, Biologist of the Mind: Beyond the Psychoanalytic Legend* (London: Fontana Paperbacks, 1980).

Tate, T., *Modernism, History and the Great War* (Manchester and New York: Manchester University Press, 1998).

Taylor, J.B., 'Obscure Recesses: Locating the Victorian Unconscious', in J.B. Bullen (ed.), *Writing and Victorianism* (London and New York: Longman, 1997), pp. 137–79.

Thomas, G.M., *Treating the Trauma of the Great War: Soldiers, Civilians, and Psychiatry in France, 1914–1940* (Baton Rouge, LA: Louisiana State University Press, 2009).

Thomson, M., 'Status, Manpower and Mental Fitness: Mental Deficiency in the First World War', in R. Cooter, M. Harrison, and S. Sturdy (eds.), *War, Medicine and Modernity* (Stroud: Sutton, 1998), pp. 149–66.

'"Savage Civilisation": Race, Culture and Mind in Britain, 1898–1939', in W. Ernst and B. Harris (eds.), *Race, Science and Medicine, 1700–1960* (London and New York: Routledge, 1999), pp. 235–58.

'Neurasthenia in Britain: An Overview', in M. Gijswijt-Hofstra and R. Porter (eds.), *Cultures of Neurasthenia: From Beard to the First World War* (Amsterdam and New York: Rodophi, 2001), pp. 77–95.

'Psychology and the "Consciousness of Modernity", in Early Twentieth-Century Britain', in M. Daunton and B. Rieger (eds.), *Meanings of Modernity: Britain from the Late-Victorian Era to World War Two* (Oxford and New York: Berg, 2001), pp. 97–115.

Psychological Subjects: Identity, Culture, and Health in Twentieth-Century Britain (Oxford and New York: Oxford University Press, 2006).

Tomes, N., 'Feminist Histories of Psychiatry', in M. Micale and R. Porter (eds.), *Discovering the History of Psychiatry* (Oxford and New York: Oxford University Press, 1994), pp. 348–83.

Tylee, C., *The Great War and Women's Consciousness: Images of Militarism and Womanhood in Women's Writings, 1914–64* (Basingstoke: Macmillan, 1990).

van Bergen, L., *Before My Helpless Sight: Suffering, Dying and Military Medicine on the Western Front, 1914–1918*, trans. L. Waters (Farnham, Surrey, and Burlington, VT: Ashgate, 2009).

Waddington, K., *Medical Education at St Bartholomew's Hospital 1123–1995* (Woodbridge, Suffolk: Boydell Press, 2003).

Watson, A., *Enduring the Great War: Combat, Morale and Collapse in the German and British Armies, 1914–1918* (Cambridge and New York: Cambridge University Press, 2008).

Wessely, S., 'Neurasthenia and Fatigue Syndromes: Clinical Section', in G.E. Berrios and R. Porter (eds.), *A History of Clinical Psychiatry: The Origin and History of Psychiatric Disorders* (London: Athlone, 1995), pp. 509–32.

Whitehead, I., 'The British Medical Officer on the Western Front: The Training of Doctors for War', in R. Cooter, M. Harrison, and S. Sturdy (eds.), *Medicine and Modern Warfare* (Amsterdam: Rodopi, 1999), pp. 163–84.

Doctors in the Great War (Barnsley, South Yorkshire: Leo Cooper, 1999).

Winter, J., *Sites of Memory, Sites of Mourning: The Great War in European Cultural History* (Cambridge, New York, and Melbourne: Cambridge University Press, 1995).

The Great War and the British People, 2nd edn (Basingstoke: Palgrave Macmillan, 2003).

Remembering War: The Great War between Memory and History in the Twentieth Century (New Haven, CT, and London: Yale University Press, 2006).

'Shell Shock', in J. Winter (ed.), *The Cambridge History of the First World War. Volume III: Civil Society* (Cambridge and New York: Cambridge University Press, 2013), pp. 310–33.

Wiener, M., *Reconstructing the Criminal: Culture, Law and Policy in England, 1830–1914* (Cambridge: Cambridge University Press, 1990).
Young, A., *The Harmony of Illusions: Inventing Post-Traumatic Stress Disorder* (Princeton, NJ: Princeton University Press, 1995).

UNPUBLISHED

Fitzpatrick, K., 'Primum non nocere: War-Related Functional Nervous Disorders, Treatment and Diagnosis at the Royal London Hospital 1914–1918', Master's dissertation, Institute of Historical Research, London (2009).
Loughran, T., 'Shell-Shock in First World War Britain: An Intellectual and Medical History, c. 1860–c. 1920', PhD thesis, University of London (2006).
Poynter, D.J. '"The Report on Her Transfer Was Shell-Shock": A Study of the Psychological Disorders of Nurses and Female Voluntary Aid Detachments Who Served Alongside the British and Allied Expeditionary Forces during the First World War, 1914–18', PhD thesis, University of Northampton (2008).

WEBSITES

BBC News, 'TV's Jon Snow Rejects "Poppy Fascism"', 10 November 2006: news.bbc.co.uk/1/hi/uk/6134906.stm. Accessed 6 January 2017.
Denham, J., 'Charlene White Hits Back after Racist Abuse for Not Wearing a Poppy', *Independent*, 13 November 2013. www.independent.co.uk/incoming/charlene-white-hits-back-after-racist-abuse-for-not-wearing-a-poppy-8937123.html. Accessed 6 January 2017.
The Long, Long Trail, 'The Royal Army Medical Corps of 1914–1918', http://www.1914-1918.net/ramc.htm. Accessed 6 January 2017.

Index

aboulia 46

Abrahams, Adolphe 13, 34 n. 35, 87, 48 n. 112

abreaction 168, 187

Adler, Alfred 133

alcohol 96

alcoholism 29, 71, 99, 201, 217

Allbutt, Clifford 60

altruism 194, 196–7, 203. *See also* conscience, duty.

animals, "shell-shock" in 95, 135–6, 184

amnesia 14, 122, 145. *See also* memory. "analytic".

  definition of 8, 110, 165

  school 79

  influence of school 230

  theories 111–12, 147, 165, 177, 183–4, 210

  therapies 6, 117–18, 158–9, 164–73, 210, 226

  relation to physiological theories 188, 190–3, 198

anthropology 31, 50, 191, 194 n.55, 195

anti-German sentiments 1–2, 22, 60 n.22, 136, 204–5, 228

anxiety, in "shell-shock" 83, 86–7, 106, 142, 162 n.52

anxiety neurosis 87, 59 n.20, 129–30, 132, 134, 167 n.77, 170, 172, 199, 210, 218. *See also* hysteria, neurasthenia.

aphasia 40, 62

Armstrong-Jones, Robert 30–1, 34, 47–8, 74, 112–13, 154, 156 n.28, 175, 187, 205

Aristotelian Society 30, 225

assimilation, process in psychological medicine 8, 65, 106, 110–12, 215, 226–9. *See also* modification, "translation".

asylum 5, 28–33, 47, 211, 214

  psychiatry 28–31, 70, 74, 108, 155, 187, 191

Babinski, Joseph 63–5

battle casualties 11–12

Bet-El, Ilana 180

Bethlem Hospital 211

biological modes of explanation 38, 42, 49, 54–5, 67, 72–6, 78, 128–9

  in theories of "shell-shock" 135, 157, 182–209

Bousfield, Paul 108, 217 n.22–23.

Brain 21, 86, 95

British Journal of Psychology 21, 30–1

British Medical Journal 136, 190, 201, 205, 227, 230–1

British Institute of Philosophical Studies 221

British Neurological Society 30

British Psychological Society 30, 189, 197, 219–21, 225

British Union of Fascists 179

Brock, Arthur 70–1, 201

Brown, Walter Langdon 133, 188 n.33

Brown, William 39, 133, 165–6, 168, 187, 217–18, 221

Bryce, Lord 203

Cambridge, University of

  psychology laboratory 31

  postgraduate diploma in psychiatry 33

Campbell, Harry 30 n.17, 207, 34 n.35, 48 n.112

Cannon, Walter B. 184–7, 190

Carver, Alfred 95, 48 n.112, 217 n.22–23

"Case A1" 160–1, 163–4

Cassel Hospital 211

Chambers, William Duncanson 108, 155

character, concepts of 46, 68–9, 71–2, 74, 104, 108, 145, 147, 150–3, 158 164–5, 171–4, 177–80, 194–8, 220, 226. *See also* national character.

Charcot, Jean-Martin 63, 121, 124

chemical warfare 2

child